D1126590

THE PSYCHIATRIC HOSPITAL AS A SMALL SOCIETY

The Psychiatric Hospital as a Small Society

William Caudill

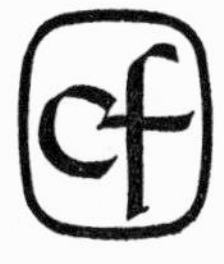

Published for The Commonwealth Fund
BY HARVARD UNIVERSITY PRESS
Cambridge, Massachusetts · 1958

Library of Congress Catalog Card No. 58–7253

Manufactured in the United States of America

For approximately a quarter of a century THE COMMONWEALTH FUND, through its Division of Publications, sponsored, edited, produced, and distributed books and pamphlets germane to its purposes and operations as a philanthropic foundation. On July 1, 1951, the Fund entered into an arrangement by which HARVARD UNIVERSITY PRESS became the publisher of Commonwealth Fund books, assuming responsibility for their production and distribution. The Fund continues to sponsor and edit its books, and cooperates with the Press in all phases of manufacture and distribution.

Published for The Commonwealth Fund

BY HARVARD UNIVERSITY PRESS

Distributed in Great Britain

BY OXFORD UNIVERSITY PRESS, LONDON

To the patients and staff
of psychiatric hospitals,
with the hope that this work
may be of use to them

Foreword

I have often heard the critical question: "Why do so many patients in mental hospitals not get well?" I believe it is equally interesting, and possibly more profitable, to ask why so many *do* get well. The full answer to these questions, I believe, would exceed my knowledge by far and also the knowledge of present-day psychiatry. The obvious answer would be that such improvement or recovery is owing to the excellence of psychiatric treatment; such a statement does not satisfy me. The truth is that there are very few disorders which can be treated by specific methods of therapy; unfortunately most organic treatments are crude and not based on good theory, and most psychotherapy is effective only in the hands of the best therapists and is extraordinarily restricted to a small segment of the suffering population for powerful socioeconomic reasons. One possible answer is that many patients come to mental hospitals from rather horrible conditions, which presumably have something to do with their mental and emotional disorders. In the mental hospital to which they are admitted, they find less horrible conditions. Even those institutions which are far from perfect are protective "asylums."

What are these less horrible conditions in mental hospitals and what is their impact on patients? What helps? Is it psychotherapy? Is it the organic treatments for those patients who receive them? Is it good nursing? Is it the so-called auxiliary therapies? Is it all these activities together which help? Or, are there other variables not known to us which might be helpful? Could it be that patients do something for each other and get each other well? Undoubtedly, such questions have occurred to many psychiatrists in their daily practice and in their research and teaching. These were some of the questions which a group of psychiatrists—

Helen Gilmore, Eugene Brody, Edward Stainbrook, myself, and others—posed when the responsibility of running a small psychiatric hospital, the key unit of a university department of psychiatry, was turned over to us. The answers to these questions seemed of considerable practical importance for the welfare of our patients, for the training of our resident physicians, and last but not least from the viewpoint of any theory outlining our therapeutic activities. The department and hospital were in a state of transition at that time. From an attitude of therapeutic nihilism, we moved toward a more positive orientation. The enthusiasm of our group was great and had been strongly influenced by the stimulating ideas of psychoanalytic theory and practice. This was also the time when Stanton and Schwartz's first papers appeared, when the revolutionary ideas of Maxwell Jones and T. P. Rees in Great Britain began to emerge, and when the progressive practices of the Menningers began to reach us through the teaching of Kubie and Knight. I felt that the addition of a social scientist to our staff would aid us greatly to make pertinent observations on the wards of our hospital, which then would help us with the problems which I have just indicated. I thought such observation should be carried out twenty-four hours a day if possible. Should such observations be made in a candid or in a concealed fashion? Should the observer be known as a social scientist or should he make his observations from the point of view of a patient, unknown to other patients and to the therapeutic and administrative personnel of the hospital? I believe I was the only psychiatrist in our group who felt that such concealed observation would be of superior value. After considerable search for the right person, I was introduced in 1949, by Professor Lloyd Warner, to Doctor William Caudill, a young and gifted anthropologist, who agreed with me on the feasibility of the project and consented to enter the hospital as a "patient." To admit Doctor Caudill as a patient under a pseudonym was not difficult. He had only to exaggerate, as would be the case with most persons, certain aspects of normal behavior. Caudill lived on the wards of the hospital for about eight weeks. During this time, he received "psychotherapy" from a resident, who found out only after his discharge who Doctor Caudill really was. During his "hospitalization" Caudill kept a meticulous research diary in which he made a great many extraordinarily interesting and, from a human point of view, moving observations; some of these findings were previously reported.[1]

[1] Caudill, William; Redlich, F. C.; Gilmore, H. R.; and Brody, E. B. "Social Structure and Interaction Processes on a Psychiatric Ward," *American Journal of Orthopsychiatry* 22:314–334, 1952.

Our most important expectation was to obtain maximally objective and detailed information by a scientifically trained observer. To our surprise we found that Caudill did not remain objective. He became a member of the patient society and identified with the patients. Temporarily, Caudill really became a "patient." It seems, at least to me, that the data collected during this period are less valuable, less clear, than the data reported in this book, which were collected openly by Doctor Caudill in a second study done at a considerably later date.

There are many reasons why we do not recommend a repetition of the first type of study. Eugene Brody and I indicated, in a paper on interdisciplinary research, some of the ethical reasons why we think this approach is apt to violate the basic principles of a trusting relation between patient and therapist.[2] From discussions with Doctor Caudill, I know that he feels similarly. I also might add that I now believe it is unwise to expose the staff to an experience which was so upsetting to them. One of the few exceptions was Doctor Caudill's "therapist," a kindly and mature man; he felt he learned a great deal from his experience, although it was disturbing to find out his patient was not ill. The patients were favorably impressed by the episode and appreciated the intent, feeling it was carried out in their interest and that it might possibly tell the psychiatrist what really goes on in their lives while they are in a hospital. All in all, however, I doubt that this particular approach warrants repetition; it did not achieve the results we hoped for.

Essentially, the data which constitute the basis for this particular book were obtained by the open observations of Doctor Caudill in the same unit where, a year and a half earlier, he had worked as a concealed observer. The aim of this book is identical with that of the first study: to explore the hospital as a social system. The principal methods described in this book consisted first of direct and open observation of the patients' life on the ward. These observations—and Doctor Caudill spent a great deal of time on the ward—supplied the bulk of the data. Caudill, incidentally, suggests that psychiatric residents should spend much more time with patients; that for a limited time they should live on the wards.

The second important segment of his observations consisted of very detailed observations of administrative and clinical staff conferences. The third approach was through the ingenious device of a pictorial test interview, using pictures of hospital life patterned somewhat after Henry

[2] Redlich, F. C., and Brody, E. B. "Emotional Problems of Interdisciplinary Research in Psychiatry," *Psychiatry* 18:233–239, 1955.

Murray's Thematic Apperception Test. These pictures were shown to patients, and to clinical and administrative personnel, with the request to comment on the content of the pictures, and helped to elicit their views and attitudes about facts and problems of a mental hospital.

Caudill makes a good case for the use of an anthropologist in a psychiatric setting. He feels—and I completely agree with him—that such a social scientist could make important observations of the total system of a hospital and report them in conferences and seminars. I might add that such a task is not an easy one for the social scientist, or for the clinicians and administrators who do not like being subjected to such social analysis and feel threatened when social science yardsticks are applied to them. Similar feelings are also aroused when psychiatric yardsticks are applied directly to the staff by the psychiatrist. If the social scientist does not proceed with the greatest tact and skill, he is apt to produce turmoil and confusion instead of easing communication and aiding harmonious administration. In this respect, too, Doctor Caudill was a pioneer. He overcame the shock of the concealed-observer study and was able to overcome many of the difficulties inherent in interdisciplinary collaboration. I have often thought that he, as well as many of my psychiatric colleagues—after this experience—should have received medals for injuries to their narcissism in the service of science.

Caudill speaks convincingly of mutual advantages of collaboration between dynamic psychiatrists and anthropologists. Both disciplines deal directly with people—one primarily with individuals in a therapeutic context and the other with groups in a scientific context—and both are able to maintain a dynamic viewpoint. The anthropologist deals with psychodynamic functions as they occur in life, under extremely varying social and cultural conditions. This is a very important supplement to the psychiatrists' and psychoanalysts' observations in the therapeutic hour. Throughout the book, Caudill is aware of the subtleties and complexities of human behavior and shows a real appreciation of the psychoanalytic method of observation.

There is no doubt in my mind that psychiatrists and clinical psychologists, psychiatric social workers, psychiatric nurses, and other ward personnel have much to learn from such a social scientist. Some of his messages will require a rather careful and slow assimilation before they can be really accepted and utilized. After the reader has finished this book, however, he probably will be convinced that the hospital is a small society which affects the behavior of the people who make it up. It has a definite caste system of physicians, psychologists, social workers, nurses, administrators, clerical workers, attendants and craftsmen, and, last but not least, the patients. One of the outstanding features of such a hospital is what social scientists call blocked mobility. The implications of such a blocked mobility system are carefully outlined in the book. Such a system is an authoritarian system. It is characterized by strong paternalism, or possibly maternalism. There is, even in our best mental hospitals, an uncomfortable similarity between our institutions and prisons, albeit very permissive prisons. The permissiveness, however, is that of the nursery, sometimes at the price of human dignity. I often wonder whether some of the rules and regulations of most mental hospitals exist because the patients are infantile or because we infantilize them.

Doctor Caudill is dealing with such problems. He couches his detailed and convincing examples in terms of transactions between persons and groups. He outlines the mutual and often conflicting roles and role expectations of individuals and groups. He describes unanticipated consequences of administrative decisions, mood sweeps, and collective changes in the situation. To me, the most interesting statements—exceeding what I know from my clinical experience as a psychiatrist—were Caudill's observations about the patient role and patients' supporting each other. He distinguishes, following Parsons, the personal role from the sick role and demonstrates conflicts between them and their consequences in everyday living on the ward and in therapy. These are strikingly new facts about the impact or lack of impact of psychotherapy as seen through the "third eye" of the social scientist. To anyone who still wishes to believe that the patient's life in a mental hospital is made up just of five psychotherapeutic hours or three minor electrocutions a week, this book will deal a shattering blow. For example, Caudill's observations raise the question in a convincing manner of the relevance of social "ground swells" in the hospital society to the therapy of individual patients.

To the social scientists, some of Caudill's theoretical formulations will be of great interest; to psychiatrists, some of his practical conclusions about the vagueness of roles of the psychiatrist and his professional colleagues, particularly the psychiatric nurse, will be very valuable. Caudill points to the conflicts between administrators and therapists, to problems of multiple subordination, to consequent job dissatisfaction, and to apathy and inertia in the hospital society. The cure of such social ills is not rushing into frantic activity and total push therapy, but a thoughtful analysis of the hospital social system and a clarification of social roles. Once this is achieved—and we are just at the beginning of such an endeavor—we may find that many of our present hospital practices are not entirely rational and effective. Beyond that, we may come to the conclusion that our mental hospitals have become anachronistic institutions.

To face such self-imposed investigation is not an easy task. Since the time of the work reported on in this book, a great many changes have occurred in the hospital, and some of the important changes are directly related to Caudill's work. Reading Caudill's book today, nobody would recognize that the small world of confusion he describes is the Yale Psychiatric Institute. Under the leadership of Theodore Lidz and Stephen Fleck, our hospital has developed toward a therapeutic community where teamwork has become more of a live concept and where more seasoned therapists carry out tasks for which they are better equipped by intensive previous training and experience. The main reason for such a development is the humble and sincere spirit for investigation which is exemplified by this book. This spirit is also the reason why we feel that we have not reached the end of the road.

F. C. REDLICH, M.D.
Professor and Chairman
Department of Psychiatry
Yale University School of Medicine

Preface

Although this book is mainly a report of research done in one small psychiatric hospital, it represents for me the precipitate of my work in a number of psychiatric hospitals in the United States and Japan, as well as the development of my thinking on some aspects of the wider problem of the part played by social and cultural factors in the course and treatment of disease.

It seems to me that this book has been a long time in the writing. Its roots lie in my background as a social anthropologist and in a long-standing concern with the study of culture and personality. My interest in work in the psychiatric hospital began in 1950 when, as a concealed observer, I lived as a patient for two months in order to experience at firsthand something of the meaning of life on a ward. This study has been reported earlier (Caudill, *et al.,* 1952) and is not of direct concern here, although later in this preface I wish to give my views on the method of this earlier study in contrast with the open observation which was used in the study presented in this book. The field work for this book was done in 1951–1952, while I held a teaching and research position in the Department of Psychiatry at Yale University. The organization of material and quantitative analysis were done at Harvard University from 1952 through 1954. The ideas contained in the chapters which were written during these years show the influence of the excitement I found in the work of my colleagues in the Department of Social Relations, and the stimulation and comparative perspective received from my consulting work and contact with on-going research in state and private hospitals in Boston. During 1954–1955 the materials for this book lay fallow while I did a year of research in Japan which included six months of work in Japanese psychiatric hospitals. Upon my return from

Japan, I resumed my teaching at Harvard and also began a nonmedical candidacy at the Boston Psychoanalytic Institute under a grant from The Commonwealth Fund. Over the summer of 1956, ten of the chapters were written in final form (Chapters 1–3 and 6–12) and the less complete these were at the time, the more they show the further influence of my work in Japan and my training in psychoanalysis. The remaining four chapters (Chapters 4, 5, 13, and 14) were completed by the end of the summer of 1957.

Thus, as I look at the book as a whole, it seems to me that overlying what I believe to be the soundness of the basic data are the changes that have taken place in my thinking and style of writing over the years. For example, I think I would now stress, with more assurance, certain psychodynamics of Mr. Esposito's personality that are not touched upon in Chapter 3 as it stands. At the same time, I would retain all that I have said about the course of his hospitalization. There are also comparative materials, such as those from Japan, that are not here in the detail I should like, as well as a forefront of ideas, as yet inadequately worked through, which is not represented. Still, there must be an ending, and I feel satisfied that what is written here conveys much of what I want to say about my understanding of a psychiatric hospital.

As mentioned, this book is about the second of two studies I did in the same hospital. In the first I acted as a patient, and my identity was concealed. The second and fuller study, reported on here, was begun a year and a half later, and in it I presented myself openly as a research anthropologist. From the published accounts of both studies the reader may judge which was the more successful. In the report of the first study (Caudill, *et al.,* 1952) mention has already been made of the ethical problems posed by such a study, along with the suggestion of the feasibility of alternative procedures. I have no wish to rationalize my actions in this earlier study. I did it, and I learned much from it. I do not recommend others' doing it because I feel the price is too high. The ethical questions here are rather tricky—some of the purposes of almost any research project on human behavior are concealed from the subject, client, or patient, and this is too involved a topic for a preface. Certainly one factor, however, is how comfortable—morally and emotionally—a person is about the matter of concealment. Once in the situation, I felt decidedly uncomfortable.

I believe I was naïve when I undertook the task of living as a patient. I had no strong opinions pro or con about the method. I did have a strong desire to learn by experience what life was like on the wards, and it was this rather than any wish to pry into secrets that provided my motivation. And yet the aura of the forbidden clings to such a study, and while I did not knowingly have such wishes, perhaps these were there unknowingly. Much is made of concealment these days, what with hidden role players in the experiments being carried out in several of the social sciences, and the question of the degree of frankness to be maintained with the patient in the sound recording of interviews and other material in psychiatry. Subsequent to my own experience with concealment, I have been somewhat startled at times at the aplomb with which plans for concealment in experiments and interviews are proposed as a matter of course. In my own case, whatever other factors were involved, I was taking the role, in a sense, for real.

What I learned from the concealed study had less to do with "facts" and more to do with "feelings." I became sensitive to such things as the difference in the meaning of "time" for the patient on the ward in contrast to the time kept by the busy staff member. I became aware of the immediate importance for patients of their communication with each other—during the day, at night, from one ward to another. On the whole, the experience taught me much about hospital life, and if, in reporting on the second study in this book, I have convincingly portrayed some aspects of the life of patients, it is in part because of the earlier study when I was, for a time, in the situation myself.

After the first study I was concerned about the one-sidedness of my work. I felt I knew a good bit about the organization of life on the wards, but very little about the operation of the hospital at the staff level. Besides, as I have said, I felt uncomfortable about the concealed study and wished to find out if similar data could be obtained more openly. More generally, I was eager to determine if scientific procedures could be worked out for studying the entire system of the hospital over time. I therefore decided to do the second study upon which this book is based. In this I hoped to correct the one-sidedness of the earlier study and to check my own observations and those of other investigators.

During the second study I spent a great deal of time with the various groups of staff and patients as they went about their life in the hospital. I believe I was able to work out methods of observation, interviewing, and analysis—as presented in the following pages—which provided data equal in richness to those of the earlier study. In addition, the methods of the second study yielded a wider range of data over which it was possible to exercise a high degree of control. Personally, I feel more satisfied, both intellectually and emotionally, with the material in this book. It must also be pointed out that, in comparison with the earlier study, the amount of time and energy expended in the present work was twentyfold.

I enjoyed my work in the psychiatric hospital reported on here, and I look forward to doing further studies such as this one—the next of which I plan to do in a small hospital in Japan. I hope that perhaps the reader will find enough of clarity in this book to share in some measure with me the intellectual and emotional satisfaction I found in writing it.

William Caudill
Cambridge, Massachusetts
September 1957

Acknowledgments

It is impossible to acknowledge in detail all the people and institutions that have helped me to bring this work to completion. I am particularly grateful for the continued support of The Commonwealth Fund, of the Department of Psychiatry at Yale University, and later of the Laboratory of Social Relations at Harvard University. I am also deeply indebted to the patients and staff of the hospital in which I worked, and to the students in various seminars at Yale and Harvard, who helped me to develop many of the ideas presented in this book.

I especially wish to thank Dr. F. C. Redlich for his advice and personal support throughout this research. I am indebted to Dr. Edward Stainbrook for the many hours we spent together working over the data, and hence for his real contribution to the material presented here. While I was at Yale, Dr. Fred Strodtbeck generously found time for frequent discussions on questions of method, and I am most grateful to him for this help as well as for the stimulation I received from our conversations during long walks on week ends. I also wish to thank Dr. Eugene Brody for his sustained interest in the research. At Harvard, I particularly received guidance from Professor Talcott Parsons, Professor Clyde Kluckhohn, Dr. Florence Kluckhohn, Professor Robert Freed Bales, Dr. George Mandler, and Dr. John Spiegel. I owe a great deal to Dr. Alfred Stanton for his encouragement over the years. It is also a pleasure to acknowledge the influence of Dr. Charlotte Babcock and of Dr. Leo Berman on my work. None of the above persons is, of course, to be held responsible for the ways in which I have handled ideas or factual materials in this book.

For the research assistance without which this work could not have been completed I wish to thank Miss Dorrian Apple, Miss Nancy Hatch, and Miss Mieko Imagi. I also wish to thank Mr. Paul Lambert for the careful attention he gave to the drawing of the hospital-life pictures used in interviewing. I am very grateful for the excellent secretarial assistance provided at various times by Mrs. Constance Ives, Miss Audrey Knowles, Mrs. Esther Smith, and Mrs. Barbara Michaels.

I wish to acknowledge the kindness of the editors and publishers of the following journals and books in which articles by myself have appeared, for permission to use parts of these materials. Materials have been taken from: "Perspectives on Administration in Psychiatric Hospitals," *Administrative Science Quarterly* 1:155–170, 1956. "Social Process in a Collective Disturbance on a Psychiatric Ward." In Greenblatt, M.; Levinson, D. S.; and Williams, R. H. (editors). *The Patient and the Mental Hospital,* Glencoe, Illinois: The Free Press, 1957. "Social Structure and Interaction Processes on a Psychiatric Ward" (with Redlich, F. C.; Gilmore, H. R.; and Brody, E. B.), *American Journal of Orthopsychiatry* 22:314–334, 1952. "Some Covert Effects of Communication Difficulties in a Psychiatric Hospital" (with Stainbrook, Edward), *Psychiatry* 17:27–40, 1954. I also wish to thank the Social Science Research Council for allowing me to use parts of an unpublished paper entitled "Some Effects of Social and Cultural Systems in Reactions to Stress," which I prepared for a meeting of the Committee on Preventive Medicine and Social Science held in New York in November 1955.

I wish to thank the authors and publishers of the following articles and books for granting permission to use excerpts from material copyrighted by them:

Watts, Alan W. *The Way of Zen.* New York: Pantheon Books, 1957

Eliot, T. S. *Four Quartets.* New York: Harcourt, Brace and Company, 1943

Sivadon, Paul D. "Techniques of Sociotherapy," *Proceedings of the Symposium on Preventive and Social Psychiatry,* April 15–17, 1957, Walter Reed Army Institute of Research, Washington, D.C. (in press)

Rapoport, Robert N. "Oscillations and Sociotherapy," *Human Relations* 9:357–374, 1956

Bales, Robert F. *Interaction Process Analysis.* Cambridge, Massachusetts: Addison-Wesley Publishing Company, 1950

Bales, Robert F. "Task Status and Likeability as a Function of Talking and Listening in Decision-Making Groups." In White, L. D. (editor). *The State of the Social Sciences.* Chicago: University of Chicago Press, 1956

Spiegel, John P. "The Resolution of Role Conflict within the Family," *Psychiatry* 20:1–16, 1957

Belknap, Ivan. *Human Problems of a State Mental Hospital.* New York: Blakiston Division, McGraw-Hill Book Company, 1956

Stanton, Alfred H. "The Study of the Psychiatric Hospital as a Therapeutic Society," *Centennial Papers, Saint Elizabeths Hospital,* Washington, D.C., 1956

Redfield, Robert. *The Primitive World and Its Transformations.* Ithaca: Cornell University Press, 1953

Firth, Raymond. *Elements of Social Organization.* New York: Philosophical Library, 1951

Kroeber, A. L. *Anthropology.* New York: Harcourt, Brace and Company, 1948

Sapir, Edward. *Selected Writings of Edward Sapir.* Edited by Mandelbaum, D. G. Berkeley: University of California Press, 1949. The article referred to in Chapter 14 was originally published as "Psychiatric and Cultural Pitfalls in the Business of Getting a Living," *Mental Health,* Publication No. 9 of the American Association for the Advancement of Science, 1939 (out of print)

Stunkard, Albert. "Some Interpersonal Aspects of an Oriental Religion," *Psychiatry* 14:419–431, 1951

Contents

Shen-hsiu:
The body is the Bodhi Tree;
The mind like a bright mirror standing.
Take care to wipe it all the time,
And allow no dust to cling.

Hui-neng:
There never was a Bodhi Tree,
Nor bright mirror standing.
Fundamentally, not one thing exists,
So where is the dust to cling?

—From the teaching of Hui-neng (637–713)
in Alan W. Watts, *The Way of Zen.*
New York: Pantheon Books, 1957

We shall not cease from exploration
And the end of all our exploring
Will be to arrive where we started
And know the place for the first time.

—T. S. Eliot, in "Little Gidding,"
Four Quartets. New York:
Harcourt, Brace and Company, 1943

Section I

PROBLEM AND SETTING

CHAPTER 1

Nature of the Problem

This book is concerned with a search for an understanding of the broad context of the therapeutic process in a psychiatric hospital. Less abstractly, it is a book about the day-to-day personal relations of people—doctors, ward personnel, and patients. The analysis of these relations presented here came from the attempt to take seriously the idea that the hospital is a small society, and that the on-going functioning of such a society affects the behavior of the people who make it up in many ways of which they are unaware. In attempting to further such understanding, this book owes much to the stimulation of the work of Jones (1953), Stanton and Schwartz (1954), and Greenblatt, York, and Brown (1955).

To say that the hospital is a small society is to call attention to its organization as a complex system of human interaction within which the performance of technical tasks takes place. The system of human interaction in the hospital is in large part a social system, and one of the aims in the following chapters is to show that much behavior which often is characterized in personal psychological terms also finds its place as part of processes in the social system. These social processes must be identified and understood before it will be possible to utilize fully the potentialities of the hospital as a therapeutic community.

Such an approach is not proposed in lieu of the insight to be gained from a more psychodynamic analysis of behavior. Rather, if it is possible to come to an understanding of how the behavior of people is in considerable part a function of the social setting within which they act, and how such a setting operates to influence behavior in many subtle ways of which the participants are often unaware, then the knowledge of this wider social context will make insight arrived at through a psychodynamic approach all the more meaningful.

The study reported on here was carried out by the writer, a social anthropologist, in a small private psychiatric hospital attached to the medical school of a large university. At the time of the study, the hospital was in a state of transition with increasing emphasis being placed on psychodynamic principles in treatment and on the reorganization of its administrative procedures and ancillary therapeutic program. The techniques used in the research were largely those of observation and interviewing, and, altogether, about ten months were spent in gathering data. During his work, the anthropologist was assisted and encouraged by the senior psychiatrist then in charge of the hospital. The psychiatrist, Dr. Edward Stainbrook, contributed his own observations, particularly on the senior staff level, during the gathering of the data, and later worked closely with the anthropologist on the analysis of the materials. The setting and organization of the research are described in more detail in the next chapter; here it is useful to turn to a brief discussion of the aims of the research.

At the beginning, a first research aim was to obtain a description of the activities of the various role groups in the hospital, such as senior staff, resident staff, nurses, and patients. What was wanted was a picture not only of the formal and informal structure of these groups, but also of the somewhat differing values and beliefs which it was felt would be found on each level. This interest easily extended to an analysis of interpersonal relations within and between role groups and to an inquiry into how representations of hospital goals were expressed and communicated among role groups.

A second aim became, therefore, to trace through the hospital the actual flow of communication about events and the delineation of what happened in this process in terms of clarification, omission, distortion, and addition. It was felt that if the hospital was indeed a social *system,* events occurring at one point would have ramifications throughout the system.

In line with the above, a third aim was to attempt to make explicit the interrelated nature of certain series of events occurring over time at all levels within the structure of the hospital. It was believed that a certain lack of awareness of the interrelated nature of these events on the part of personnel in positions of decision making at various levels of the hospital contributed to the existence of such problems as the seemingly inexplicable recovery or deterioration of patients, the unanticipated consequences of administrative decisions, and the occurrence of mood sweeps and collective disturbances throughout the hospital.

Such an interest led to a fourth aim: a concern with the compatibility of the various subsystems of the hospital—for example, the degree of fit between the psychotherapeutic program and the administrative program. Entering into this was the need to consider the differences between psychotherapy carried on inside the hospital and psychotherapy conducted under ordinary living conditions. Because of the relatively closed nature of the system inside the hospital, it seemed that special problems would arise (and ramify throughout the hospital) with reference to such things as the control over patients' actions and the meaning of this for therapy; the pressures to utilize confidential material from patients for making administrative decisions; and the systematic influence exerted on the development of the transference and countertransference relations between doctor and patient because the individual therapeutic relationship occurred as part of an organized matrix of events making up the operation of the hospital over time.

These research aims resulted in three interrelated studies in which much the same phenomena were approached in different ways, and the various studies thus served as a check on each other. Each of these studies forms a section of this book. The first study consisted of detailed daily observations of what went on at various levels of the hospital and how the events occurring on these levels were interrelated (Chapters 3 through 5). The second study utilized a series of pictures of hospital life as visual questions in interviewing members of all role groups in order to determine the patterning of the similarities and differences in their perceptions of life in the hospital (Chapters 6 through 9). The third study involved making an essentially verbatim record of consecutive daily administrative conferences over a period of five months and then analyzing a substantial portion of this material in both quantitative and qualitative fashion. Since members of four role groups attended these conferences each day (senior doctors, residents, nurses, and other personnel—social worker, occupational therapist, and so on), the conferences provided an excellent opportunity for exploring the interaction between role groups and for observing the flow of communication through one crucial point in the hospital structure (Chapters 10 through 12).

One of the things that is missing from this series of studies is a report on what was happening during the patients' psychotherapeutic hours. From the indirect evidence of the behavior of patients on the wards, the reports of therapeutic progress given by the residents at the daily administrative conferences, and the behavior of the residents themselves, it is felt that there probably is a type of "ground swell" affecting psychotherapy in the hospital where a majority of the patients on a ward will be doing well or poorly at a particular time. In the work presented here, an attempt was made to use the notes dictated by residents on the therapeutic progress of their patients, but in only a few cases were these data even reasonably adequate. One such case is analyzed in Chapter 3. In view of the way events were interrelated in the hospital, as indicated in the following chapters, where it is believed that fairly convincing evidence is given to support the contention that the hospital really is a small social system, it would seem that a next research task would be to include in the observations what happens on a daily or perhaps weekly basis in the psychotherapy of patients. The gathering of such data will be fraught with many procedural difficulties, the more so because the data should also include what happens, on the one hand between the senior psychiatrist and the resident in the supervision of psychotherapy, and on the other hand between patients on the ward in relation to their therapeutic hours.

As the data for this book were being analyzed, a fourth study developed. It soon became obvious that the patterns and processes which were appearing in the data had a certain applicability not only to other hospitals but also to many other hierarchical settings, such as factories, schools, and families. This raised further questions about whether similar patterns and processes would be found in other cultures or, if not, what the differences would be. Such questions led to a concern with the general problem of the influence of cultural and social factors in the occurrence of disease and its treatment. These questions received some discussion and development in the writer's teaching and writing during the four years in which the data for this book were also being prepared for publication. During the same period the writer was able to widen his comparative perspective through contact with several large state hospitals in this country and through working for six months in psychiatric hospitals in Japan. Some of the ideas and implications of this fourth study are contained in the final section of this book.

As can be seen from the four studies sketched above, the primary emphasis in the following chapters is on what went on inside a small psychiatric hospital: how the events that occurred could be seen as interrelated within an on-going social system; what more general meaning this might have for understanding the effects of hospitalization on patients and staff; and the import of these phenomena for the development of a somewhat separate therapeutic technique—the use of the hospital as a therapeutic community. As such it is necessary to indicate the relation of this book to the work of others. No attempt is made, however, in the following paragraphs to present a thorough review of the literature, as this has already been done in a number of publications (Rioch and Stanton, 1953; Schwartz, 1953; Caudill, 1953a; Stanton and Schwartz, 1954; and Greenblatt, Levinson, and Williams, 1957).

At the beginning of the research one of the aims was the delineation of the formal social structure of the hospital. This formal structure becomes increasingly important in the life of the patient the longer he lives within the hospital. In the hospital reported on here, patients lived on the wards from one month to more than a year, with an average stay of about four months. In general, in psychiatric hospitals in the United States, it is well known that if a patient is not one of the roughly 50 per cent of patients who are discharged during the first year, he is likely to stay a very long time indeed. As of 1951, the average daily census in general hospitals was 470,692 patients, with an average length of stay in the hospital of 10 days. For psychiatric hospitals the average daily census was 697,521 patients, with an average length of stay of 829 days (President's Commission, 1953). As of the date of this book, things are perhaps a bit better as to length of stay in psychiatric hospitals owing to the effect of the use of tranquilizing drugs (Kramer, 1956).

Studies of the formal structure of both psychiatric and general hospitals (Smith, 1949; Woodward, 1950; Wessen, 1951; Henry, 1954; Burling, Lentz, and Wilson, 1956; and Belknap, 1956) emphasize the existence of a sharply defined status hierarchy in the hospital—e.g., senior physicians, residents, nurses, and attendants. As pointed out by Smith (1949), one aspect of these status levels, which is relatively unique to hospitals in contrast with other types of organizations for work, is that they are "mobility blocked." That is, under ordinary circumstances personnel can advance only within their own level—an attendant cannot become a nurse, or a nurse become a doctor. Movement from one level to another can only be achieved by leaving the system, acquiring further training, and returning in a different status. As will be seen in the following chapters, such a social structure makes for the development of somewhat separate values and perceptions of hospital life on the various levels (see Chapter 7); interpersonal relations between levels are highly formalized; and all this has important effects on the content and flow of communication through the system (see Chapter 10).

Previous hospital studies also emphasize the existence of a system of dual control—the formal administrative lines of authority and the more informal but very potent power of the physicians who do the clinical work. Given a system of dual control, hospitals are especially prone to struggle with problems of who makes what decisions, and much time is spent in trying to clarify which areas come under the authority of the hospital administrator and which under the authority of the medical staff. Particularly in a psychiatric hospital, where the patients are not usually sick in bed but are very much up and about, there are often differences of opinion over administrative and therapeutic goals and areas of responsibility in such matters as whether a patient should paint on the walls of his room, when and what he should eat, where he should (or should not) be at various times during the day, and how he is to get there (see Chapters 3 through 5).

A further aspect of the formal structure of a hospital is the extent to which it relies on systems of what Henry (1954) has called "multiple subordination," where one worker is under the authority of several independent chiefs (see also Stanton and Schwartz, 1954). For example, in the hospital about which this book is concerned, the nurse on the ward *could* have orders issued her independently by the head of the hospital, the supervisors of therapy, the referring physician, the head resident, the supervisor of nurses, and the patient's resident physician. Whether a nurse *should* have orders about a particular patient coming to her from so many sources, such as the somewhat delicate problem of the referring physician, was another matter, the discussion of which consumed much time at the daily administrative conferences (see Chapters 8 and 11). In this sort of situation the nurse has a difficult time resolving potentially conflicting orders, which is probably one reason why nurses are so insistent that things be put in writing.

If the formal structure of the psychiatric hospital is unwieldy for communication purposes, it is made more workable by the existence of informal channels of communication. An outstanding attribute of this informal structure is the personalized channel of communication set up by each doctor. These informal channels are developed—often over coffee in the ward kitchen—through frequent casual conversation with nurses and attendants with whom a doctor is especially congenial. This serves a useful function for the particular persons involved, but the over-all result is a large number of informal authority and communication networks which are covert and are not likely to be openly identified.

One interesting phenomenon which seems to be related to the characteristics of the formal and informal social structures is that hospitals are particularly subject to mood sweeps. These are made the more discomforting because few persons can identify where or why they began. Owing to the barriers to communication in the formal structure and the hidden nature of the informal structure, emotion arising from an event seems to be transmitted from person to person more quickly than cognitive knowledge about the event (see Chapter 5). This process is analogous to that observed in some unpublished work by Deutsch[1] when subjects were asked to identify the content and feeling tone of a somewhat controversial magazine article from which, in a series of experiments, varying proportions of the words had been deleted. The article was a report on a coal strike, and the author was arguing against the position taken by the labor union. In the cases of the deletion of every fifth and every fourth word, the subjects were still able to identify both content and feeling tone. With the deletion of every second word, however, content could no longer be recognized, but the subjects could still say how the author felt about whatever it was he was writing about. In this example it seemed that fewer cues were necessary for the communication of emotional information than of cognitive information. In human interaction the transmission of these two kinds of information depends upon somewhat differing types of cues; it is important to realize that the particular types of social structures to be found in a psychiatric hospital systematically affect the flow of both emotional and cognitive information and the balance maintained between them.

Further consequences of the hierarchical structure of the psychiatric hospital are the sharpness of the boundaries between social roles and the formalization of certain interpersonal relations as in the traditional relations between doctor and nurse, doctor and patient, nurse and patient, and so on. For the individual person, however, a social role is much more than a set of behaviors and attitudes required of him because he occupies a particular status position. While the same role may be taken by a wide range of personality types, there is always a link between personal motivation and social role, and the concept is used here as a bridge between the processes of intrapsychic life and those of social interaction (see Ackerman, 1951). As will be evident in the following chapters, it is necessary to keep track of both the individual attributes of people and their relative positions in the status and role structure of the hospital over time in order to understand some of the processes that characterize hospital life. Whatever the personal motivation for playing a role in a particular way, however, there is always considerable pressure for con-

[1] The author is indebted to Professor Karl W. Deutsch of the Massachusetts Institute of Technology for this information. In general, see Deutsch, 1952.

formity (see Chapter 10), and in the last analysis it is within the role that power inheres and from the role that action stems. Given the social structure of the hospital, the final demand is always: "You must act as a therapist, or a nurse, or a patient; you cannot act solely as Dr. Ryan, or Miss Nugent, or Mrs. Lasswell."

The doctor's role in the hospital is fairly well defined, although his obligations as therapist and as administrator are sometimes in conflict. This is a source of confusion because the general assumptions upon which the relationship between doctor and patient is built (Henderson, 1935; Fromm-Reichmann, 1950; Parsons, 1951) are not necessarily in line with the assumptions underlying the formal structure of the hospital. This problem will be given a good deal of attention at various points in this book (see Chapter 3).

The nurse's role in the hospital is much less clear than the doctor's—especially about how she should act on open wards where she is in interaction with less disturbed neurotic or psychotic patients. She also has the problem, as pointed out by Wilson (1950), of having a great deal of responsibility in certain areas without commensurate authority, and to complicate matters she is subject to a system of multiple subordination, as already indicated in the discussion of Henry's (1954) work. Perhaps one of the main problems in the nurse's role is that she has very little time to spend with patients—as Bachmeyer (1943) points out, somewhat over 50 per cent of the work done by professional nurses is nonprofessional in character. Equally, Devereux and Weiner (1950), writing on the occupational status of nurses, indicate that the nurse is caught between progress notes, ward rounds, and the alternate swabbing of floors and throats, and usually has neither the time nor the opportunity to give very much emotional support to the patient. Moreover, such emotional support as she is able to provide is too often viewed both by the nurse herself and by the hospital in general as ancillary to her role and almost unprofessional. Devereux and Weiner go on to say that one of the basic conditions of the ability to give human warmth is the security of the person called upon to dispense it, and that the professional status of nurses today is vague and lacking in security. As will be seen in Chapters 8 and 9, this situation obtained among the nurses in the present study, many of whom said that they preferred to work on the locked wards where there was "more real nursing"; they were unsure of themselves on the open wards, where they defined their role more as a domestic and policing one. Much thought is currently being given to such problems by the nursing profession (Brown, 1948; Peplau, 1952; Robinson, *et al.,* 1955; and Schwartz and Shockley, 1956).

The patient's role in a psychiatric hospital is probably least clear of all, with the exception of his relation to the therapist. The patient's life in the hospital, however, is made up of much more than his psychotherapeutic hour, and just how he should act during the remaining twenty-three hours is quite unclear. In thinking about the patient in the hospital, it is useful to make a distinction between the "sick role" and the "patient role" (Parsons, 1951). A sick role is a general category within which society defines a person as in need of medical attention. This is not entirely a matter of "having" a somatic or emotional illness. It is quite possible to die of an illness without ever having been sanctioned as sick by the society in which one had been living (Ackerknecht, 1947). The sick role has as much a social as a physical or emotional reference. The patient role is more specific than the sick role and is entered into by sick persons when they commit themselves to a relation with an individual or institution defined by the society as one which will help them. Most patients (but by no means all) enter the hospital already in the sick role, and the group of other patients on the ward has a great deal to do with bringing pressure to bear on the new arrival to take on the patient role (see Caudill, *et al.,* 1952). Equally, if the patients as a group come to hold the opinion that the institution, or the doctor, is not of sufficient help in their illnesses, there may be a movement among the patients to abrogate the patient role, but to retain the sick role (see Chapter 5). This sort of phenomenon seems in considerable part to be caused by the state of the whole hospital system at a particular time and is not adequately explained by reference to problems such as those of diagnosis or of psychological resistance. This was well illustrated some time ago in the work of Dembo and Hanfmann (1935) in a state hospital where they investigated one hundred consecutively admitted patients (exhibiting a wide range of neuroses and psychoses) for their psychological attitudes during the first week of hospitalization. Six major types of reactions were categorized and were found to be largely independent of the diagnostic classification, but to correlate with certain social factors in the patient's background, such as first admission, readmission, level of education, and the sexual roles of men and women in our culture. The work of Rowland (1938, 1939) and Devereux (1944) is also pertinent in this regard.

The main problem of this book, the meaning for both staff and patients of the context of the psychiatric hospital, received attention in the psychoanalytic literature some thirty years ago with the work of Simmel (1929). Simmel emphasized that the family situation was re-enacted within the hospital structure. He also pointed out the differences between psychotherapy carried out within the hospital as contrasted with outpatient treatment: he felt that within the hospital the doctor-patient relationship extended far beyond the doctor's office and that the inpatient was far more inclined to act out his conflicts than the outpatient. This latter was believed to be so because of the proximity of the doctor in the hospital; the patient, in trying to avoid the direct expression of hostility toward the doctor, usually displaced it onto the ward personnel or other patients. Interestingly enough, in terms of this book, Simmel also felt that life should be as comfortable as possible for the patient in the hospital, since if life was made difficult, the patient might obtain relief from his conflicts by the feeling that he was suffering in the hospital and hence would not be as ready to work with his doctor.

Much of profit is to be gained from Sullivan's (1931) early work, the research implications of which still need emphasizing. He established at Sheppard a special receiving service in which "it was proposed that a study be made of the therapeutic possibilities of carefully organized personal environments." In many ways this is the focus of the present book as well, except that an additional attempt is made to see how such personal environments fit into the larger social systems of the ward and the hospital in general. Sullivan eliminated the regular ward nurses, substituted attendants trained by himself, and was able to achieve some remarkable social recoveries with hebephrenic patients.

There has been considerable attention in the literature to the psychoanalytically oriented inpatient treatment done at the Menninger Clinic; such treatment is coupled with a use of the social environment to provide the patient with opportunities to achieve short-run obtainable goals that will develop his self-esteem and give him a sense of accomplishment (Menninger, 1937). Along different lines, favorable results have been reported at Boston Psychopathic Hospital when the environment was changed to allow the patients a measure of self-government and fuller communication with the staff (Hyde and Solomon, 1950; Greenblatt, York, and Brown, 1955).

Paralleling the work presented in this book in many ways is the report of the collaboration between Alfred H. Stanton, a psychiatrist, and Morris S. Schwartz, a sociologist, who studied a small private psychiatric hospital specializing in the treatment of psychoses by intensive psychotherapy (Stanton and Schwartz, 1954). In line with the remarks made earlier in this chapter on the flow of, and balance between, emotional and cognitive information, Stanton and Schwartz report how, repeatedly, the increased agitation and dissociation of a patient can be linked with an on-going disagreement about how the case shall be handled between two persons (such as therapeutic physician and administrative physician, or administrative physician and charge nurse) who exercise authority over the patient. The excitement of the patient is especially noticeable when neither of the two persons in authority nor the patient is consciously aware (or willing to admit openly) that there is a disagreement. In such a situation there is little transmission of cognitive information, but a good deal of emotional interchange goes on—at conscious and unconscious levels. Such a "split social field" as Stanton and Schwartz call it, makes for a considerable amount of free floating emotion which, since its source remains covert, may attach itself to many secondary and inappropriate contexts: the patient may burst into tears over the cold morning coffee, the nurse may distribute the nighttime sedation on the ward more with feelings of getting the patients out of the way than helping them to go to sleep, and the doctor may find himself in a heated argument at lunch with his superior over financial policy.

Stanton and Schwartz go on to point out that when such a disagreement is brought into the open and resolved between the persons in authority, the patient quickly improves. A further equally observable phenomenon is that the mental health of the staff members also usually improves when such disagreements are resolved. This latter point, as well as the fact that such processes are not confined to three-person social systems but can involve the total hospital, became apparent in the study of the dynamics of a collective disturbance reported in Chapter 5 of this book. The point to be made here is that the administrative process and the therapeutic process can become intimately related both consciously and unconsciously. At least this is true for the psychiatric hospital, and probably for the general hospital as well.

This question of the binding influence of a social system on unconscious as well as conscious processes needs emphasis and much further exploration, as to date social scientists have not paid much attention to unconscious processes, whether in the study of communities, factories, hospitals, or small groups. Psychiatrists have studied these phenomena chiefly with reference to the two-person system of psychotherapy, and only recently with reference to the dynamics of the family as an on-going small social system (Henry and Warson, 1951; Spiegel, 1954, 1957;

Parsons and Bales, 1955; and Ackerman and Behrens, 1956). Some years ago the writer became aware of this problem through a study of the sort of social organization that patients on an open ward created among themselves (Caudill, *et al.,* 1952). On the ward much primitive "instinctual" behavior, which would not be directly used for social purposes in the outer world, became enmeshed, and was so used, in the subculture and role system of the patient group. Hence, psychotherapy and administration carried out in the hospital had to contend with such behavior not only caused by regression but also supported by the social organization and values brought into being by the interaction of patients on the ward. Later, in further work reported in this book, it became evident that the staff were also involved in these processes, both in three- or four-person groups and in terms of the operation of the entire small hospital under study.

It is, of course, one thing to explore the unconscious meaning of interaction in the privacy of psychotherapy and quite another, requiring perhaps more courage, to ask staff to engage in a somewhat related type of scrutiny of their daily behavior. Especially this is true when the traditional structure of the hospital serves to make the interpersonal sources of such processes difficult to identify and hard to discuss freely. Partly for such reasons, there has been a growing dissatisfaction with the traditional administrative structure and therapeutic procedures of psychiatric hospitals, and some hospitals have undergone radical reorganization in an effort to reach the goal of becoming a therapeutic community. Outstanding in this regard is the work done by Maxwell Jones (1953) at Belmont Hospital in England.

It is interesting that a good deal more work emphasizing the social structure of hospitals and the concept of a therapeutic community has been done in child psychiatry than in adult psychiatry. Apparently, in our culture it is easier to recognize the existence of the influence of one's fellows among children than among adults. These studies have been reviewed by Rioch and Stanton (1953). Many of the studies on the organization of institutions for young children have used the model of the family as a basis for orientation. One of the classic descriptions of this kind is that by Anna Freud and Dorothy Burlingham (1944). The institutional organization was changed from an ordinary ward in which the nurses worked collectively with all the children to one in which each nurse took the role of a substitute mother for a group of four or five children. After an initial rather frenzied period of two or three weeks, the children blossomed under the new program. For somewhat older children, the model of a home has been used, and some of the most complete clinical studies in this area have been carried out by Bettelheim (1950) and by Redl and Wineman (1951). The work of Szurek and his colleagues with children is similar in many respects to the approach in this book, in that he emphasizes the significant effect upon the behavior of patients of conflicts between staff members (Szurek, 1947; and Sheimo, Paynter, and Szurek, 1949).

Owing to the current excitement over the results obtained through the use of tranquilizing drugs (chlorpromazine, reserpine, etc.) and the renewed hope of finding specific biochemical changes in certain psychotic disorders (particularly the schizophrenic reactions), it is probably useful to re-emphasize that results in these areas, by bringing the patient to a point where he can be worked with more effectively, serve to increase the need for further understanding of the patient's psychological conflicts and interpersonal difficulties. Any disease has psychological and social as well as organic concomitants, and the more variables that can be concretely identified, the more effective the study of the multiple aspects of the disease process can become.

The mention of the patient's psychological and interpersonal difficulties in the study of the multiple aspects of the disease process serves to introduce a conceptual problem that became evident early in the gathering of data for the research reported on in this book. In both the making of observations and the later analysis of material, the focus of attention was (1) sometimes on a single person; (2) sometimes on a small group of people—either belonging to one role group, such as patients on the ward, or to several role groups, such as the interrelations between patients, nurses, and doctors; and (3) sometimes on the processes going on throughout the entire hospital. Interest in a single person or a single event might be termed an interest in the *self-action* of the person or event, while interest in the interrelations of several people or events could be characterized by the well-known term, *interaction*. A term for the processes going on throughout the entire hospital, or a substantial part of it, was more difficult to find. Especially this was so since it was desired to keep track of the individuality of people and events while seeing them as part of a wider context of occurrences. The term chosen to denote these processes seen as part of a wider context was *transaction*.[2] At this point, the following example will indicate why

[2] This concept is taken from the philosophical work of Dewey and Bentley (1949). It appears in writings of Cantril (1950), Frank (1951), and Kilpatrick (1952) in the field of psychology. Spiegel (1954, 1957) has used it in psychiatric

the need was felt for a term that was broader than interaction and that denoted a multiplicity of interrelated events occurring over time in the hospital.

As the observations in the hospital progressed, it became evident that many of the actions taking place on the ward on a given night were related to the particular *combination* of nurses and doctors who were on duty—the kind of "field" that they formed. However, in the hospital under study, as in most hospitals, the particular combination of persons on duty was a purely chance occurrence because the administrative scheduling of nurses and physicians was carried out independently by the nursing supervisor and the chief resident. Some of the implications of this fact appear in the following chapters, but the point can best be made here by means of a hypothetical example. Suppose that on the ward there is a schizophrenic patient, Miss Jones, who has a phobia about fire engines, and one evening a fire engine with the siren on goes by the hospital. Also suppose that Miss Jones' anxiety is aroused to the level where she cannot handle the problem with her own psychological resources. At this point she has, in a sense, a choice: she may become excited, with certain attendant physiological changes such as crying, incontinence, exhaustion, and sleep; or she may turn to other persons for support which, if given in a way she can receive it, may at least lessen the depth of her excitement. She may turn to the other patients, to the nurse on duty, or to the doctor on call. It is here that the problem becomes complicated, as there is need to know both the general structure of the integration (and its balance at this particular moment) between patients, nurses, and doctors in the hospital, and the attributes of the individual persons filling these roles as these are mutually perceived by Miss Jones and the specific individuals concerned.

It may be that Miss Jones has not formed usable close relations with other patients, and, ignoring the ramifications of this fact, the question then centers on her contacts with the staff personnel on duty. Perhaps Miss Jones knows, and patients usually make it their business to know such matters, that her own doctor, Dr. Rolfe, is on call. Things may go smoothly *if* Miss Jones can get through to Dr. Rolfe because she is willing to ask the nurse on duty, Miss Nicholas, whom she likes and trusts, to telephone him. If another nurse, whom Miss Jones dislikes, is on duty,

studies of the family and in a more general theoretical development (Spiegel, 1956). Grinker (1953) discusses the concept with reference to psychosomatic disorders. Its use is related to similar ideas in communication theory as developed by Ruesch and Bateson (1951), Ruesch (1953), and von Foerster (1953).

things may go differently *even though* Dr. Rolfe is on call, since he can be reached only through the nurse.

The various permutations of this problem—involving combinations of specific individuals in hierarchical role arrangements and the influence exerted on these by the state of equilibrium or disequilibrium in the total hospital system—need not be worked out here. It is sufficient to indicate at this point that such phenomena go beyond what is usually meant by interaction and are better characterized by some other term, such as transaction.

The above discussion about Miss Jones implies a theoretical concern with the linkage between the related open systems of physiology, personality, meaningful small groups, and wider social structures. Only a brief reference to these ideas is possible here, and they are taken up again in Chapter 14. As to the notion of open systems: in a rough way most physical systems (e.g., a mechanical clock or a telephone circuit) are closed, while biological (e.g., the human body) and cultural (e.g., the family in everyday life or the grouping of patients on a ward) systems are open in that their existence depends on reciprocal interchange with other systems, and this process tends to be of a self-regulatory nature. Once wound, all the clock can do is run down, but the body and the personality are continually adapting to each other and to pressures arising from the family and community, or, in the hospital, from the various groups of patients on the ward and the operation of the administrative and therapeutic programs. In speaking of the difficulties that might arise in either closed or open systems, the emphasis in this book is not so much on a dysfunction of a specific *part* of a system (e.g., the mainspring of a clock or a broken arm), as on a dysfunction in the *pattern of the relations* between parts (as in metabolic disturbances, a neurosis, or interpersonal problems in a hospital).

Some of these ideas can be indicated in the example of Miss Jones and the fire engine. As envisaged, the situation started when the integrative capacity of her personality was placed under stress, and then led into the possible alternate links with other systems. The initial disruption might, however, just as easily have begun in a different system and then ramified. Things might have started when Miss Jones had an acute attack of abdominal influenza; or there might have been a collective disturbance among the patients on the ward; or the nursing staff might have been up in arms over a change in policy made by the senior staff; and so on.

This way of thinking about the effects of linked systems is not confined to the hospital, but is equally applicable to questions of health and illness in everyday life. However, such processes can be very advantageously studied in a hospital, where a higher degree of control is possible over certain variables, and data can be gathered with relatively greater ease on what is happening in social, psychological, and perhaps even physiological systems to produce effects on the patterning of relations between staff and patients.

Further than this, one would anticipate that in trying to come to terms with problems of health and illness, the patterns of relations between people in everyday life, and between staff and patients in a hospital, would vary from one culture to another. The contrast between the nature of the Japanese family and its place in the general culture of Japan and the nature of the family in the culture of the United States, makes the problems of a person in distress very different in the two situations, particularly regarding to whom he can turn for help and what he can expect.[3] These expectations about interpersonal relations are carried along by a person when he enters a hospital, since a patient does not take off his culture with his clothes (or at least not the more important internalized aspects of it). And the organization of the hospital itself is influenced by, and forms one special manifestation of, the general culture of which it is a part. These cultural influences affect personnel and patient selection, administrative and therapeutic procedures, and site and architecture.

The wider questions referred to in the preceding paragraphs will be returned to in the concluding section of this book. The focus of attention in the following chapters is on the theoretical and practical understanding to be gained from the detailed analysis of one small psychiatric hospital.

[3] There are, of course, important regional and social class variations in family organization and general culture in Japan and the United States.

CHAPTER 2

Setting and Organization of the Research

SETTING

The hospital in which this study was done was, as mentioned in the preceding chapter, in a state of transition. It had its inception some twenty-five years ago as a research and teaching unit attached to a medical school. At that time the main emphasis of the hospital was on descriptive psychiatry—the diagnosis and classification of psychopathology. With the entrance, some years prior to the beginning of this study, of a new head of the hospital, the emphasis shifted to a greater concentration on psychodynamic principles in treatment. With this change there also was a turnover in the senior physicians in the hospital, and this resulted in a different type of training for residents, with an attendant change in the kinds of relations established by residents with their patients. The same nurses and other therapeutic personnel were, however, retained from the previous organization of the hospital, and they were bewildered by the new policies. It was several years after the inception of these changes that the study reported here took place. Since the time of the study, the hospital has moved on to a thoroughgoing integration of its therapeutic and administrative programs and is now functioning smoothly as a psychoanalytically oriented small psychiatric hospital.

What it is hoped, then, to bring to life in these pages, lies in the past. Of the hospital at the time of the study, little remains: the patients are gone; the residents are gone; many of the senior staff and nurses are gone; and there have been changes in the physical aspects of the wards. Yet, in a general sense, the problems raised by the study of this hospital remain and are to be encountered in many psychiatric hospitals throughout the country. It is toward the further understanding of such problems that this book is directed.

Although attached to a medical school, the hospital that was studied was organized as a self-supporting, nonprofit institution because there were no funds for subsidy. Thus the weekly rates were high. At the time of the research, a standard rate of $133 per week was charged each patient, plus professional fees for psychotherapy and other forms of treatment. The financial and broad administrative policies of the hospital were the part-time responsibility of a business manager, who reported directly to the dean of the medical school.

The policies of the hospital with respect to treatment, training, and research were the responsibility of the chairman of the department of psychiatry in the medical school. Under the chairman of the department was a senior psychiatrist who was the head of the hospital and was in charge of its actual operation. The residents attached to the hospital were under the direction of the head, and the psychotherapy done by the residents was supervised by three part-time senior staff members. During the year in which the study was carried out, there were five psychiatric residents and a chief resident. The chief resident acted as the direct representative of the head of the hospital, and because of his position in this regard he will be classified with the senior staff in the following chapters.

The nursing staff was under the direction of the head of the hospital and included a supervisor and assistant supervisor of nursing, and some fifteen nurses (five of whom were charge nurses, while the remainder were staff nurses). Because of the small size of the hospital, the psychiatric aides were of less importance than in most hospitals, and they will appear infrequently in the data. In addition to the nurses, there were four female aides, who worked on the women's locked ward; divinity students in training at the university theological school were used as aides on the men's locked ward. There were no aides on the open wards. During the two daytime shifts the attempt was made to have two nurses on duty on each of the locked wards and one nurse on each of the open wards. It was not always possible to carry out this plan because of personnel shortages. In addition, each of the locked wards had two aides on duty during the daytime. On the night shift the ward personnel were reduced to about half of the number available in the daytime. Other therapeutic personnel in the hospital included a psychiatric social worker, a group activities worker, and an occupational therapist.

The hospital accommodated fifty patients and was divided into four wards—two locked wards (one for men and the other for women) and two open wards. During the day, men and women were together on the open wards. There was usually a census of about thirty-five patients in the hospital at any one time, and they were fairly equally distributed among the four wards. In general, there was a slightly greater proportion of women than men. The patients' diagnoses were broadly those of severe neuroses, character disorders, and psychoses of recent onset. In age, the patients were mostly young adults from twenty-five to forty-five years, and came from upper middle or higher social class backgrounds, although a few patients of lower social class background were present and supported financially by governmental or social agencies.

Treatment was mainly carried out by the residents, who did individual psychotherapy, although electric shock and insulin subcoma were also used. A few patients were in treatment with senior staff psychiatrists, and in these cases a resident took over the administrative management of the patient, while the senior psychiatrist did the therapy. The expected stay of a patient in the hospital was about four months, but frequently was much longer.

With the exception of those patients in treatment with senior psychiatrists, the residents took responsibility for both the therapeutic and administrative care of their patients. A resident usually had three or four psychotherapeutic hours with each of his patients during the week and discussed the progress of these patients with his supervisor once a week. The administrative care of patients was channeled through a fifteen- to twenty-minute administrative conference each morning. The personnel attending this conference were the head of the hospital, the chief resident, the residents, the supervisor of nurses, the charge nurses, the psychiatric social worker, the activities worker, and the occupational therapist.

The patients, in addition to their psychotherapeutic hours, participated in the activities and occupational therapy programs, and those patients who had going-out privileges were able to use the facilities of the city within which the hospital was located.

METHOD

As mentioned in Chapter 1, the methods used were largely those of observation and interviewing. The details of the more specialized techniques that were used, such as the picture interview and interaction process analysis, will be given in the appropriate chapters.

At the time of the study, the writer held an academic post as a social anthropologist in the medical school to which the hospital was attached.

In the course of his work in the hospital he made it clear to both patients and staff that his interests and role in the study were those of a research anthropologist, and he avoided being drawn into decision-making situations. The aims of the research were presented to both patients and staff in a series of meetings at the beginning of the study in much the way they have been outlined here—as an attempt to describe and gain a wider understanding of the context of events occurring in the daily work of the hospital. The writer concentrated on obtaining observations of ward life, recording the discussion at the daily administrative conferences, and carrying out an interviewing program. During the observational phase of the study, the head of the hospital was particularly helpful in providing the writer with information about what was happening at the senior staff level. After the gathering of data was completed, the head of the hospital also worked closely with the writer, particularly on analysis of the observational data.

Altogether, the writer completed over three hundred hours of observation on the men's locked ward, and over three hundred hours of observation on the open wards. Each of these periods represented about eight weeks of work carried out during all days of the week—thus observations were made over the week ends as well as on weekdays. The analysis of this material provided the first of the three studies mentioned in the preceding chapter. Prior to, as well as during, this same sixteen-week period, the writer made an essentially verbatim record of more than one hundred twenty consecutive daily administrative conferences, not all of which are used in the analysis in this book. Toward the close of the observational period, after the writer had been working on the wards for about three months, he began an interviewing program with the patients and staff which continued for seven months. This interviewing program was carried out by means of a series of pictures specifically drawn for the study and representing everyday life situations in the hospital. While this technique was similar to that of the Thematic Apperception Test, it was used more as an interview in which the pictures served as visual questions. Interviews were obtained from over half the patients who were in the hospital during the observational study, and from all the nurses, residents, and senior psychiatrists. This material was used in an analysis of the attitudes held by persons on any one level toward the everyday events of hospital life. It was also possible to determine how the various groups evaluated their own roles, and the roles of others, in the social structure of the hospital.

In addition to the role of research anthropologist, the writer felt it would be useful for him to have a minor functional role in the hospital so that it would be easier for people to identify him; hence, he explicitly associated himself with the activities program in terms of being a person who was available to take patients out of the hospital on various excursions once the activity had been planned and passed upon in the regular administrative channels. It is one thing, of course, to decide what one's roles will be, and quite another thing to put these into action. As mentioned earlier, before the study began, the writer held a meeting with each of the separate role groups in the hospital—senior staff, residents, nurses, and patients—in which he took considerable care to explain what he was going to do and to answer any questions people might have. As the study progressed, however, his work came to mean different things to people in the various role groups, and this was only to be expected.

It seemed to the writer that throughout the study the senior staff retained their initial conception of him as a research anthropologist who, for purposes of furthering his work, also had a minor role in the activities program.

The resident staff, on the other hand, with whom the writer became quite close, often told him how they saw him on the ward, and their view of him was at variance with the role he had originally conceived of taking. The residents tended to see the writer, even in his capacity as a rather passive observer, as having a therapeutic role on the ward.

The nursing staff had little understanding of the writer's research interests and tended to look upon him as a useful adjunct to the activities program in terms of a person available to take patients out. They tolerated—with some ambivalence—his note-taking and observing, which they felt at first as threatening to their own position in the hospital, although these feelings lessened as the study went on and there were no repercussions.

The patients also had little understanding of the writer's research role and looked upon him as a staff member who was connected in some vague way with the activities program and was available upon occasion to take them out. Equally, the patients soon came to place him as a generally handy social man about the ward, and he spent much time playing bridge and badminton, doing crossword puzzles, and so forth.

At the very beginning, not only the patients, but all levels of the staff, tried to use the writer as a source of information and to involve him in the decision-making processes of the hospital. For example, the patients on the locked ward requested him to bring up the need for a television set at the administrative conference. He replied that he would not do this because, although he might with some effort be able to get the television set for the ward, this action would greatly interfere with his research work and he felt that ultimately more benefit would accrue to the patients from his research than from the immediate goal of procuring a television set. He said, however, that he would be able to escort the patients on various activities, once these had been cleared through routine channels in the hospital. As he was careful not to become part of the decision-making process, his role in this respect soon came to be accepted by the patients and staff.

In terms of a fairly typical day in the hospital, the writer would arrive on the ward at about 7:45 a.m., just shortly before breakfast, and would stay on the ward until time for the daily administrative conference at about 9:00 a.m. He would attend this, and then either return to the ward or work in his office until time to go to a morning case conference. He usually had lunch with the residents, worked on the ward in the afternoon, had supper with the residents, and worked on the ward in the evening until about 9:00 p.m., at which time he retired to his office elsewhere in the building and, from his written notes, dictated the material for the day. Altogether, he usually spent about six hours a day on the ward, three of which involved detailed note-taking of what was going on, while the other three were spent in more active participation with the patients.

There was very little distrust of the writer by the patients on the ward. After an initial period of about a week, during which they were somewhat concerned over his note-taking, they came to accept it as a matter of course. The writer feels this was partly because he showed the patients his notes whenever they wished to see them, and partly because he was able to establish a rather passive but positive relation with most of the people on the ward.

The writer would not want to give the impression that his methods of observation on the ward were fixed from the beginning. At the start he attempted to keep track of a great many areas of interaction for later quantitative analysis. In order to do this he spent most of his time writing. After having followed this procedure for about three weeks on the men's locked ward, he began to feel that he was missing a considerable amount of important material, as he found that when he would stop his note-taking, people would interact with him very freely and tell him many things he wanted to know. He came to feel that he was not using the most valuable research instrument he had, his ability to get along with patients, and therefore he modified the course of his work on the wards so that he spent about half his time in detailed note-taking and the other half in participant observation.

Equally, the research had to adjust to the vicissitudes of the operation of the hospital. After about five weeks of observation on the men's locked ward, where he began his work, the writer found that, owing to the transfer of patients to the open ward and the lack of new admissions on the men's locked ward, his subjects were rapidly evaporating. Faced with the possibility of having only three or four patients to work with on the locked ward, he decided to shift his observations to include the open wards.

SUMMARY OF DATA OBTAINED

In summary, the data available after ten months of work were derived from: (1) two months of detailed observation on the men's locked ward; (2) two months of detailed observation on the open wards; (3) five months of recording daily staff administrative conferences; (4) four months of recording the twice weekly clinical case conferences; (5) a running account of senior staff interaction during the period of observation, obtained from the head of the hospital; (6) an account of the supervision of residents, obtained through irregular interviews with senior staff supervisors; (7) daily progress notes dictated by residents of their psychotherapeutic hours with patients; (8) daily nursing notes on patients; (9) informal interviews with nurses and residents; and (10) formal interviews using the series of pictures of hospital life.

It would be ideal if all the data were of the same quality. They were not. For one thing it was necessary to rely on the material that would be gathered by the hospital itself in the course of its ordinary work. This had both advantages and disadvantages. The advantages lay in that the material was gathered by someone other than the writer and therefore provided a check on the material he gathered personally. The disadvantages lay mainly in that the material might not be in sufficient detail or of the type that was wished.

For example, as pointed out in Chapter 1, it would be useful to know what went on in the daily psychotherapeutic hours with patients. One reason for this, which will become more apparent in Chapters 5 and 12, is the hypothesis that progress in therapy is not solely a matter of the relations between the doctor and patient, but that, in general, psychotherapeutic work in the hospital follows a certain "ground-swell," so that many patients may be doing fairly well at one point and somewhat less well at another. One way of getting at such phenomena would be to make sound-recordings of all the psychotherapeutic sessions as of any one day, and to analyze these over time. This would obviously be an extremely expensive, difficult to put into effect, and cumbersome procedure, which would probably produce too much data. In any case, in the exploratory study reported here, the best that could be done was to rely on the daily progress notes dictated by the resident therapists. These proved to be very useful in certain cases, as will be seen in Chapter 3 in the case of Mr. Esposito, and to be totally inadequate in others.

The writer is under no illusion that what was dictated in the progress notes bore anything but a shadowy resemblance to whatever the reality of the psychotherapeutic hour was. The material was useful, however, in that it provided a projection of what the therapist felt was important in the hour and what he either consciously or unconsciously may have been stressing. The adequacy of such material varies, of course, according to the extent of the dictation and how soon after the hour the notes were recorded. In the best cases there was an average of a full page of single-spaced typed material dictated during the same day (as was usually true for the material analyzed in Chapter 3). In such instances the analysis that can be done is quite exciting. In many other cases the progress notes were of much less value because they were short and the resident had waited for some days or weeks before doing his dictation.

The nursing notes on the patients had the great advantage of being kept regularly each day. They tended to fall into a rather stereotyped pattern in terms of both form and content, but despite this fact some interesting things could be done in the analysis of these notes (as indicated in Chapter 3).

In the analysis of data and the writing of this book the writer has, of course, made extensive use of his observations on the wards and in the administrative conferences, as well as of the formal and informal interviews he carried out.

MANNER OF PRESENTATION

This book is organized in terms of the four studies outlined in the preceding chapter. These are indicated by the major headings in the Table of Contents as Interrelations, Perceptions, Administration, and Implications.

A major restriction was, of necessity, placed on the study and the manner of presentation. This book is concerned with what occurred inside the hospital and not with the relations of the hospital to the world of which it was a part. The writer is well aware of the importance of the relation of the hospital to the community and of the influence of the patient's family and friends, the referring physician, and the courts and the law (Clausen and Yarrow, 1955). Equally, there is the question of the influence of the culture in general upon events in the hospital. For example, the effects of the relative social class positions of doctors, nurses, and patients upon their professional and personal interaction (see Chapter 9; and Schaffer and Myers, 1954; Hollingshead and Redlich, 1953). One must, however, for practical purposes break into such a continuum of relations, and the subject matter of this book lies largely within the hospital.

In the following chapters, partly for descriptive purposes, life in the hospital has been divided into three broad areas: therapy, administrative care, and human relations. Most of the work of the hospital can be placed within these three areas. Broadly speaking, the work of the doctor finds its greatest emphasis under therapy; a large portion of the work of the nurses and aides falls under administrative care; while the day-to-day relations of the patients on the ward are included under human relations. These areas are, however, something more than arbitrary categories, in that a certain set of values surrounds each of them. For example, the doctor most often sees himself in the role of therapist and is quite discontented if too much of his time is taken up with administrative duties; in addition, he frequently feels uncomfortable in the area of human relations with patients. The nurse, on the other hand, tends to see herself as carrying out administrative orders and directs most matters which she defines as therapeutic to the doctor. She, too, often is uncomfortable in human relations with patients. The patient, on his part, usually structures his contacts with other patients in terms of human relations, but feels uncomfortable if the doctor or nurse leaves the therapeutic or administrative role.

These three areas of life figure prominently in each of the major sections of this book. Thus, in the next section on Interrelations, Chapter 3 can be thought of as starting from a focus on therapy, Chapter 4 from administration, and Chapter 5 from human relations. At the same time, the focus of interaction in the next section increasingly widens from a single doctor-patient relationship in Chapter 3, to a small group on the ward in Chapter 4, and finally includes the entire hospital in Chapter 5.

Because of the emphasis placed in this book on the interrelated nature of events, a convention will be followed throughout in the citation of material. It is hoped that the reader will meet a number of real people in these pages and will wish to follow them from one chapter to the next. Thus the same names (which are, of course, fictitious) will be used for the same individuals in all cases. In order to make this procedure simpler, the names of all senior staff will begin with *S,* as Dr. Sutton, Dr. Scott, and Dr. Shaw. The names given the resident staff will all begin with *R,* as Dr. Rolfe, Dr. Reynolds, and Dr. Ramsay. The names of the nursing staff will all begin with *N,* as Miss Nugent, Miss Noyes, and Miss Nicholas. The names of the other therapeutic personnel, as the occupational therapist and the activities worker will begin with *W,* as Miss Winston, Miss Wright, and Miss Wells. The names of male patients will begin with vowels, as Mr. Ashton, Mr. Erskine, and Mr. Onofrio. The names of female patients will begin with one of four consonants, *F, P, L,* and *M,* as Miss Prescott, Mrs. Lasker, and Miss Miller.

In the following chapters the reader may feel as if life in the hospital was very difficult indeed, when actually things at other points than those being subjected to scrutiny were going along with tolerable smoothness. This, in part, is the inevitable problem of studying something in order to find out how it might be made better. Not only on such a practical level, but on a theoretical level as well, the very focusing on a phenomenon makes it stand out, and other phenomena recede into the background. In another sense, the analysis presented here may suffer from the same terminological difficulties as are found in the literature of psychodynamics when the attempt is made to describe the functioning of a reasonably adequate personality. No matter how well the person may be, he sounds rather sick when described in psychodynamic terms, and the same may be true for attempts to describe the social dynamics of a hospital.

Section II

INTERRELATIONS IN THE HOSPITAL

Daily Observations at Various Levels

CHAPTER 3

Influence of the Hospital on the Doctor-Patient Relationship

As part of looking at events within a wider context than usual, one interest of the study was on following in detail the experiences a patient had at the time of admission and during his first few weeks on the ward. This chapter concerns the stay of eight weeks in the hospital of a patient who will be called Mr. Francis Esposito. Although material was gathered on Mr. Esposito from the time of his admission, he became of special interest to the anthropologist when, about half way through his hospitalization, he began to paint pictures on his wall. This was not an unusual type of activity for a psychotic patient, and attention was initially focused upon the administrative question of how the patient's painting on the wall would be handled by the staff. There was some resistance to the painting in terms of the administrative routine of the hospital, but, in general, the staff viewed the painting as a harmless diversion and attached little significance beyond this to it.

Attention was next drawn to the fact that the patient was a plasterer by occupation. It was observed that he was reluctant to paint on paper or cardboard when these were offered to him, and he stated explicitly that he preferred to paint on the wall. The anthropologist began to wonder what this meant to him, in general and in terms of his occupation.

Another aspect of Mr. Esposito's painting was that it seemed to be related to similar actions on the part of other patients on the men's locked ward. Although Mr. Esposito started his painting earlier, and continued it later, there was a period of several weeks when Mr. Ashton and Mr. Innes were also engrossed in painting. In addition, Mr. Esposito had formed a flirting relation with Miss Lewis on the open ward. Miss Lewis had pretensions of being an artist and she also was painting at this time. The juxtaposition of these events raised questions about the meaning of Mr. Esposito's painting with reference to the relations between patients in the immediate ward situation.

Finally, the anthropologist heard that the patient had told his therapist on rounds: "I talk to the wall." This clue led to the exploration of the relation of Mr. Esposito's painting to his therapeutic progress. All the above events suggested that perhaps there was more to Mr. Esposito's painting than just a harmless way of amusing himself. It will be easier for the reader to follow the material and its analysis if the discussion starts at the beginning, with Mr. Esposito's admission to the hospital.

Mr. Esposito was a forty-nine-year-old, unmarried, Italian-born, construction worker. Four years prior to the present admission, he had spent several months in another psychiatric hospital. This previous hospitalization followed several fainting spells and periods of apprehension while at work. From the record it would appear that this earlier disturbance was accompanied by increased drinking. Several years ago he had visited his family in Italy following his father's death. Upon his return he had trouble in sleeping, and this difficulty continued into the present situation.

Two days before the present admission he had a heated argument with his employer, who wished him to work overtime. He did the additional work but remained excited over the matter. While at the home of relatives the next evening, he became dizzy and confused, fearful of the people about him, and blacked out. He came to after a minute and pleaded to be taken to a hospital, but refused to go with anyone but the doctor who had previously treated him for an eye injury. This doctor brought him to the emergency room where he was admitted at 1:30 in the morning. In essence, then, here was a patient who was very fearful of being hurt by people around him, had difficulties with authority relations, and had trouble in sleeping. These points are stressed as they are important in understanding Mr. Esposito's first few weeks on the ward.

On the ward the patient was cooperative for the first twenty-four hours and then went into an intermittently disturbed state for the next two weeks, during which time he had many noisy, denudative, masturbatory episodes. As a result of these he was frequently placed in seclusion. Following this his behavior changed and came to be characterized by the staff as clowning, silly, and inappropriate. At this point the patient was regarded as inaccessible to psychotherapy, and his behavior was looked upon as the result of a schizophrenic process. In going over the material, it was felt that, although Mr. Esposito very probably was schizophrenic, such an explanation was not sufficient to account for many of the specific details of his behavior.

Analysis of the material seemed to indicate that Mr. Esposito's eight weeks' stay in the hospital could be divided into three periods: (1) The first two weeks of hospitalization. During this period the patient gave evidence of wanting help on his immediate problems, but the therapist, while showing an immediate liking for the patient and giving him support in his organic symptoms, was more centrally occupied with obtaining a history and making a diagnosis. These latter activities were, of course, legitimate concerns on the part of the therapist, who, since he was a first-year resident, would be required shortly to present an initial diagnosis and history to the staff. (2) A second period of two weeks. This was marked by the therapist's increased interest in treating the patient more directly, but at this time the patient had lost much of his initial motivation for treatment, although he still showed his initial reciprocal liking for the therapist. (3) A third, and final, period of four weeks. In this period little psychotherapy was attempted. The therapist restricted himself to administrative care, and the patient focused his attention largely on himself and on the other patients. At the close of this period the patient was discharged. Each of these three periods will be discussed in turn.

FIRST PERIOD

The general framework within which it was useful to view Mr. Esposito's first period was to consider that when a patient enters a hospital there are at least five sources to which he may turn for satisfaction of his immediate needs: (1) his physician, (2) the nurses and aides, (3) the use of the physical space of the ward in ways that he finds most comfortable, (4) the other patients, and (5) himself—as this is related to his psychological resources and the manipulation of his body. A patient's use of the last source, himself, may vary from relatively integrated activity such as reading and exercising, to less integrated activity such as hallucination and self-mutilation. It is important to point out that the ordinary communication system of a psychiatric hospital is designed to provide information about patients from the first two sources—the relation to the physician, and to the nurses and aides. The ordinary hospital system is less adequately designed to provide information about how the patient uses the physical space, the other patients, or himself. During his first week in the hospital, Mr. Esposito attempted to utilize these five sources, but often he did not obtain the kind of response he was seeking from the first three sources, and hence he frequently turned to the use of himself and the other patients.

Mr. Esposito's actions during his first two days on the ward seemed to parallel closely the events which led to his hospitalization. He had an argument with another patient—a "big fellow" whom he saw as having authority on the ward; he was frightened by people around him; and he had an attack ending in loss of consciousness. During these first few days he seemed grateful for the routine care of the nurses and for the presence of the doctor—particularly in terms of the doctor's attention to his physical symptoms. To help himself meet these problems, Mr. Esposito also seemed to have brought certain other patterns of behavior into the hospital with him. In his regular life, he had been in the habit of going to bed for a few hours upon his return from work and then having a late evening meal, following which he visited and drank with Italian cronies until midnight. In the hospital he went to bed in the afternoon, was awake at night, and read a good deal. At the same time, he attempted to learn the hospital routine and cooperate with it. Much of this is reflected in the nursing notes for the first few days:

(First night, upon admission to ward) Walked in accompanied by Dr. Ryan at 1:30 a.m., quiet, appeared bewildered. To bed. Asked for towel, wanted to get washed before going to bed. Administrative care waived. Seconal 0.29 mgs. at 1:45 a.m. Offered no conversation. To sleep immediately. Slept well.

Later in the morning of the first day the patient had a recurrence of the same kind of "seizure" which precipitated his coming to the hospital.

(First day) Patient was very startled when called for breakfast. Jumped up from bed with a glassy stare. . . . Was observed holding his hand up with fingers spread far apart and shaking it while he stared at it. This was soon followed by a seizure when the patient developed a rapid bodily movement, with his one hand hitting the table and the other striking the chair, legs also twitching. He was helped to his room and put to bed. Appeared very frightened by every movement in the room, but was told that he was in the hospital and that the doctors and nurses wouldn't hurt him. Dr. Ryan was called and he saw the patient for some time. . . . Patient asked for his glasses and did some reading in the early evening. . . . Patient was quiet, seemingly grateful for attention. Read for short periods of time alternately in living room and own room. Complained early in evening about his foot. Asked what time everybody went to bed and retired cooperatively.

(Second day) No recurrence of seizures. Patient seemed in good contact. . . . Went to x-ray, was relaxed. Even slept while waiting for technician. Seemed to understand technician's instructions perfectly. Cooperated well.

Began reading toward bedtime. . . . Was awake at night. Hot milk was given at 1 a.m. . . .

In these notes of the first two days it can be seen how the patient received help from the doctor, who came to the ward when the patient asked for him, and how the patient also received support from the nurses and aides in terms of routine care. The patient also seemed to have made good use of his own defenses: the moment he came into the hospital he asked for a towel in order to wash; later he asked for his glasses and did a certain amount of reading; he slept much of the time during the day and was awake at night. This fairly adequate defense system, perhaps of a somewhat obsessive-compulsive nature, was important because at a later date these defenses broke down under stress into regressive alternate smearing and cleaning-up of feces when the patient was in the seclusion room; at this later time, however, such regressive behavior seemed to come "out of the blue" because earlier the staff had not made themselves sufficiently aware of the nature of the patient's immediate defenses.

In the therapeutic hours for the first few days the therapist concentrated on diagnosis and history, and only casually touched upon the events occurring on the ward. He paid particular attention to the patient's organic complaints and scheduled tests for him, and it seems likely that the patient received considerable support from these actions. In his interview on the first day, the therapist also noted the cooperative behavior of the patient. The therapist dictated in his progress notes:

(First day) He answered questions with pertinent answers and is oriented as to time, place, and person. . . . He seemed rather frightened but reassured that he was in a hospital where he could be taken care of. He said he had sufficient savings to remain in the hospital for a reasonable length of time. At that time he indicated he could stay as long as a year if necessary. . . . When he signed the commitment papers, his handwriting was very slow and methodical but legible. He seemed to know what he was doing and he read the commitment paper before he signed.

A complete and thorough physical examination revealed no significant abnormal findings. . . . On detailed questioning there is no history of convulsions or blackout spells in the mother, father, or the two sisters or two brothers. . . . When I pressed him a little bit about his alcoholism, he admits that he drinks quite heavily. . . . In view of this history . . . the diagnosis of epilepsy is most probable. . . . Further organic work-up will be done in the nature of skull series, electroencephalogram, psychological tests, and lumbar puncture.

After seeing the therapist on his first day, Mr. Esposito returned to the ward, where he had an upsetting experience with another patient.

The therapist discussed this with him on the following day, but tended to view it in terms of its origin in the past, whereas the patient immediately brought the discussion back to the present. Of this interview on the second day, the therapist dictated:

(Second day) The patient was in bed resting when I saw him. He said that he was very tired, that he was able to sleep very little. . . . Apparently at the lunch table he was upset by Mr. Erskine (another patient). . . . Mr. Esposito said that Mr. Erskine told him on one occasion to shut up or keep quiet, but indicated that he had not said anything to Mr. Erskine to provoke this. I asked him if this upset him, and he indicated that it probably did. His hands were shaking as he told me this, palms were quite moist, but his pulse was about 80. He said sometimes this big fellow, meaning Mr. Erskine, seemed like a patient to him and sometimes he seemed like someone who worked here. He said he had been sleeping poorly for about three years, ever since his return from Italy. I pressed him on this to see if he had had a disturbing experience in Italy. He indicated no, the family was well. He complained bitterly about severe sweating at night, saying that this had been going on for several weeks now, and that last night he had sweated very profusely.

The time from the third to the eighth day was marked by the daily repetition of a pattern of events during which Mr. Esposito became progressively more agitated, and his defenses deteriorated. His daily pattern consisted in the following: a morning hour with the therapist, who continued to explore the patient's previous life; an afternoon nap; relations with the other patients in the early evening; and a disagreement with the nurse at night, after which the patient would become excited and would finally be placed in seclusion.

The evening of the third day also marked a change in Mr. Esposito's cooperative behavior on the ward. Concerning the therapeutic hour on the morning of the third day, Dr. Ryan dictated: "The patient was dressed and came to my office this morning. . . . I got him to talk a little bit more about his past. . . ." Mr. Esposito complied with this request by Dr. Ryan, but quickly brought the conversation back to the present. During the afternoon of the third day Mr. Esposito slept until he joined the other patients for supper. After supper he borrowed a cigarette from Mr. Ashton—a manic patient with whom he later became quite friendly—and laughed and joked with him. That night, Mr. Esposito's fourth in the hospital, he was awake and standing at the window of his room. The nursing notes read:

(Fourth night) Had repeat sedation at 2:20 a.m. Fifteen minutes later was found out of bed standing at porch door in room. Unsteady on feet, seemed confused and irritable. Asked to stay in bed by nurse, which he said he'd try to do. Had wanted a cigarette earlier which was refused. Up once during this, would not keep pajamas on, lying on top of covers without pajamas remainder of night without sleeping.

The main interest in this piece of behavior is, as will be seen later, that it became repetitive. On subsequent nights the patient again asked for a cigarette and was given repeat sedation instead, whereupon he refused to go to sleep and became excited.

On the morning of the fourth day, the therapist inquired about the episode during the preceding evening. Dr. Ryan dictated:

(Fourth day) The patient was dressed but not shaven when he came to my office. He looked much better and said that he felt good today. He was aware that he did not sleep well last night, and when I asked him about the incident of taking his pajamas off and lying in the bed nude during the night, he said that he knew he tore the pajamas off as he felt they were too small and too tight, but he seemed to be rather vague about this. The nurses indicated that he was somewhat confused. We talked about the patient's family in Italy. . . . Today he seemed to talk rather freely, and we seemed to have a good relation. . . . Though there may well be organic brain pathology here, there certainly is a significant emotional disturbance in which some superficial psychotherapy should be of definite value.

There are a number of things of interest in this therapeutic hour that became increasingly important in the progress of the patient's illness. First, the doctor again avoided the present and pressed for past history. Second, the doctor's own cultural values may have entered into his feelings around the fact that the patient was unshaven. Third, Dr. Ryan had previously thought of the patient's illness as organic in origin, but in the therapeutic hour on this day he felt there might be some question about this. In subsequent therapeutic hours there was a tendency for the therapist to vacillate between an organic and a functional diagnosis, depending upon whether or not the discussion between therapist and patient had been productive.

Following his usual pattern, on the afternoon of the fourth day Mr. Esposito put on his pajamas and went to sleep. Later in the evening, however, he again had an "anxiety attack." Knowledge of the circumstances surrounding this attack is vague, but, as on the previous evening, the events seemed to involve a disagreement with the nurses. The nursing notes indicated:

(Fourth day) At 4:00 p.m. patient cried out. Patient found lying on his bed, lower extremities rather rigid, trembling all over. Color poor, pulse 110, respiration 122. Complained of chest pains. Very confused. One hour later he removed his pajamas, took cord out of pajamas, threw cord on floor in a straight line and tried to walk on cord. Walked about room nude, ate supper in his room, nude, sitting on the chair. At 5:50 p.m. patient ripped screen off porch door and commenced hopping about on one foot. Taken to seclusion at 6:25 p.m.; threw wet towel at the nurse on his way to seclusion. Ordered nurses to get away from him. Pounding on walls in seclusion. Put his ear to screen as though listening to some imaginary person. . . .

The following morning, the patient's fifth day in the hospital, he was seen in the seclusion room by Dr. Ryan, who questioned him about his excitement during the preceding evening. The therapist dictated:

(Fifth day) I saw the patient in the seclusion room this morning. He was nude but protected himself with the hospital gown. He was taken to seclusion and on the way threw a towel at one of the nurses. I asked him about this, and he says that he remembers it quite well. He said he doesn't know what happened, he said that something made him mad. He remembers one of the nurses saying something to him before he got upset. This is questionable as probably he was upset before that. . . .

It is interesting here that the therapist refused to see the possibility that the patient's disturbance was connected with his immediate interpersonal experiences on the ward. Rather, as will become apparent a little later, the therapist's thoughts were mainly in terms of the possible organic basis of the psychosis. Concerning this fifth therapeutic hour, Dr. Ryan continued:

(Fifth day, continued) He remembers that, thinking back, this has happened two or three times in the past year. It occurred twice when he was working. He claimed the scaffold was too low, whereas it had previously been adjusted properly. He went home at this time and was confused. In response to my questioning, he did think that he was drinking a little bit more during these spells, but not a great deal more. I asked him a little bit about his drinking, and he says he doesn't know why he drinks and that it is very difficult to explain. I asked him if he felt depressed and sad when he started to drink, but he did not respond to this. He said that he usually drinks with men friends and occasionally with women friends. I asked him if he had any particular girl friend. He denied this, and denied that he was going out with any women at the present time. . . .

It is possible that what the patient was trying to tell the therapist here was that the same things happened to him on the ward with the nurses as happened to him on the job with people who had authority over him. However, the therapist ignored this possibility and went on to ask the patient about his drinking and heterosexual relations. At this point in the patient's hospitalization he was experiencing difficulty in: (1) communicating satisfactorily with his therapist, (2) achieving a good relation with the nurses, and (3) utilizing the physical space of the ward in a way comfortable for him. He was, therefore, increasingly turning to (4) his relations with other patients, and (5) the use of himself. Dr. Ryan closed his notes on the fifth therapeutic hour by dictating:

> (Fifth day, continued) This episode again introduces the strong possibility of an epileptic fugue state, although such diseases as Alzheimer's can certainly begin in this manner. . . . The lumbar puncture revealed normal protein, and the skull series was normal. The EEG report is not back as yet.

It can be seen how the therapist again returned to an organic diagnosis when the discussion with the patient had not been too rewarding.

In the afternoon of the fifth day Mr. Esposito returned to the ward, slept, had supper, and talked at length with Mr. Ashton, the manic patient, about restaurants, opera, and preferences in phonograph records. As on previous nights, Mr. Esposito was awake late; he requested a cigarette, which was denied. The nursing notes read:

> (Sixth night) Awake at midnight asking for a smoke to enable him to go to sleep. When asked to go to room escorted by nurse, he started hopping and so was walked out to seclusion. After getting into seclusion, asked again for smoke, saying he wouldn't stay there. Started pulling on penis. Chloral hydrate 8 cc. given. Lying on mattress, partially nude, noisy, masturbating, apparently hallucinating.

The sixth day being Sunday, Mr. Esposito did not see his therapist. He was returned to the ward at supper time, and he immediately related to Mr. Ashton—the two of them laughing and talking. During this conversation, the nurse asked Mr. Esposito to get dressed, as he was wearing only underwear shorts. He appeared bewildered and remarked that Mr. Ashton went around in his shorts. (Mr. Ashton was wearing whipcord tennis shorts.) When Mr. Ashton went to the gym, Mr. Esposito asked for his glasses and read quietly.

While Mr. Esposito's diagnosis was schizophrenia, and Mr. Ashton's was manic-depressive psychosis, it became very clear from the observations on the ward at this time that Mr. Esposito was almost directly imitating much of Mr. Ashton's behavior—and hence adding a manic "flavor" to his own symptomatology. Also at this time, during a manic phase of his illness, Mr. Ashton was much impressed by the help patients could give each other. In conversation with the anthropologist on the ward, Mr. Ashton said that Mr. Esposito had put a lot of pressure on him to stop talking and swearing so much. On the other hand, Mr. Ashton said that Mr. Esposito used to disturb the ward at night by singing and laughing, but that Mr. Esposito had said last night that he would try to stop his singing if it bothered Walt (Mr. Ashton) and Joe (Mr. Erskine). Mr. Ashton went on to say that Mr. Esposito had been in seclusion a great deal recently, and that the patients had all told him that seclusion wasn't so bad—that they had all been there. Mr. Ashton said this was something of a little white lie, but they had said it so that Mr. Esposito wouldn't feel badly about being in seclusion.

Continuing his usual pattern, on the sixth day Mr. Esposito rested in bed from 9:30 to 10:30 p.m. Later he was awake again and was taken to seclusion. The nursing notes read:

(Seventh night) Awake, and at times singing to himself. Taken to seclusion at 11 p.m. Pajamas dropped to floor, and patient refused to tie them securely about waist. . . .

On the seventh day, the hour with the therapist took place in seclusion while the patient was eating lunch. Dr. Ryan dictated:

(Seventh day) . . . The patient had been put in seclusion during the previous night because he had apparently become upset. He had been associating a great deal with the patient Ashton, who has been playing his phonograph, and both of them have been laughing and carrying on quite loudly. The patient remarked about the odor of the room, spitting in the corners and saying that he wanted to return to his own room. We talked a little bit about his going back, and he said that he had to see Walt (Mr. Ashton). He said that Walt made him laugh, and then he giggled and laughed very loudly.

(At this point Mr. Esposito's lunch was brought into seclusion) . . . He mentioned that he was afraid that maybe he was poisoned. I asked him if there was anyone he knew who would want to poison him, and he indicated that he liked everybody but maybe somebody didn't like him. I asked him if he was afraid that the hospital was trying to poison him, and he said that that was possible but that he could not be sure. I asked him if he was afraid that we were doping him, and he said that that could happen here. I asked him if he had ever taken any dope, and he vehemently denied this. I reminded him that alcohol was something like dope, and after thinking for awhile he agreed with this. I asked him why he drank, and he said that he did not really know. Referring to dope, he said that he wouldn't take dope because he was really dopey enough, and he laughed a great deal at this pun he had made. I asked him if he felt like this when he drank, and he indicated after a moment that he does sing and carry on like this when he is drunk.

He then asked me if he could shave, and I agreed it would be a good idea. He said that he felt okay and that he wanted to return to his room. I told him why he was here in seclusion—that when he gets upset, he upsets other patients, particularly when he is noisy. He indicated that sometimes patients made a lot of noise and yet they are left where they are, but that when he makes a lot of noise, he is removed to seclusion. And he said very strongly that he disliked this room. . . .

Today's behavior seems to be quite schizophrenic; there are paranoid ideas here . . . and there is also a little perseveration in his speech. . . . The EEG was negative, but certainly does not rule out epilepsy. I am undecided at present.

There are a number of important points in the therapist's report of this hour. First, the patient was apparently receiving considerable satisfaction of his immediate needs from the other patients, particularly Mr. Ashton, and wished to return to the ward to continue these relations. The therapist did not attempt to evaluate the emotional meaning of these relations with the other patients, but viewed them more as evidence of psychotic symptomatology and as presenting administrative problems. Both the latter points are, of course, valid, but the emotional meaning of the relations for the patient was not explored. Second, it seems likely that the patient was trying to communicate with the therapist by telling him that "he was afraid maybe he was poisoned . . . and . . . that he liked everybody but maybe somebody didn't like him." The therapist seemed to miss this attempt at communication and went on to remind the patient that "alcohol was something like dope." The patient seemed to be trying again to communicate in asking if he could shave and return to his room. In a sense, it would seem the patient was saying: "I realize this behavior isn't getting me anywhere, and I want to shave and act like a good patient because I want to get help from you." The therapist and the patient seemed to have misunderstood each other a second time, as the therapist responded by pointing out the administrative reasons why the patient was in seclusion, and the patient resisted this line of thought. Finally, the therapist seemed to have considered this hour a rather difficult one as, at its close, he returned to his thinking about an organic diagnosis. The therapist's concern over the patient's diagnosis was reinforced at the administrative conference the next morning when he reported:

Dr. Ryan: Mr. Esposito is in seclusion. There seems to have been a change in him. He has what I have been calling a fugue state lately during which he will tear off his pajamas. Yesterday morning he was dancing around nude in seclusion complaining that the odor was very bad. He had lunch in seclusion and was balancing the cups and saucers on his knees, and giggling. He wanted to see Mr. Ashton as they like to play music together. This looks very much like schizophrenic behavior to me and not so much like epilepsy.

Dr. Shaw: If there is epilepsy here, we will have to disentangle the schizophrenic behavior from it.

Returning to the material on the seventh day, after the hour with the therapist, Mr. Esposito was taken back to the ward where, according to the nursing notes:

(Seventh day) . . . He talked and laughed with his good friend Mr. Ashton, and they made plans to have Scotch and soda upon dismissal. (Later) . . . The nurse spoke firmly to him telling him he'd be put out in seclusion again if he didn't behave and quiet down. . . . Mr. Esposito immediately calmed down and remained cooperative the remainder of the evening.

At this point it seemed that Mr. Esposito had begun to realize he could not communicate his needs through excitement. He therefore shifted his approach to his therapist, as indicated in the therapeutic progress notes of the next few days. He became "submissive, quiet, calm, clear, and clean shaven." Dr. Ryan seems to have responded very positively to this shift in Mr. Esposito's behavior, and communication improved between doctor and patient. Evidence for these developments comes from Dr. Ryan's dictation of the therapeutic hours on the eighth and ninth days:

(Eighth day) When I saw him he was very submissive, insisting that I take a more comfortable chair and so on. . . . He was much quieter. He was in his room, dressed in his pajamas. He told me about his Army experiences when I questioned him about this. . . . I indicated that we should talk more about this. . . . This afternoon his behavior seems quite normal.

(Ninth day) Today the patient was calm, quite clear, and was clean shaven for the first time. . . . I asked him about his experiences with religion as a child. He said that he was frightened by a bearded priest when he went to confession. He said that he didn't like the church; it smelled bad. He didn't want to tell the priest what he was thinking about and he ran away, and thereafter he had real dislike for the church, though he went when his mother asked him to. He indicated that during a previous hospitalization he was directed to go to church and went once to the Catholic and once to the Protestant church. He seemed to like the latter better. He did not seem to have any guilt about going to church. He said that people should never force one to do something against one's will. I remarked that that happened sometimes in his work, and he took this up quite readily and indicated yes, that many times people feel that they know some things that they don't, and insist on bossing others around. Today he was very clear and very alert, more talkative than usual, and I will be unable to make a diagnosis of his psychosis at this point. In the afternoon he had psychological testing, the neurosurgeon saw him and felt there was no evidence of organic brain disease at this time.

The session on the ninth day was a very complex one because it apparently represented a blending of many things that were never disentangled. Mr. Esposito was again telling Dr. Ryan that "many times people feel they know some things that they don't and insist on bossing others around" which could very well be a reference to his feelings about being placed in seclusion. Equally, the description of his early experiences when he was frightened by a bearded priest at confession, did not want to tell what he was thinking, and did not like the church because it smelled bad (he had said the same of the seclusion room), all sound like oblique references to seclusion and to the doctor-patient relationship. At the same time, however, these references seem to be a mixture of present and past, the current situation blending with memories that may have been stirred up by Dr. Ryan's questioning.

As indicated in the therapeutic progress notes for the ninth day, Mr. Esposito had had a rather full and successful day: his hour with the therapist, an appointment with the neurosurgeon, and psychological tests. In general, his behavior had "seemed quite normal." During the evening, however, an unfortunate incident occurred that resulted in his again being placed in seclusion. The nursing notes for the evening of the ninth day indicated:

(Ninth day) Reasonably quiet during afternoon and early evening. Ate well and in normal fashion at supper. Unscrewed the top of the water fountain; inability to put top back on, and resulting mess, caused patient to become quite upset. When nurse entered the ward, shook fist at her and said: "Do you want me to kill you? . . ." Began mopping the entire corridor; wandering about disturbing other patients.

(Tenth night) Taken to seclusion about 10:30 p.m. Noisy. Began banging on door. Taking feces from rectum. Washing hands and face for about five minutes. Taken back to room. Quiet for about half an hour and then banging again. Out at 6 a.m. and spent much time washing hands and face and drank some water. Agitated at this time, stating that he wouldn't go back to that room. "My room is outside." Went back and started cleaning seclusion with a pillow case. Then started usual banging to get out. Was not allowed out again. Excited, cursing, profane, and threatening. Face flushed, perspiring. . . .

The foregoing material shows quite clearly the breakdown, and attempts at reintegration, of Mr. Esposito's defenses as manifested in washing and cleanliness. These worked well for him when he first came into the hospital, but neither the therapist nor the ward personnel seemed to be consciously aware of the defensive usefulness of such behavior or its meaning to the patient. Thus, the ward personnel reacted to Mr. Esposito's "mopping the corridor" after breaking the water fountain only as bizarre and troublesome behavior without recognizing its value to the patient. The patient was simply removed to seclusion, where he continued to utilize his defenses in a less integrated manner—alternately smearing feces and cleaning them up.

The next morning, and Mr. Esposito's tenth day in the hospital, this situation was discussed at the administrative conference as follows:

Dr. Rolfe (who had been on duty the preceding evening): Mr. Esposito was banging this morning and—

Miss Nicholas (breaking in): He is still banging.

Dr. Shaw: Did we have fire and water last night?

Miss Nicholas: Just water. (In reference to Mr. Esposito's breaking the fountain.)

Dr. Ryan: Was Mr. Esposito disturbed before this incident?

Miss Nicholas: I don't know.

Dr. Ryan: The attendant should watch Mr. Esposito and put him in his own room when he sees signs of his beginning to be disturbed. I feel that Mr. Esposito is not really disturbed but is simply unhappy at being in seclusion. At present he has his hand wrapped up in a blanket and in his banging against things he says he will pay for whatever he breaks, but that he doesn't like being in there, and that he's going to keep banging until he gets out.

Dr. Sears: How is the order written on Mr. Esposito?

Dr. Ryan: Mr. Esposito may be put into seclusion at the discretion of the nurses.

Dr. Rolfe: It looks like a disturbance at being in seclusion rather than an actual dynamic disturbance.

Miss Nicholas: Mrs. Netter had him out of seclusion once each hour with her, and then he would swear and holler and curse so much that she would have to put him back in.

Dr. Ryan: Yes, that's true, but he was swearing and hollering because he had to go back into seclusion, and I feel that if he were to be put into seclusion for a few minutes and then taken out when he was quiet, things would go much better.

Miss Noyes: Mr. Esposito was so disturbed last night that I certainly don't think he should be on the ward, and I don't think that he should stay on the ward this morning either.

Dr. Ryan: He's asking to get out and is making it so uncomfortable for us that he will get out.

Dr. Shaw: The patient will have to show us that he can be calm and demonstrate his rationality before we let him out of seclusion.

Dr. Ryan: Mr. Esposito wasn't banging when I saw him a little while ago, and he said that he would give us a half hour and then would go back to banging.

Dr. Shaw: If he keeps this up he will be harder to manage on the ward, and he will become anxious about being put into seclusion. This is a problem you (Dr. Ryan) will have to work out with Mr. Esposito.

Dr. Sears: I think it would be a good idea to put Mr. Esposito in for an hour and then take him out. I mean have Dr. Ryan personally be present when he is put in and then take him out and see how he is at the end of that time.

Dr. Ryan: Mr. Esposito has never been in seclusion all day during the daytime.

Dr. Sears: It might be a good idea to work it out on an hour-to-hour basis and have you be there.

Dr. Rolfe: I am wondering about sedation and why this couldn't be used. I understand Mr. Esposito is going to be given an EEG this afternoon, and I wonder what effects sedation would have after an EEG?

Dr. Reynolds: What contra-indications are there for sedation?

Dr. Ryan: What indications are there for it?

Dr. Reynolds: Well, the patient has been disturbed a little bit lately.

Dr. Ryan: We want to get an EEG that is undisturbed by the effects of sedation.

Dr. Shaw: This is a difficult problem and one that will have to be worked out with the doctor.

There were a great many points of interest in this administrative conference, not all of which can be considered in detail. Perhaps the most important point was that Dr. Ryan found himself caught between the staff, who felt Mr. Esposito should remain in seclusion, and the patient, who felt he should not be in seclusion. As a result, Dr. Ryan became defensive both of himself and the patient. Equally, the patient found himself caught between Dr. Ryan, who now felt the patient should be out of seclusion, and the nurses, who felt he should remain there. This situation was exacerbated by two other things. First, Dr. Ryan's order was written in such a way that Mr. Esposito could be placed in seclusion at the discretion of the nurses. Second, Mr. Esposito's situation was involved in a broader, but not openly stated, disagreement between the nurses and the residents—the nurses felt that in general the residents were too permissive with patients (see Chapter 5). This attitude was behind Miss Noyes' statement: ". . . I certainly don't think that he should stay on the ward this morning either."

It is interesting that this disagreement among the staff should have coincided with the increased excitement of the patient. This would seem to be a fairly exact replica of the situation described by Stanton and Schwartz (1954), where two persons with power over a patient disagree about how the case is to be handled, and the patient participates in this disagreement by increased agitation and dissociation.

A few other points should be mentioned in passing. For example, the placing of the burden of proof solely on the patient, again with the implication that the patient's behavior stems much more from qualities somehow inherent in him, and with little reference to the interactional field, as was implied in Dr. Shaw's statement: "The patient will have to show us he can be calm and demonstrate his rationality before we let him out of seclusion."

Coupled with the above was a simple lack of information on the part of the senior physicians, as evidenced by Dr. Shaw's belief that Mr. Esposito "will become anxious about being put into seclusion." The patient had been anxious about this for some days. In addition, the seniors twice avoided points at issue—once in reference to Mr. Esposito's banging, and once on the matter of sedation—by referring the problem back to Dr. Ryan as something he would have to work out with the patient. This resulted in Dr. Ryan's becoming increasingly defensive, so much so that a simple misunderstanding in communication occurred at the end of the discussion where Dr. Rolfe was concerned about the effects of sedation *after* an EEG, and Dr. Ryan interpreted this as a suggestion that sedation be used immediately and *before* the EEG.

Following the administrative conference just discussed, Dr. Ryan went down for his therapeutic session with the patient, about which he dictated:

> (Tenth day) The patient was in seclusion this morning banging loudly on the walls and on the door and asking to be let out. When I was with him he quieted down and told me that he just could not stand it in that room, that it was dirty and that there was not enough air. I told him that I would see about getting him out. This was discussed at meeting, and it was decided that I should be present when he was put into seclusion and try to be present to evaluate him after an hour or so on letting him out. . . . The patient returned to his own room and dressed and came to my office with me. I asked him about the episode last night in which he dismantled part of the water fountain. He doesn't know why he did it, that it was just something he had to do. I asked him about this, and he said it reminded him of a missing water fountain in his home town in Italy. There were two fountains in the town, and people said that someone stole one of the fountains, and it was never brought back. This tale went back to when he was a young child. He said that when he returned to his home town on a trip, that it was an unchanged town after all these years, and that nothing new was being done there. The roads, the people in the streets, and the buildings were just the same.

In this session it is possible to see again the same things that were contained in the therapeutic hour on the ninth day. The patient was somewhat more successful in communicating his desire to get out of seclusion. He also seemed to be blending the past and the present together when he said that his home town was "an unchanged town after all these years and that nothing new was being done there." It is possible, in the light of earlier material, that this was a reference to the immediate therapeutic situation as well as a reference to the patient's childhood.

SECOND PERIOD

Mr. Esposito had now been in the hospital for almost two weeks, and it was at this point that what has been called the second period of his stay began. During this period Mr. Esposito's behavior changed considerably, and he was reported by the nurses on the ward as "subdued and irritable" with a "tendency to ask if it is all right to do this or that."

He continued to develop his relation with Mr. Ashton, who made a cigarette box in occupational therapy and gave it to Mr. Esposito on his birthday. These changes are reflected in the nursing notes. For example:

(Twelfth day) Patient seems subdued, less excited. Relatively few requests, little laughter, little loud or profane talk. Tendency to ask if it is all right to do this or that.

(Fourteenth day) Appeared to get angry at times, and then would smile and joke with patients. Asked if he had to sign his name to read the paper, the books, etc.

(Sixteenth day) Patient had birthday today. Congratulated by the group. Looked quiet and friendly. Went to OT at 2:45. . . . Quiet, good-humored, friendly. . . . Very happy at remembrance of his birthday when cake and candles brought in, and he received gifts from the patients. Laughed, and was very appreciative.

(Twenty-first day) Restless, in and out of bed. Slept very little. Did not ask for any sedation. Very irritable. Reading. When asked if he would like his glasses, he replied very sharply: "No, I wanna spoil my eyes. They spoiled already."

The second period was also characterized by an upswing in the therapist's interest coupled with a withdrawal of the patient away from active therapeutic work. For example, concerning the eleventh day, Dr. Ryan dictated:

(Eleventh day) I saw the patient in occupational therapy, and he was washing his hands. He indicated that he did not want to come upstairs to talk with me, that he wanted to continue working. He then changed his mind and said that he would stop working, that he wanted to come upstairs with me. He continued washing his face many times, washed his mouth with water, saying that he was trying to get the dusty taste out of his mouth. He folded and arranged his apron very carefully. He danced around the room and made loving gestures toward Mr. Erskine . . . and then waltzed out of the room with me and came up to my office. . . . He indicated that he was just playing when I asked him if he was upset. He said no, that he did not think so, and got rather disturbed at my accusing him of this, and asked me if I thought that he was upset. I told him I thought his behavior was a little peculiar. He said that he did not know. I told him I was interested in his outburst of yesterday in which he said that he hated all Italians and Catholics. I asked him more about this, and he said that this was the way he felt. He said he had been observing people for thirty-odd years and that he felt that he knew a little bit about them. He also said that some people are good and others bad, and that in most of his dealings it turned out that people had been bad to him. He told me of a fellow he had lived with for some time, who had turned out to be very authoritarian and directed him to do this and that work for various people. One night they had a fight about this. He told me about another man he knew and said that they also got into the same sort of relation, and that then he would go out and drink. I asked him about his feelings concerning these people and whether his drinking might be responsible for, or a result of, these relations, but he didn't seem to make much of a connection here. . . . I really feel that this man could use superficial supportive psychotherapy, trying to point out the inconsistency in his behavior and what it may mean, and trying to help him adjust a little bit more in his feelings toward Catholics and Italians.

There are at least three things of considerable interest in this session. First, there is evidence that the patient had begun to withdraw from active participation in therapy. He indicated he did not want to talk to the therapist. He once again stated his position: that he had been observing people for thirty years, and in most of his dealings "it turned out that people had been bad to him." This almost seems like a direct reference to the hospital situation, but it was not explored by the therapist. Second, Mr. Esposito seemed to have been able to reintegrate his old pattern of defenses which he had when he entered the hospital. That is, he was again able to use a somewhat obsessive concern over cleanliness and neatness as a defense, rather than more excited and regressed behavior. Third, Dr. Ryan had changed his approach to the patient, partly in response to pressures placed on him elsewhere in the system, and now felt that the patient "could use superficial supportive psychotherapy."

In order to see Dr. Ryan's rather sudden shift of interest in the patient within a wider context, it is necessary to note two things: (1) the general air of tension and confusion over administrative policy which was current at this time; and (2) the pressure placed on Dr. Ryan by the senior staff with the implication that he was not working well with his patients. These two things were not unrelated, and both quickly had an effect on the relation between Dr. Ryan and Mr. Esposito.

One indication of the general confusion over policy was the position taken by the nurses in the administrative conferences, and commented on at length among themselves on the ward, concerning the need to have doctors write their orders very explicitly so that the nurses' position would be as unequivocal as possible. In this connection, it is interesting that the observations on the men's locked ward at this time showed a general opinion on the part of the patients that one had to plan far in advance to get a privilege, and there was much discussion about how one could get it in writing.

It is within this context that the nursing notes reported: "Mr. Esposito asked if he had to sign his name to read the paper, the books, etc." Mr. Esposito's actions here probably had a double reference: first to the general situation on the ward, and second to his own particular difficulties in communicating with Dr. Ryan. For example, the therapeutic session on the morning of the twelfth day included the following events, which were noted by the therapist:

(Twelfth day) I met the patient in occupational therapy this morning. . . . He came to the office with me and handed me a slip of paper on which was written the name of a book. . . . He said that he wanted to buy it, and asked me if it was all right. I told him that it looked like a very complex book, but that it was perfectly all right if he wanted to buy it. I suggested that he get it from the library. . . . He also handed me a slip on which he had written several things: a request for going to the gymnasium to work out, a request to go to the movies, and to go to church. . . . He surprised me somewhat with his church request. . . . I said I would try to arrange it. . . . We talked a bit about reading in general, and apparently he has been doing more reading than I had thought. . . .

The next morning in the administrative conference, following a general discussion over the policy of letting patients go out of the hospital, Dr. Ryan said he would like to let Mr. Esposito go to the gymnasium, and also go to church, as he felt that both these things would be therapeutic. Dr. Shaw, however, said to postpone this decision, as Mr. Esposito would be coming up for discussion at a staff conference during the day.

At the staff conference on Mr. Esposito, most of the discussion centered around the part played by alcohol in Mr. Esposito's pathology. The question was whether this was an acute alcoholic psychosis. The feeling was that if the patient was now dried out and was still psychotic, then the alcohol had only helped to produce the paranoid picture. The feeling was that Mr. Esposito would be able to recompensate. It was suggested that there were two things for the therapist to treat: his alcoholism and his hostility. It was suggested that Dr. Ryan try to get Mr. Esposito to see what alcohol did for him. It was also decided to carry Mr. Esposito in treatment for at least two more weeks, and to assess whether to transfer him to a state hospital.

The additional pressure placed on Dr. Ryan in the administrative conferences at this time can be seen in the following excerpt:

Dr. Ryan (who had been on duty the night before): Mrs. Pomeroy was admitted last night and wanted to make a phone call. Rather than deny this request directly, I told her it was against the hospital rules and policy.

Dr. Scott: Why didn't you want to say no directly to the patient?

Dr. Ryan: Well, I thought I could sidetrack the issue or do it directly, and I preferred to sidetrack it.

Dr. Scott: You've been here for quite a while and you know enough about the hospital now that you don't always have to say yes to a patient in order to form a relation. People have been saying no for years and still forming relations. I suggest that you try this. Of course if you don't want to take the responsibility—

Dr. Ryan: We'll talk about this later.

Dr. Scott: That's your problem.

(Later in the conference)

Dr. Ryan: Mr. Esposito does fairly well on the locked ward now, and I think it would be all right to let him visit on the open ward.

Dr. Shaw: I don't think that Mr. Esposito would be able to handle this by himself on the open ward.

Dr. Ryan: All right. There also is the request to go to church. It's very hard to get Mr. Esposito to make requests because he is so afraid of crossing the boundary of what is allowed him in the hospital.

Dr. Shaw: Well, from the point of view of available personnel it probably won't be possible to let Mr. Esposito go to church, and even if this weren't the case I don't feel that dynamically it would be wise.

Dr. Ryan: All right.

It seems likely that the patient was becoming involved here in the pressure being placed on Dr. Ryan, and that it was not only Mr. Esposito who was confused about the boundaries of what was allowable, but also Dr. Ryan and the staff. It is also interesting that the request to go to church was denied partly on "psychodynamic" grounds, although really very little was known about the patient's actual dynamics.

It was in such an atmosphere that Dr. Ryan became concerned with movement in the patient—with his psychological movement in the therapeutic hours and with his physical movement in the hospital. With regard to the latter, Dr. Ryan requested that Mr. Esposito be transferred to an open ward, that he be permitted to participate more fully in occupational therapy, that he go for walks outside the hospital, and so on. This led to a number of distortions in communication. One such began during the next therapeutic session Dr. Ryan had with the patient following upon the rather stormy administrative conference referred to above. Dr. Ryan dictated:

(Fourteenth day) . . . I asked him how he thought he'd like it on an open ward, and after some discussion he said that it might be worth while there because he could rest better. I then tried to relate his present thoughts about his reactions to authority to his childhood reactions to his parents, and tried to relate his resentment concerning authority to his present drinking sprees. He was very quiet during this period and seemed to be thinking. I told him that it seemed that he did not like other people to tell him what to do, and he said that he actually did like to have other people tell him what to do, but they had to be certain good people. He means people who are authoritative and really know what they are talking about.

In view of this session, and of the interaction between Dr. Ryan and Drs. Scott and Shaw in the preceding administrative conference, it seems reasonable to suggest that another complication had perhaps been added to the communication process. It has been previously noted that Mr. Esposito had not been too successful in communicating his immediate problems to Dr. Ryan. Now, on the other hand, Dr. Ryan had had additional pressures placed on him so that his own conflicts with authority were being brought to bear on the therapeutic relationship in ways of which he was not totally aware. It seems likely that the feelings involved in the statement "people who are authoritative and really know what they are talking about" were as applicable to Dr. Ryan and his feelings about Dr. Scott as they were to Mr. Esposito and his feelings about persons in authority.

A second aspect of this therapeutic session was the quite tentative quality with which Mr. Esposito is reported to have agreed with the suggestion made by Dr. Ryan that the patient move to an open ward. Indeed, the nursing notes for that afternoon read in part:

(Fourteenth day) Patient did not want to go to open ward. Stayed in room most of time talking to nobody. Then he washed and dressed carefully after 8:00 p.m.

In the administrative conference the next morning, however, Dr. Ryan said that Mr. Esposito had raised the question of moving to the open ward (whereas Dr. Ryan dictated in his progress notes that it was he who had raised the question). As in the previous conference, the discussion of Mr. Esposito followed another difference of opinion between Dr. Ryan and Dr. Scott:

Dr. Ryan: There are a couple of things. I want to let Mrs. Martin go to occupational therapy. She had been busy around the house until she came into the hospital and she has nothing to do here, and I hope we can get her interested in OT. I also think that it might be good if Mrs. Martin was allowed to visit on the open ward when the door to the open ward is locked.

Dr. Shaw: Let's try occupational therapy and see what we can do.

Dr. Scott (addressing Dr. Ryan): When Dr. Shaw and I made rounds the other day, Mrs. Martin thought that Dr. Shaw was yourself, and she seemed disoriented. I think you had better be careful in evaluating her behavior state.

Dr. Ryan: There is one other thing. Mr. Esposito has raised the question of moving to the open ward. He feels that when he gets in his room there is no door that he can close and that he can't sleep or be by himself. . . . I'd like to think about moving Mr. Esposito to the open ward.

Miss Newcomb: He was very disturbed last night for over an hour and was wandering up and down the halls apparently hallucinating.

Dr. Ryan: Oh, I didn't know that. In that case I will withdraw my request.

Having met administrative resistance in his plans to allow Mr. Esposito greater freedom, and being unable to perceive much progress in the therapeutic hours, Dr. Ryan shortly began to think of discharging the patient or transferring him to a state hospital. The withdrawal of interest at this time on the part of both the patient and therapist was evident in the therapeutic sessions which took place during Mr. Esposito's fourth week in the hospital. For example, Dr. Ryan dictated:

(Twenty-fourth day) Today the patient was quiet, uncommunicative, and rather obviously disturbed. . . . He said he slept poorly last night when I asked him, but he said that he had not been thinking about anything in particular, insisting that he doesn't think very much. . . . He says he's thinking of moving his things over to his cousin's. . . . When I asked him which cousin, he said any cousin, and I was somewhat surprised at this . . . and had the impression that he was just telling me this to satisfy me with an answer. I asked him in what way he felt badly, and he expressed some irritation and said: "Doctor, I don't know what I have to say, I don't know everything." I assured him that he didn't have to know everything to know how he felt. . . . I asked him if he was upset about staying in the hospital so long, and he said no, that he was just sleepy. Rather than prolong this I suggested that he go upstairs and rest and perhaps he would feel better later. . . .

(Twenty-fifth day) . . . I asked him about his refusal to see his landlord . . . and he said that he doesn't know why he did it but that the landlord didn't bring in what he wanted. I reminded him that he said he wanted his cousin to take his things so that he wouldn't have to pay for his room. . . . He asked me what he should do. I reminded him of how he felt about people who told him what to do, so that I didn't want to be in that position. He said that he knew I wasn't telling him what to do, but that he just asked me a question. He seemed to be somewhat excited about this, as if to say: "Why can't you ever tell me what to do?" . . . This morning he was very emotional. He expressed very strong feelings in the things that he said, the ideas he had on how his illness got started, and certainly it is useless to push him on these points. He will just have to air his feelings as he can.

It was at this time that the third period of Mr. Esposito's stay began. Coincident with the shift of emphasis on the part of the therapist, a stereotyped perception of the patient crystallized among the staff, and the patient intensified his clowning and painting on the ward. A content analysis of the nursing notes indicated that during this transition the proportion of *general* remarks about the patient's behavior ("usual playful, silly self") began to exceed that of *specific* remarks ("he tore up bits of paper and gave them to Mr. Erskine"). It is, of course, not unusual that written remarks about a patient should become more generalized the longer the patient stays in the hospital. The point here is that it was just at the time of the therapist's withdrawal of active interest that this occurred in the nursing notes. In a more static sense, during the first 28 days of hospitalization, the nursing notes contained a total of 336 remarks about the patient's behavior, of which 43, or 13 per cent, were general. During the last 29 days of hospitalization—the third period—the notes contained 194 remarks, of which 51, or 26 per cent, were general.

At the administrative conferences discussion of Mr. Esposito's behavior contained much benign humor—for example, a suggestion that he participate in a swimming class called forth the remark that he was "a floater, not a swimmer." It was also during this time that the resident who had been on call the preceding night reported the following the next morning in the administrative conference:

Dr. Reynolds: Mr. Esposito was shouting a good deal last night, and I asked him if he wanted to go to seclusion. He said that everyone else was making noise and why couldn't he. He asked me: "Am I sick?" and I said: "No, you feel fine!"

There was general laughter at this in the conference, partly with regard to the situation, and partly at the very direct use of suggestion by the resident. Some six days later, however, as indicated in the observations on the ward, Mr. Esposito was very angry over not having been called for supper and repeated over and over again the phrase: "They make me say I'm well."

Also at this time the patients increasingly encouraged Mr. Esposito in his clowning role, as was evident from the ward observations:

Mr. Esposito took a sport shirt and wound it loosely around his head. Mr. Ashton asked him: "Francis, are you being a sheik? Where's your horse?" Mr. Esposito laughed and said: "I never had a horse." He then lighted his cigarette from Mr. Ashton's cigarette. Mr. Ashton said: "Francis, you didn't quite get that light." Mr. Esposito beamed, took off his costume, and brought out his drawings, which he showed around.

(On another occasion) Mr. Erskine mentioned to Mr. Esposito that he had ordered a box of paints for him. Mr. Esposito sort of clapped his hands with joy and ran over as if to embrace Mr. Erskine. Mr. Erskine said: "Now, now, Francis, let's not have you making love to me." Mr. Esposito then wandered about shouting he could probably get paints elsewhere. Mr. Ashton broke in and said: "When a guy tries to do something for you, Francis, you ought to thank him for it and not be angry at him." Mr. Esposito said he wasn't really angry at Mr. Erskine or making fun of him. Mr. Esposito then raised his hands over his head and bowed down as if salaaming, while calling Mr. Erskine his landsman. Both Mr. Erskine and Mr. Ashton then said: "Now, Francis, you've got to be a good boy."

That this sort of behavior was something of a role for Mr. Esposito would seem to be indicated by the fact that at times when he would withdraw from the group, or when the other patients were off the ward, he would usually be found quietly sitting or reading in his room. Also, though there was a sharp decrease in formal therapeutic activity as Mr. Esposito entered the third period of his hospitalization, he retained his attachment to Dr. Ryan and continued his attempts to communicate indirectly. This he did through painting on the wall and through gathering wild flowers for Dr. Ryan on excursions to the woods with the activities worker.

THIRD PERIOD

The third period of Mr. Esposito's stay lasted four weeks, or half of the total time he spent in the hospital. The beginning of the period was marked by an intensification of Mr. Esposito's painting on the wall which was to continue throughout the four weeks. Mr. Esposito's painting can be thought of as serving at least three functions: (1) it was a continuation of his efforts to communicate with his therapist by other than verbal means; (2) it gave him an additional way of relating to patients and staff within the clowning role he had begun to play on the ward; and (3) it was a pattern of behavior which helped to confirm the staff in their now stereotyped view of Mr. Esposito as a clowning, harmless schizophrenic. At this point, the diagnosis seemed to function less as a useful classificatory tool, and rather more as a security operation on the part of the staff by means of which they could feel there was little the hospital could do further for the patient. This very possibly had the reciprocal effect of bringing the patient to sense that he was now considered more as a case than as a person. The vigor with which Mr. Esposito attacked his painting during this period might hypothetically be considered an unconscious attempt to retain his individuality in the face of a dim awareness that he was being treated in a stereotyped fashion by all three groups with whom he was in relation—his therapist, the nurses and aides, and the patients.

Although Mr. Esposito's painting occupied a major portion of his time during his last four weeks, there were only a few references to it in the brief therapeutic notes dictated by Dr. Ryan during this period. Some days after Mr. Esposito started his painting, the first reference to it in the therapeutic notes occurred:

(Thirty-first day) . . . I asked him about his getting up and drawing things on the wall at night, and he said that he really doesn't know why he does it. He said he never did it at home because there he could be up and around and was able to go out, but here he was not able to do this. He said that he does not see things here and denied hearing voices telling him what to do. . . . All in all the interview was successful in reducing his disinclination to talk. He was much more able to communicate with me. However, the content of the material did not change one iota. . . .

(Thirty-sixth day) . . . He has been drawing pictures on paper pasted on his wall. (The paper was supplied by the nursing staff who objected to painting directly on the wall. Mr. Esposito pasted the paper on the wall and continued his activities.) These pictures are in very vivid contrasting colors, mostly of people, as if he were drawing a Madonna's head. I told the patient I thought he needed more hospitalization, and he said okay with a shrug of his shoulders. I told him he could either go to a state hospital or stay here and that there was a significant difference in money. . . .

Following the therapeutic session on the thirty-sixth day, Mr. Esposito went on an outing in the woods with the activities workers and the anthropologist and carefully selected wild flowers for a bouquet which he gave to Dr. Ryan. This seemed to be another way of communicating with the therapist in a non-verbal fashion. Mr. Esposito succeeded to some extent in this communication because during the next therapeutic session on the fortieth day Dr. Ryan responded more fully to the patient's drawing. The therapist, however, did not go on to explore this in further sessions, and the matter was dropped:

(Fortieth day) The patient began painting with water colors in his room today using weird colors, disconnected figures, and rather peculiar and primitive combinations of people. He seems to be enjoying himself in expressing his feelings in this way. He laughs a good deal when he is painting and says that this is the first time that he has done anything like this. He enjoys showing his things to other people and seems to be getting a great deal of pleasure from it. I expressed my agreement with what he was doing, telling him it was a good way to express himself. I asked about his hernia, and he said he was doing a picture of what a hernia is and how it is repaired. I told him I didn't think we should repair it right now as long as it wasn't bothering him a great deal. I told him that I approved of his painting and doing these things that allow him to express himself.

(At the next hour, on the forty-fifth day) . . . There has been little change in the past five days. He continues to socialize a little better. He has been playing games with the rest of the group and spending a good deal of time in his room doing water coloring. . . . I indicated that it might be helpful to him to carry the things that he learned here home with him—that is, ceramics, water coloring, drawing, and so on, but he seemed to feel that this cannot be done in a room by himself. I indicated to him that this really could be done. . . .

As can be seen from the context of Mr. Esposito's drawing a picture of how to repair a hernia, he was attempting to use this activity as a means of communication and as a way of mastering the arousal of anxiety. A further attempt at non-verbal communication occurred during the ward observations on the forty-ninth day when Dr. Ryan made his morning rounds:

(Ward observations, forty-ninth day) At 9:10 a.m. Dr. Ryan came on the ward and said hello to the group. Mr. Esposito came up to him and started revolving like a pinwheel and then raising his right hand above his head and making little pointing movements with it. He asked Dr. Ryan what this was. Dr. Ryan said that he couldn't guess. Finally Mr. Esposito said that this was the ceiling in the lobby of the reception ward (which has a sun and clouds painted on it). Dr. Ryan asked Mr. Esposito if he remembered this from the first time he came in (seven weeks ago) and Mr. Esposito said yes, that he did. Dr. Ryan and Mr. Esposito then went into Mr. Esposito's room and talked from 9:15 to 9:25.

On the same day as the above observations occurred, the anthropologist talked with Dr. Ryan at lunch. Dr. Ryan said that Mr. Esposito had told him at rounds that morning: "I talk to the wall." The anthropologist asked if anything further had come up about Mr. Esposito's drawing, and Dr. Ryan said he thought the pictures provided an outlet for Mr. Esposito but did not have any real meaning for him. Dr. Ryan went on to say that the plans were to discharge Mr. Esposito within a week and to try and make arrangements for him to be seen on an outpatient basis, as this would be much less expensive for him.

Actually, it was Mr. Esposito's felicitous phrase, "I talk to the wall," as reported by Dr. Ryan, that caused the anthropologist to re-examine his data and led to the analysis presented in this chapter. Up to that point the anthropologist had not focused his attention particularly on Mr. Esposito, and had thought of him in much the same way as did the hospital personnel.

That Mr. Esposito must indeed have felt he was "talking to the wall," not only with regard to his therapist but also with regard to the ward personnel, can be seen in the events on the ward that immediately followed his contact with Dr. Ryan on rounds:

(Ward observations, forty-ninth day, continued) Dr. Ryan left the ward on his rounds at 9:30 a.m. . . .

10:15 a.m. Mrs. Nye came on the ward and had a pleasant short conversation with Mr. Ashton and Mr. Erskine. She then went in and talked to Mr. Innes who had been isolating himself in his room. She came out of Mr. Innes' room and asked Mr. Esposito: "Do you want to go visit on the open ward?" Mr. Esposito said: "Yes."

10:17 a.m. Mrs. Nye went off the ward. Mr. Esposito went into his room. . . .

10:35 a.m. Mr. Ashton asked an attendant: "Take me down to the open ward please." Mr. Ashton and the attendant left the ward. A few minutes later the attendant came back. . . .

11:00 a.m. Mr. Esposito came out of his room and asked one of the attendants: "I want to go to the open ward." The attendant said: "No." Then he said: "I will go out and check." Mr. Esposito said to the other attendant in a very excited voice: "You're not supposed to check. You're supposed to take me any time I want to go. Doctor's orders." (This was true. The order read in the nurse's order book: "Patient may be on open ward ad lib during day and evening; patient *should* be on the open ward as much as possible.") The attendant made no response to this excited outburst by Mr. Esposito. Mr. Esposito turned around and went back to his room where he began painting again on his Madonna on the wall.

11:12 a.m. Mr. Esposito came out of his room and got a light for his cigarette from an attendant. Mr. Esposito then said, complaining: "Why do I lose so much time; do you want me to jump down?" The attendant said: "Beats me, I don't know why you can't go down."

11:15 a.m. Mrs. Nye came on the ward. Mr. Esposito asked Mrs. Nye: "Can I go down to the open ward?" Mrs. Nye said: "It's very near dinner time, Mr. Esposito." Mr. Esposito put up a fuss at this, so Mrs. Nye said: "Okay, I'll take you down." Mr. Esposito was very irate and said: "I want to go down when I feel like it, and I don't want to go down now." Then he changed his mind, and an attendant took him to the open ward.

At the close of the third period, after being in the hospital for eight weeks, Mr. Esposito was discharged, and arrangements were made for him to see a psychiatrist on the outside from time to time. The final note dictated by the therapist summarized very well many of the events that have been discussed, but it failed to indicate the significance of the context of hospital life for this schizophrenic patient. As such, this final note read like hundreds of others to be found in the case records of almost any psychiatric hospital:

Final note. Diagnosis: (1) schizophrenic reaction, paranoid type; (2) chronic alcoholism. The schizophrenia is manifested by paranoid ideas, particularly concerning the power of people over him, strong fears of people in authority, extreme suspiciousness of people with money, Catholics in particular, and inappropriate behavior noted on several occasions, such as "plastering the wall" with his hands at night, washing the floor with a mop, dismantling the water fountain, on one occasion in seclusion having thoughts of being poisoned, spitting in corners, and balancing his dishes and tray. External precipitating stress is uncertain, but it was apparently tied up with a sudden increase in his alcoholic intake and the suspicion of strongly charged matters in the relations in his family. Predisposition is not definitely known. This particular episode is one of a series of similar episodes that have occurred in the past, only one of which required hospitalization. Even between acute episodes, the patient is characterized as rather queer, withdrawn, moody, and seclusive by his friends. Degree of incapacity is mild between attacks and is total during the acute attacks.

In the hospital the patient was at first anxious and later became rather hostile toward me, toward the nurses, and toward the hospital in general for imposing restrictions on his activities. In the final third of his hospital stay he became much more friendly with the patients, entering into group activities quite easily and expressing feelings of affection toward the hospital, toward the nurses, and toward me. During the hospital stay he gained some insight into his feelings concerning the part that the family had played in his acute disturbances, his reactions toward authority in general and people who hold authority positions such as his employers, his strong anti-Catholic feelings, and his strong feelings about money and its power. He still maintained a desire to blame his disorder on his various bodily disturbances, such as his epigastric hernia, and seemed to feel that these must have something to do with his recurrent disturbances.

The recommendation of the hospital was that the patient should be discharged into the community to work . . . and an attempt will be made to establish the patient in routine psychiatric treatment on an outpatient basis.

DISCUSSION

It was noted earlier that the events in Mr. Esposito's case were seen here through a different lens than usual. Like any lens, this one created its own distortions. It is hoped, however, that through presentation of this case within a wider context, the reader has gained a sense of the systematic interplay of variables other than those considered in more orthodox approaches to the events of hospital life.

It may not have seemed so, but the choice of the case of Mr. Esposito for analysis here was dictated by the fact that it was such a *simple* one. This was so because it was possible to focus on one patient whose relations to other persons in the hospital never became a matter of intense personal interest for a particular staff member or for another patient. The problems in the case were fairly clear and uncomplicated and ranged over a wide variety of topics. In other cases that were followed out in a similar manner, the ramifications in the material quickly became much more complex. For example, this was true in the case of the interrelations over time between Dr. Reynolds and her patient Mr. Osgood, and Dr. Shaw and his patient Miss Prescott. Dr. Reynolds and Dr. Shaw had a long-standing difference of opinion about how administrative procedures could be used to therapeutic advantage, and this difference of opinion was accentuated when Mr. Osgood's progress in therapy arrived at a point where he tentatively reached out for heterosexual contact and developed a friendly relation with Miss Prescott. From this point on, an analysis of this four-person system would have to include the continuing interrelations of: (1) Dr. Reynolds and Mr. Osgood, (2) Dr. Shaw and Miss Prescott, (3) Mr. Osgood and Miss Prescott, (4) Dr. Reynolds and Dr. Shaw, (5) Dr. Reynolds and Miss Prescott, and (6) Dr. Shaw and Mr. Osgood. One can see how such a situation would become much more complicated to follow than the relatively simple case of Mr. Esposito. To have presented such other cases in anywhere near the detail that has been used for Mr. Esposito's would have been to make a book instead of a chapter out of the analysis.

The complications in analysis just referred to are related to the reverberations which must be followed out when events are seen as part of a transactional system. Thus, the material from one day's therapeutic interview would have to be followed both backward and forward in time as it impinged upon, and was influenced by, events that occurred in other subsystems of the hospital. This is much less true for psychotherapy carried on outside the hospital. There, the doctor-patient relationship is not as likely to be *systematically* subject to pressures from other sources because the doctor and patient are not usually part of the same network of personal relations. Within the relatively closed system of the hospital, however, any action of either doctor or patient resulting from the therapeutic hours quickly comes into contact with the desires and feelings of other people to whom both the doctor and the patient have obligations and responsibilities. This difference in the immediate effect of reverberations from treatment carried on inside, as opposed to outside, the hospital is analogous to the effect of a rock tossed into a bathtub of water, as against a pebble thrown into a lake. In the one instance the ripples quickly meet a barrier and turn back upon themselves, while in the other the ripples gradually widen and are dissipated.

In the presentation of Mr. Esposito's case, despite its length, there have been many facets of the material that could not be explored. It may well have been, for example, that significant organic disorder was present although all tests were negative. It may also have been that the therapist's initial concentration on the past stirred up submerged conflicts in the patient. If this was true, these underlying conflicts were added to the patient's immediate problems before the latter had been at least temporarily resolved. The main point here is the simple but important one that during the early stage of his hospitalization the patient's increasing agitation was not solely owing to some unknown psychopathological process, but could be related, in ways that often went unnoticed, to his difficulties in communicating with people around him. Whether or not a sustained awareness of, and acting upon, the kind of problems that have been outlined would indeed have prevented Mr. Esposito from reaching his disorganized state in seclusion is an open question. It is important, however, to point out that there were many avenues of approach to the patient which were ignored and which might have proven useful.

In concluding this discussion, it is useful to refer in summary form to five broad areas of concern to which attention has been directed.

First, at the beginning of the chapter it was pointed out that a patient had at least five sources to which he might turn for satisfaction of his immediate needs upon entering a psychiatric hospital: (1) his physician, (2) the nurses and aides, (3) the use of the physical space of the ward in ways he found comfortable, (4) the other patients, and (5) himself—as this was related to his psychological and physical resources. In terms of these five sources, Mr. Esposito, during his first period in the hospital, was only partially able to reach his therapist, and he could not use the physical space of the ward comfortably or make contact with the nursing staff. This had little to do with the general feelings of the therapist or the nurses, all of whom were by and large positively oriented toward Mr. Esposito, but had rather more to do with the nature of the hospital system. The therapeutic and administrative routines, as these were set up within the structure of the hospital, operated in such a way as to cut off Mr. Esposito's access to several of the sources from which he could have obtained help with his immediate problems. He perforce focused on the other patients and himself for need-satisfaction and tension-reduction, but since these sources were unable to provide support adequate to enable him to maintain his behavior at a fairly integrated level, he utilized them in a progressively less integrated fashion.

In the second period of hospitalization, the partial communication between Mr. Esposito and his therapist gradually declined, and this source of help was largely lost to him. Throughout this period the therapist's interest in the patient was strongly influenced both positively and negatively by pressures from other subsystems in the hospital.

During the third period, Mr. Esposito devoted the majority of his attention to maintaining and pleasing himself and to his relations with the other patients. The role Mr. Esposito came to play in this third period was influenced not only by the way in which he was accepted by the patients on the ward, but also by the attitudes that crystallized among the staff toward him. In this connection, it was also of importance that Mr. Esposito's fairly useful pattern of defenses, such as reading and compulsive cleaning, was largely ignored when he first came into the hospital. These defenses rapidly deteriorated during the first period of hospitalization, but Mr. Esposito was later able to reintegrate them as part of his role as a clown on the ward.

In general, the entire system of the hospital seemed to become involved in Mr. Esposito's case in ways which were not always recognized or readily apparent, and this problem was directly connected with the organizational structure and communication network existing at that time within the hospital.

Second, the point was developed that the doctor-patient relationship became involved with other subsystems in the hospital. Thus, the pressures placed on Dr. Ryan by the senior staff exerted a significant influence on the emotional meaning of the patient for Dr. Ryan. This phenomenon is often identified as countertransference in the work of the hospital, although such a use of the term is rather loose. Similarly, the administrative aspects of the relations between Dr. Ryan and Mr. Esposito became a matter of explicit disagreement between Dr. Ryan and the nurses. This masked a more underlying disagreement, only indirectly expressed through the person of Mr. Esposito, between the residents and nurses over administrative policy.

The wider context of the development of transference and countertransference phenomena needs to be emphasized. It was recognized quite early in psychiatry that psychotherapy was a complex interactive experience for both therapist and patient. The process by which the patient placed the therapist in the role of emotionally significant persons in the patient's past came to be called transference, and the working through of this relation became an important part of therapy. Somewhat later, the term countertransference came to stand for the needs and emotions aroused in the therapist by the patient which were inappropriate to the relation and might interfere with the goals of treatment. Beyond such basic conceptions, however, psychiatry has not gone very far in considering how these relations could be embedded in, and related to, other systems of interaction—particularly as to psychotherapy carried out in a psychiatric hospital. It would appear that within the hospital the course of events in psychotherapy will be influenced not only by transference and countertransference behavior based on the past learning of therapist and patient, but also upon the utilization of the psychotherapeutic relationship to obtain relief from tension arising out of the participation of therapist and patient in other aspects of the work of the hospital. Anger, for example, may be directed toward the patient because the patient represents an anxiety-evoking person for the therapist, and not because the patient's behavior threatens to awaken anxiety-laden fantasies in the therapist. Rather, the anger may be caused by the fact that the therapist's personal security in the hospital is threatened by his being held responsible for the behavior of patients over whom he cannot exercise any very high degree of control. Especially this might be true if the therapist felt that his therapeutic and administrative duties were in conflict. A partial answer to this problem is, of course, the delegation of therapeutic and administrative functions to separate physicians (see Morse and Noble, 1942; and Fromm-Reichmann, 1950). This procedure was carried out in a number of cases in the hospital under study, and worked very well in some instances but created new problems in others.

Third, some thought was given to the meaning of diagnosis as a security operation. Within a hospital, diagnosis may be thought to serve two functions: on the one hand, it is a useful way of classifying a patient in terms of the etiology and symptoms of his illness; but, on the other hand, it also is a way of disposing of a patient by labeling him. For example, if a patient's behavior comes to be continually explained by the "fact" that he "has" schizophrenia, then the chances of the patient's being relegated to a chronic hospital career are increased. In this latter case, diagnosis may be thought of as a security operation, meaning that uncertainty about a patient is removed by labeling him and that many communications from him may now be safely ignored.

In connection with the above, it was seen that when Mr. Esposito had a good day the therapist thought of his illness in "functional" terms, but when he had a bad day "organic" factors became uppermost in the therapist's mind. In addition, there was an implicit tendency toward thinking of psychotherapy as a method of treatment that is helpful for patients with functional illnesses, but that is of little use for patients with organic illnesses. This is, of course, a misconception. It was also noted that the therapist was supported in his concern over whether the patient had schizophrenia or epilepsy when, at the administrative conference, it was pointed out that if it was epilepsy, the schizophrenia would have to be disentangled from it. Without in any sense denying the great usefulness of proper diagnosis as a tool, it would seem that the extension of classificatory categories until they become, as it were, self-acting entities, puts unnecessary difficulties in the way of thinking about human behavior (see Frank, 1951).

Fourth, the material on the development of Mr. Esposito's clowning role suggested that the hospital often does much to help create a role for a patient and that the course of the patient's illness is strongly influenced by such a role. Thus, in his first period, Mr. Esposito's symptomatology took on a "manic" coloring because of his relation to Mr. Ashton, and the stabilization of his clowning role in the third period would seem to be the counterpart of the crystallization of a stereotyped attitude toward him on the part of the doctors, nurses, and patients. In such a case, a patient's patterned behavior cannot be sufficiently apprehended within the usual meaning of terms such as "symptom" or "defense," but must also be thought of as an adaptation to the relatively circumscribed situation in which he is placed. Such an adaptation can be thought of as a role, or focal point, brought into existence by the ongoing transactions between persons in a social field (see Grinker, 1953; Spiegel, 1954). This is stated in this manner, not with the idea of substituting one type of jargon for another, but in the attempt to avoid the dichotomy implied in the use of the terms structure and process. The particular clowning role Mr. Esposito played in the hospital had not existed before his admission, nor was it ever formalized (or even explicitly formulated as such) at any point in his stay, but there certainly came to be a focusing of a pattern of attitudes held by the staff and patients about Mr. Esposito, and a pattern of attitudes held by Mr. Esposito about the staff and patients. This difficulty, inherent in the terms structure and process, will be returned to in Chapter 10 in discussing the administrative work of the hospital over time.

Lastly, it was noted that, particularly during his third period, Mr. Esposito gained most satisfaction from his relations with other patients and that this was partly owing to the nature of the hospital situation at the time. It is probably not useful for a patient to concentrate his relations in one role group, and on an *a priori* basis it seems likely that a patient who has been able to develop successful relations with all groups (doctors, ward personnel, patients, and so on) would have a more productive and less stormy course in the hospital. This suggests a continuum varying from patients who have successful relations with all groups to patients who do not have successful relations with any group. Using the three role groups of doctors, ward personnel, and patients, this continuum has been divided into eight categories, and a rough breakdown has been attempted of the total 36 patients observed during the research con-

TABLE 3–1. Schematic summary of patterns of relations established by patients within the hospital, and rating according to administrative problems presented and therapeutic progress

Category	Patient had established good relations with:	Number of patients[1]	Rating according to: Administrative problems presented by patient	Therapeutic progress of patient
I	Doctor, ward personnel, and patients	4	Low	High
II	Doctor and ward personnel	2	Low	Average
III	Doctor	7	Average	Average
IV	Ward personnel	2	Average	Average
V	Doctor and patients	12	High	Average
VI	Ward personnel and patients	0	High	Average
VII	Patients	6	High	Low
VIII	Nobody	3	High	Low

[1] These numbers represent a rough breakdown of the total 36 patients evaluated according to predominant category occupied.

cerning the predominant category they occupied. This breakdown can be seen in Table 3–1. The judgments there represented were checked with the head of the hospital. In a rough way, 4 of the 36 patients seemed to have established successful relations with all three role groups (category I). All 4 patients were considered to have made a good therapeutic recovery. For example, Mr. Onofrio was frequently cited with pride by both patients and staff. He came into the hospital as a very sick paranoid schizophrenic with a well-developed delusional system, and left to go to a good job. He had an excellent relation with his doctor, the ward personnel became very fond of him, and he was of central importance to the patients on both the locked and open wards in that he mediated arguments and took initiative in organizing activities.

Two of the patients seemed to fall into a second category in that they had achieved a meaningful relation with their doctor and with the ward personnel, but not with the patients. For example, Mr. Eggan was an adolescent schizophrenic who made a close relation to his doctor and to the attendants on the locked ward, but because of his youth was unable to relate to the majority of the patients, who were older. In general, patients in categories I and II presented a minimum of administrative problems, probably in considerable part because they had established successful relations *both* with the doctors and the ward personnel.

A third category was formed by those 7 patients who had made a relation to their own doctor, but not to any of the other groups. These patients were generally withdrawn on the ward and did not participate to any great extent in the life of the hospital. For example, Mr. Edwards was able to have a very helpful relation with his doctor, but was almost unknown to the ward personnel or patients. He would occasionally cause administrative difficulty by purchasing liquor outside the hospital, which he would bring back to his room and drink, but since he was not in contact with the other patients this behavior often went unnoticed by them and did not spread to others.

A fourth category comprised 2 patients who had only been able to establish relations with the ward personnel. For example, Mr. Oliver, an adolescent with a background in several foster homes, was able to develop a close relation only to the attendants on the men's locked ward. He was the only patient who knew the names of all of the many divinity students working as attendants. Upon his discharge the attendants somewhat covertly, but with the sanction of the therapist, got together and found a room for Mr. Oliver and helped him with his plans for an education.

Administratively speaking, a patient in either categories III or IV was interesting because, although his behavior might disturb the ward personnel since his relation was solely to his own doctor, or his behavior might disturb the doctors since his relation was only to the ward personnel, he was essentially isolated from the other patients and the effects of his actions did not spread readily throughout the ward. Hence, such a patient usually presented no more than average administrative difficulty.

Patients in categories V through VIII did, however, cause considerable administrative difficulty. In this regard, the 12 patients in category V were interesting because they were able to form helpful relations with the doctors and other patients, but not with the ward personnel. Thus, these patients were viewed uneasily by the ward personnel, who saw the doctor and patient as sharing a relation about which they knew very little. This uneasiness was heightened by the fact that when such a patient's behavior presented an administrative problem, the ward personnel felt that this problem might spread because of the patient's relation to other patients on the ward. When such patients were discussed at the administrative conferences, the doctor was frequently placed on the defensive, the subjects of transference and countertransference often arose, and the patient was seen as a source of difficulty on the ward.

A situation similar to that in category V would logically obtain in category VI, where patients had established helpful relations with ward personnel and other patients, but not with doctors. None of the 36 patients observed during the study fell into this category, although a number of patients who had been in the hospital at other times did do so. Such patients would be viewed uneasily by the doctors because of the relatively unknown nature of their relations to the ward personnel and the other patients.

A seventh category consisted of patients who had been unable to achieve a relation either with the doctor or with the ward personnel, but had integrated themselves into the patient group. There were 6 patients in this category; and this is, of course, where Mr. Esposito belonged during his third period. Administratively, these patients were seen as a source of almost endless trouble, and in contrast to patients in most of the foregoing categories, patients in category VII usually did not remain in the hospital for very long. Such patients were seen as having influence over the other patients, but not being easily amenable to control by either the doctors or the ward personnel.

An eighth, and final, category contained 3 patients who were unable to make a significant relation with any of the three role groups. These patients usually were transferred or discharged shortly after their admission. Mr. Innes was such a case. He was brought to the hospital by the police with the story that he had attempted to murder some of his relatives. Unfortunately, he was placed in a room which had previously been occupied by a patient with a similar history, and many of the previous patient's symptoms also came to be attributed to Mr. Innes. It was later learned that the behavior which precipitated Mr. Innes' entrance into the hospital was not so lurid as it had been pictured, but the initial attitudes of both ward personnel and patients remained unchanged because Mr. Innes, a muscular man with a heavy red beard, chose to play a silent role on the ward. He refused to speak to anyone except an outside physician he had previously known, who visited him regularly in the hospital. There was evidence which indicated that Mr. Innes was not as frightening a person as he seemed, but this was lost in the general attitude that developed toward him. Mr. Innes stayed in the hospital only a short time.

The reader should not be left with the impression that patients remained constantly in one category. In the case of Mr. Esposito, for example, during his first few days on the ward he would probably be placed in category II as having a helpful relation with the doctor and ward personnel. However, as his first period in the hospital developed, he was unable to reach the nurses but maintained a partially satisfying relation with his doctor, and increased his relations with the patients. This would place him in category V, where he remained until his third period, at which point he shifted to category VII.

Such a movement of a patient from one category to another could be turned to therapeutic advantage. For example, it was mentioned earlier that Dr. Reynolds had brought her patient, Mr. Osgood, to a point of attempting to make contacts with women near his own age (at this time he would be in category V), and during his efforts to do this he was relatively uncommunicative in his therapeutic hours for a period of several weeks (shifting to category VII). The therapist felt threatened because the patient was not working in therapy. Given the conception developed here, however, it might have been that therapy was still going on, but within a somewhat different context. This therapeutic context, now centered on the ward, could be followed by the therapist, but this would necessitate fuller communication about life on the ward than was occurring at the time the study was made, and would also require a close working relation between the therapist and the ward personnel.

In general, it can be seen on Table 3–1 that of the total 36 patients observed, 27 had established patterns of relations that would probably result in therapeutic benefit (categories I–VI), while 9 had not done so (categories VII–VIII). In the administrative area, one would expect the care of 15 of the patients to proceed smoothly (categories I–IV), whereas 21 of the patients would probably present greater difficulty (categories V–VIII).

This chapter has centered around a discussion of a case which illustrated a number of problems in the area of therapy within the hospital, and of how such problems were influenced by factors arising in other areas of hospital life. The next chapter turns to an example of communication difficulty in the administrative area.

CHAPTER 4

Misunderstandings in Administrative Decisions

Information requiring administrative decisions is continually moving up and down in the hospital system, and this chapter is concerned with some of the misunderstandings that can arise during this process. The observations reported here attempt to trace the events that led to the bewilderment of the nurse on the open ward when she was greeted by laughter from the patients following a meeting in which the chief resident had told the patients they could see television twice a week after hours as they had requested in a petition. The events leading to this incident concern: (1) how the petition got started on the ward, (2) how it was discussed at the staff level, and (3) once a decision had been reached, how this was communicated to the patients.

Thus, this chapter is focused on a small group of patients and a few members of the staff as they worked to reach a solution to one specific administrative question. As such, this chapter is transitional between Chapter 3, which was mainly concerned with a single doctor-patient relationship, and Chapter 5, where the attempt is made to see the entire hospital in operation over time.

The kinds of questions raised by the account given below of the course of the television petition are directed partly at the confusion that can occur when what is, in the short-run situation, a purely administrative matter is approached as if it were a topic for psychotherapeutic discussion. The confusion which arises when this is done suggests the question of the separation of administrative and therapeutic functions in the hospital, which was alluded to at the close of the preceding chapter. Such a separation was not part of the general policy of the hospital, and there are a number of things to be said against as well as for this type of organizational procedure. Beyond this there is the question of whether or not very different, and perhaps opposite, processes are involved in administrative and therapeutic tasks. The exploration of this question would lead into a discussion of the relative advantages of an "authoritarian" or a "democratic" emphasis in the work of the hospital, and of whether or not opposition from patients or staff should be met head on and the attempt made to utilize it creatively rather than to try to avoid or suppress it. The questions raised in this paragraph will receive some discussion at the end of this chapter after the observational material which suggested them has been presented.

In connection with the present chapter, the reader may also wish to look at the interview material on administrative matters in Chapter 9 and at the quantitative treatment of the administrative conference data in Chapters 10 and 11.

THE COURSE OF THE TELEVISION PETITION

The observations of the patients during the time of the television petition were made on the open wards. The men's and women's open wards adjoined each other at right angles, forming an "L" shaped arrangement. Each ward had a large day room or, more accurately, living room in which male and female patients intermingled. The time of these observations was roughly a month after Mr. Esposito's discharge (see Chapter 3), and the reader will again meet some of the same people who appeared in the preceding chapter. For example, Mr. Ashton and Mr. Erskine had, at this point, been transferred from the locked to the open ward because of their therapeutic progress.

Origin of the Petition

The situation started one evening on the ward when Miss Farrell circulated a petition which contained the request to see television after hours. Inasmuch as Miss Farrell was soon to be discharged, this was one of several attempts on her part to retain the security of participation in the patient group. The petition, however, was picked up by the patients on the ward and used as a lever to dislodge Mr. Erskine from his monopolization of the television set. Mr. Erskine was talked into signing the petition himself by the other patients, but he was aware of the hostility toward him expressed by the petition, and his anxiety was increased.

Later the same evening after the petition had been signed by most of the patients on the open ward, Miss Farrell gave the petition to Mr. Ashton with the request that he turn it in to the staff. Mr. Ashton, however, kept the petition in his room for a week because, while he rather disliked Mr. Erskine's overbearing and patronizing behavior, he was unable openly to express the aggression against Mr. Erskine that would have been signified by turning the petition in to the staff. Finally, Mr. Ashton gave the petition to his own therapist, Dr. Rolfe, who transmitted it to the chief resident, Dr. Shaw, with the consequence that, a week after its origination, the petition came up for discussion in the administrative conference.

It is useful here to turn to the observations and "listen in" on some of the discussion among the patients about the television issue during the week before the petition reached the staff. It should be noted in these observations that Mr. Ashton said that he had given the petition to Miss Wright when actually he was still keeping it in his room. It seems likely that Mr. Ashton said this in order to assert himself against Mr. Erskine:

(On the ward at supper) There was much conversation about the petition last night which was started by Miss Farrell. Mr. Ashton and Mr. Erskine talked back and forth, Mr. Erskine wanting to see the fights and Mr. Ashton wanting to see the drama, Studio I. The two fight programs and Studio I all occur after hours in the hospital, and hence special permission must be obtained to see any of them. Mr. Ashton and Mr. Osgood both put considerable pressure on Mr. Erskine, saying that they wanted to see Studio I on Monday night, and the fights on either Wednesday or Friday nights. Mr. Erskine wanted to see the fights on both nights, and not to see Studio I at all. Mr. Edwards sided with Mr. Erskine for the fights and against Studio I. The following conversation took place:

Mr. Erskine: I think they ought to make TV every night until 11 o'clock.

Mr. Ashton: No, because the nurses have a hundred and one things to do, and that's their busiest time of day.

Mr. Erskine: Well, there's an attendant available from 6 o'clock.

Mr. Osgood: The attendant doesn't do anything. He doesn't have any medication to give.

Mr. Erskine: Well, I doubt that the fights will be taken away from us.

Mr. Ashton: Would you abide by a vote? One night for fights, and one night for Studio I?

Mr. Erskine: I would fight like hell for the fights. There are three or four other plays that come on at regular hours during the week that one could see.

Mr. Osgood: There's only one decent one during the week.

Mr. Erskine: I'll go get the TV book and look it up.

Mr. Edwards: The best thing that TV puts out is the fights, and I look forward to the fights.

Mr. Erskine goes and gets the TV program book and comes back and reads from it, naming the plays which are presented during the week.

Mr. Osgood: You haven't hit a good one yet.

Mr. Erskine: We should have handled that whole situation about Studio I differently.

Mr. Ashton: Well, Liz Farrell just passed the buck to me. She gave me the petition and told me to give it to someone. I gave it to Miss Wright as I thought that would be the way to handle it. (Mr. Ashton had done no such thing; he still had the petition in his room.)

Mr. Erskine: You should have asked the doctor on call. Actually that way we probably could see Studio I anyhow as Miss Neal doesn't come around to turn off TV until 10:30 anyway. I don't feel we should give up the sporting events because there are so few of them. . . .

After supper a bridge game started, and Mr. Erskine rode Mr. Ashton very hard about the quality of his playing. After the bridge game broke up the men went over to the women's living room. Miss Farrell came in and began to talk about her petition. Mr. Ashton threw it back to her saying:

Mr. Ashton: Don't you put it off on me, that was your business.

Miss Farrell: Well, I'm not a full-fledged member of the group any more.

Mr. Erskine: My little boy Edwards is with me against Ashton and the women.

As is indicated in the foregoing, the petition was an expression of resentment against Mr. Erskine, who was placed on the defensive. As the week progressed, Mr. Ashton became more able to express his aggression openly toward Mr. Erskine, and this reached a peak at the end of the week, when Mr. Ashton gave the petition to Dr. Rolfe and told Mr. Erskine on the ward that he was against him. These developments are indicated in the observations on the ward a week after Miss Farrell started the petition:

This evening Mr. Ashton set up a rival activity to Mr. Erskine's bridge game. Mr. Erskine had a bridge game going in the women's living room and a number of patients were kibitzing. Mr. Ashton obtained permission to order a large pizza from a nearby restaurant, and when this arrived he set up his party in the men's living room. Mr. Ashton went to the women's living room and invited several of the patients to join him, but he did not invite Mr. Erskine. Shortly, both the invited patients and Mr. Erskine came over to the men's living room and began to eat the pizza. Mr. Erskine took a piece of pizza and said to Mr. Ashton:

Mr. Erskine: Well, guy, how are you?

Mr. Ashton (speaking to Miss Lindsey and Miss Farrell): I think Joe (Mr. Erskine) will be going back to the locked ward soon.

Miss Field (speaking to Miss Farrell, who is staring at her): For Christ's sake stop staring at me!

Mr. Ashton (to Miss Farrell): After you gave me the petition I gave it to Dr. Rolfe and he will take care of the matter. I think it's going to be difficult for us to see Studio I because the nurses are so busy between 10 and 10:30.

It would be funny if it turned out that the decision was one night of fights and one night of Studio I.

Miss Farrell: It would be the men against the women.

Mr. Ashton: Well, I would side with the women and against Joe (Mr. Erskine).

Discussion of the Petition among the Staff

A week after it had been originated on the ward, the petition was given to Dr. Shaw by Dr. Rolfe, and the matter came up for discussion at the daily administrative conference. The assumption in the conference was that the petition had been circulated the preceding night, and there was uncertainty as to which of the patients was responsible for it. It was suggested that it was probably Mr. Erskine's petition, as he was frequently a source of administrative difficulty on the ward. This attitude on the part of the staff was, of course, incorrect, and it placed Mr. Erskine in the difficult position of having both the patients and the staff against him.[1] The suggestion that it was Mr. Erskine's petition led into a discussion of the psychodynamic meaning of the request for the patients, and the question of whether or not the residents should explore the implied authority conflict with those of their patients who had signed the petition. No specific decision on the disposition of the petition was reached at the administrative conference. The following excerpt gives a feeling of the discussion that went on:

Dr. Shaw: There's one other matter to be brought up. I have a petition here which is signed by the patients, who say they would like to stay up and see Studio I on Monday nights from 10 to 11 p.m. It's signed by most of the patients.

Miss Newcomb: That's not always a good play for the patients to see.

Miss Nugent: If they see the fights, then it's reasonable for them to say, why can't we see other things? However, I don't know if we can manage this in relation to the medication. Also we only have an attendant at night on

[1] The position of Mr. Erskine in this regard represents a common problem that arises in the communication process when there is inadequate information. An almost exact parallel to the situation reported in this chapter occurred while observations were being made in another hospital, a large state institution, at a later date. In this state hospital, seventeen of twenty-two patients on a men's locked ward complained that force was used by the attendants, and circulated a petition to this effect. The ward office ignored the report and the nurses sympathized with the attendants by saying that "patients shouldn't be allowed to circulate petitions." The difficulty on the ward was attributed to one patient, Mr. Johnson, who was a chronic source of trouble. Mr. Johnson was blamed for the petition, although in fact he did not sign it or originate it. In this situation a very perceptive head nurse started discussions, continuing over several weeks, with the ward personnel which helped to clear up the difficulty and resulted in a reduction in the use of seclusion from 132 hours per week to 13 hours per week in subsequent months.

duty downstairs, and Mrs. Netter can't always go downstairs to give the medication herself.

Mrs. Netter: I never know what the locked ward is going to be like. If it's quiet, it would be all right, but if it's not quiet I'd be here until midnight.

Mrs. Nolan: Mr. Onofrio works and gets up early, and if he's trying to sleep the television will keep him awake. At present he's the only one who does go to bed reasonably early.

Dr. Sears: Couldn't we put it on a situational basis? If things are bad upstairs then we wouldn't allow it downstairs, but if things are all right on the locked ward we could allow it.

Mrs. Nolan: It means a lot of extra work and demands on the nurses.

Dr. Shaw: Well, our time is up this morning. We need to think about this and make a decision.

Dr. Scott: I don't think that everyone would want to stay up. I wonder what this means to the patients and whether we shouldn't have the therapists explore this problem with their patients.

Dr. Shaw: Well, most of the patients have signed their names to the petition.

Mrs. Netter: We can try it.

Miss Nugent: The relief nurses are not here today, but they certainly might complain.

Dr. Sears: It looks like it's Erskine's petition.

Mrs. Nolan: He'll probably sit and play bridge while the late TV is going on.

Miss Nicholas: I wonder who put him up to it?

Dr. Scott: We'll have to study this rather carefully. It might turn into an every night thing, and we need to know what needs we satisfy by this.

Dr. Shaw: Well, we'll hold off on this.

Following the administrative conference, the head of the hospital, Dr. Scott, and the chief resident, Dr. Shaw, held their regular weekly meeting with the nursing staff, at which considerable resistance to the petition continued to be expressed. Some nurses first indicated their feelings in such remarks as: "The patients will want to see all the fights, and they don't even know who is fighting." Then the very real problem that late television would interfere with the change of nursing shifts was brought up. When the head of the hospital indicated that he thought that 10 o'clock might be too early to go to bed, the nursing staff resisted this point of view by responding: "Your evening starts later than theirs," and, "You're not a patient anyway."

What is of particular interest in the administrative conference and the nurses' meeting is that a simple request from the patients seemed to have set off considerable overreaction on the part of the staff, who were responding to tensions arising from other sources which were not made explicit or verbalized. Owing, in part, to the on-going state of transition in the hospital, there was disagreement and confusion between the various staff levels about administrative policy and the conceptualization of therapeutic goals. These underlying differences of opinion complicated the discussion of the television petition, but overtly the situation was phrased in terms of the problems of the patients. The patients thus became heir to many covert tensions in the hospital which had their locus elsewhere. This general process can also be seen in operation in the discussion of the individual doctor-patient relationship in Chapter 3 and in the development of the collective disturbance as reported in Chapter 5.

The overreaction of the nurses to the television petition is apparent in the following excerpt from the meeting of the senior staff with the nurses:

Miss Nugent: Several of the nurses wanted to talk about this problem of the patients' wanting to stay up late. As many of you know, the patients signed a petition, which was brought up this morning in administrative conference. They are already seeing the fights on Wednesday night. If this program is over by 11 o'clock, the open ward patients just plain don't get quiet until about 12 o'clock, but the new staff people come in and the shift changes at 11:15. . . . I cannot see why the TV should be on for one night and not for every night. As for myself, I don't think the fights are enough reason to stay up and see TV, and I would prefer not to have them see TV at all.

Mrs. Nixon: They are not satisfied with just seeing the main bout on TV. They want to see all the fights.

Miss Nicholas: It's not fair just for the men to see TV, and also I think it's really on a rather low cultural level—this wanting to see the fights.

Miss Newcomb: Studio I can be a great deal of trouble. I've watched it two or three times and the programs were really fairly scary, and I myself might be afraid to go to bed after some of them.

Dr. Scott: This is interesting, but who knows the real (i.e., psychodynamic) import of all these requests?

Miss Nicholas: I don't know where the petition started, but as soon as it was mentioned this morning I thought of Miss Lindsey. I had the feeling this morning when it came up that it was Lindsey. . . .

Dr. Scott: Does this mean that several people are supporting Miss Lindsey?

Miss Nicholas: She may have been the one who started it. . . .

Dr. Scott: Well, here it is, the impact of a request on us, and we are trying to figure out the psychodynamics of it. The impact on us, and the conflict with authority, and how should we treat this conflict. Also, the fact that it inconveniences us.

Dr. Shaw: It seems to be a unique situation. There seems to be a struggle about authority on the ward right now. In various ways Mrs. Lasker, Miss Prescott, Mr. Osgood, and Mr. Erskine, and also Elizabeth Farrell, are always having perpetual problems with authority. In the last week I've had the feeling that this conflict with authority has been much more in evidence. . . .

Dr. Scott: . . . If the problem here is, "How do the patients feel about relations to authority," and I think it is, then we ought to have the therapists bring this up in individual therapy. Taking Studio I seriously is just like taking the delusion of a patient seriously. Just as we want to know what's behind a delusion of a patient, we want to know what's behind this request, and this points up our real paucity of knowledge of what goes on on the ward.

Dr. Shaw: This came as a real surprise this morning. Nobody knew this was brewing.

Miss Nugent: This whole problem is also bound up with the bus schedule in the community and the fact that the nurses have to make their busses to get home.

Mrs. Nixon: The patients don't even know who is fighting. They just watch it because it's there.

Mrs. Nolan: At first they wanted to see the championship fights, but now they just watch whatever happens to be on.

Mrs. Nixon: Next they'll want to watch the wrestling matches until midnight.

Dr. Shaw: If the nourishment were given out before late television and not afterwards, and if this were made a policy, this might help.

Mrs. Nixon: How are you going to refuse them when they ask you for a glass of milk and some crackers?

Dr. Scott: Why not refuse them; just define the situation and tell them they can't have it.

Mrs. Nixon: Well, Mr. Ashton always comes up afterwards and wants a couple of quarts of milk and some crackers.

Dr. Scott: They give up something and we give up something in this situation. I think that's fair.

Miss Nugent: To come back to the problem of medication, suppose somebody is asking for sedation and needs it. Then this conflicts with the problem of giving out nourishment. When you say there isn't going to be any nourishment after TV, and then at 11 o'clock they come starving to the door, you can't very well deprive them.

Dr. Scott: Why is it depriving them any more than not letting them see the TV is depriving them? They are both deprivations.

Mrs. Nixon: Yes, but then there is the relation of hot milk to sedation, which TV doesn't have.

It is quite clear in the above material that the nurses were reacting to something far beyond the request of the patients to see television twice a week. However, these underlying feelings did not come out into the open. The result was that a simple administrative problem triggered off an emotional reaction all out of proportion to the importance of the initial stimulus because of the existence of latent tensions in the hospital system.

Several other points in the foregoing material should be mentioned. One is the equation of nourishment, as snacks are usually called in the hospital parlance, with sedation, and the reluctance of the nurses to see any therapeutic value in such a "nonmedical" activity as watching television. This is related to the lack of clarity the nurses felt about their role on the open wards and their preference for working on the locked wards where there was "more real nursing." These matters are discussed at greater length in the interview material in Chapter 9.

A second point in the above material concerns the emphasis placed by Dr. Scott on discovering the psychodynamic meaning of the petition for the patients and staff. This is a reasonable enough interest, but it is likely to cause confusion when it is not clear where the question of psychotherapy leaves off and the question of administrative procedure begins. There is some evidence that the process of psychotherapy and the process of administration stand in reciprocal relation to one another, and it is therefore most confusing to try to carry out both processes at the same time. This point will receive more attention in the discussion at the end of this chapter.

Not only were the nurses reacting to underlying tensions in the matter of the petition, but so also was Dr. Scott. At this time Dr. Scott was feeling that his authority in the hospital was being overridden by his superior, Dr. Sutton. It is likely that this feeling contributed to Dr. Scott's identification with the patients in regard to the petition, as indicated in the further excerpt from the meeting with the nurses given below. At the time of this meeting, however, Dr. Scott was not consciously aware of the influence of his resentment against Dr. Sutton on the way in which he handled the matter of the petition. At a later date he told the anthropologist that he believed his feelings toward Dr. Sutton had unconsciously entered into his decisions about the petition. This sort of "identification with the patients" on the part of Dr. Scott is similar in its psychological and social dynamics to the identification of the residents with the patients during the period of the paired role group response in the collective disturbance, as described in Chapter 5. In both these instances it would seem that the patients were being put in the position of acting out the forbidden impulses of Dr. Scott, as in the events given in this chapter, and of the residents, as in the events outlined in the next chapter. This is a somewhat more detailed way of again pointing to the fact that the patients are often made heir to many of the tensions existing among the staff. For example, in the meeting with the nurses Dr. Scott continued:

Dr. Scott: Why can't I say to myself that this is it, there won't be any TV, but I guess it's because I, myself, feel that 10 o'clock is too damned early to go to bed. You have to consider the going-to-bed patterns of these people before they came into the hospital. Many of them, of course, perhaps most of them, didn't go to bed at 10 o'clock.

Miss Nugent: Well, you're not a patient. You're on the other side of the fence, and that makes it different.

Dr. Scott: Yes, but some of my identification apparently is with the patients.

Mrs. Nixon: Their evening starts much earlier than yours.

Dr. Scott: That's a rather arbitrary opinion. We ought to relate the at-home sleeping habits of the patients to their behavior in the hospital. They don't go to bed early at home, probably not until a good bit after 11 o'clock.

Miss Nugent: But the reality is there. That is, they are in a hospital. They can't go to the icebox in the hospital as they can at home either.

Dr. Scott: I'd like to ask the group, do they have a great variability or consistency in going to bed in their habits? How about your going-to-bed habits? If for twenty years you've gone to bed at midnight, and then we ask a person to go to bed at 10 o'clock if we could just as easily make it later, why don't we do this? However, I guess there is a problem of practical reality.

Dr. Shaw: We start their day differently too. We give breakfast to them at 8:30 a.m., and very often those people who stay up late wouldn't get up so early.

Miss Nugent: Their day actually starts earlier than 8:30. It starts about 7:30 when they begin to get up.

Dr. Scott: Well, let's regularize what we've been doing with TV and let's keep it at once a week.

Mrs. Nixon: Unofficially, it's been twice a week.

Dr. Scott: Well, shall we say Mondays and Fridays. . . .

Dr. Shaw: I sense that the nurses feel that two nights is already too much.

Miss Nugent: I think that if we have a statement of when they are allowed to stay up, and the fact that it's explicitly made known that there will be no nourishment at all, it might be all right. . . .

Dr. Scott: Well, I'm going to make a decision. Let's make it Monday night and a choice of either Wednesday or Friday night, but no nourishment afterwards. Gee, it took a long time to kick that around.

Miss Newcomb: A simple thing like watching a TV program has to go to God and back again.

Dr. Scott: You would have preferred immediate pronouncement?

Miss Newcomb: Yes.

Miss Nugent: Just because there are two sides and you say by edict one side is going to be right, that doesn't settle anything. The whole crux of the thing is that this comes at a time of change of shift.

Dr. Scott: It relates to their attitudes toward authority.

Miss Nugent: The edict doesn't change the opinion.

Miss Newcomb: Well, you can't satisfy everyone.

Miss Nugent: The business of seeing the fights was originally for only championship fights and now it's for any old fight.

Mrs. Nolan: The last time the President spoke, they switched from the fights to the President on the TV program, and when they did this, why everybody went to bed. Mr. Owens said he couldn't understand how when the fights went off and the President came on that everybody would stay up for the fights but wouldn't stay up for the President of the United States.

Dr. Scott: That's another way of expressing their feelings to authority.

Communication of the Decision about the Petition

Since a decision had been made by fiat in order to cut off what seemed likely to become an interminable discussion, the problem then arose of how this decision was to be communicated to the patients. The reactions of the nurses and the chief resident to this problem were interesting: the nurses had considerable difficulty in conceiving of their role in the hospital as one in which they could easily communicate such a decision to the patients; the chief resident was very unclear in his own mind about the extent of his authority and how to exercise it, and, as will be seen later, his tendency to confound administrative with therapeutic actions led to a misunderstanding with the patients. Some aspects of these reactions on the part of the nurses and of the chief resident, Dr. Shaw, are indicated in the discussion which concluded the meeting with the nurses:

Dr. Scott: How are we going to communicate this to the patients?

Miss Nicholas: It might best be communicated in a group. That is, if they all signed their names to a petition, the least we can do is to tell them about it all together.

Miss Nugent: . . . Are you going to have a gripe session?

Dr. Scott: I'm personally against these gripe sessions.

Dr. Shaw: So am I, particularly if the patients feel that they are legislating something at these sessions and find out later that they are not.

Dr. Scott: The only good that these gripe sessions can do is that if you can get the patients as a group to scrutinize what is going on in their behavior, then it is productive.

Miss Nugent: You brought up one question, Dr. Scott, and that is to give the patients an explanation. This is a difficult thing for us to do. We are not accustomed to doing this. It's the same sort of problem as the one in which the patient can't eat at a decent hour because the men who bring the food over from the other side have to go off work at 5 o'clock in the afternoon. We don't tell this to the patients. I think the patients should know this. They have to fit their feelings and demands into the situation along with everyone else.

Dr. Scott: Isn't that the point? We impose authority, and then the patients have a rebellion which is justified. But if we impose the real limits of the hospital then the patients can handle them. If they don't handle them then we can, in fact, say that it is irrational.

Miss Nugent: It's extremely difficult for doctors and nurses to communicate that sort of thing to the patients. They aren't used to it.

Mrs. Nixon: Some apartment houses have restrictions like that. Lots of apartment houses I know of you can't play musical instruments after 10 o'clock.

Miss Nicholas: We would have less trouble if we would explain restrictions like that.

Dr. Scott: So we have to be aware of what we have. We are setting up structures and then showing the patient that he has to react to them. If we don't, the patient is hostile and refuses to examine his feelings. That is, if we don't give him the real reason then we don't know if his hostility is really justified or irrational. The same thing is true with me. If I stated the patients could stay up until 11 o'clock then I get real feelings of hostility from you toward me. I think that in some hospitals where things are run on a very authoritative plan, it must be a very comfortable situation—everybody knowing what they should do. Well, anyway let's . . . have Dr. Shaw communicate our decision to them formally in a session with the patients as a group tomorrow.

The next morning in the administrative conference, Dr. Shaw, who was later to hold a group session with the patients, communicated to the staff what had been discussed in the nurses' meeting the preceding day. At the administrative conference he said:

Dr. Shaw: The main thing about the TV hours that came out of the nurses' meeting was that it involves problems about the nurses' time. We have to communicate this to the patients and have them work through their reasoning. They can see Studio I on Monday, and the fights on either Wednesday or Friday. After TV there will be no nourishment because the nurses have to make their busses and get home at a reasonable time. So, after TV at night there will be no milk or fruit juice available.

As can be seen from Dr. Shaw's remarks at the administrative conference, he was thinking of two problems: first, that he had to communicate Dr. Scott's decision to the patients; and second, that he wished the patients to work through their reasoning for wanting to see television after hours. The first problem was more an administrative one, the second more a therapeutic one.

Since he did not feel at ease with administrative problems, Dr. Shaw began the meeting that afternoon with the patients by asking them to discuss their reasoning rather than by telling the patients what Dr. Scott had already decided. Dr. Shaw said: "We have received your petition and want to discuss this with you and get your views on the problem of staying up late for TV." Most of the patients took this as an opportunity to participate in the making of a decision, and felt that they had, in fact, done so when Dr. Shaw closed the meeting by saying: "Well, we'll leave it at Monday night plus a choice of Wednesday or Friday nights." After

Dr. Shaw had left the ward, the patients continued an informal discussion in which they expressed appreciation at being asked to help in reaching a decision, and pleasure over having won their point. Only one patient held it was "all a fake," and she was argued down until a staff nurse, who had just come on the ward, said: "All I know is that I was ordered yesterday you were to be allowed to see late TV twice a week." The patients broke into laughter, the nurse was bewildered, and the patients felt that they had been led to believe they were participating in a decision that had already been made.

Obviously this result was not the one intended by the hospital, and the problem would seem to be one of administrative confusion and misunderstanding in communication. In somewhat more detail, some of the events sketched in the preceding paragraph can be seen in the following excerpts from the observations of the group session which Dr. Shaw held with the patients:

At the meeting there were eleven open ward patients present, plus Dr. Shaw, and the writer.

Dr. Shaw opened the meeting by saying that the staff had received the petition and wanted to get the views of the patients on the matter. Mr. Erskine started off by getting the schedule of television programs and saying that he had made a little survey and that there seemed to be good programs on from 8 to 11 every night. Miss Lindsey broke in at this point and told Mr. Erskine that it was only the hour from 10 to 11 that they were concerned about. Mr. Erskine went on to say that there were not many sporting events on television during the winter months, and that he felt the patients should be allowed to see the fights on two nights and also see Studio I on Monday night. The women patients disagreed with him, and he took the position that he refused to have one of the fight nights discontinued in favor of Studio I.

Mr. Osgood and Mr. Isherwood attempted to arbitrate the conflict between Mr. Erskine and Miss Lindsey. After defending Mr. Erskine for a bit, Mr. Osgood gave up his position and stated that as far as he was concerned one night of fights and one night of Studio I was satisfactory. Mr. Isherwood left the meeting shortly, but before he went he said that he felt that one night of Studio I and one fight night seemed reasonable.

The following exchange then took place between several of the women and Dr. Shaw:

Miss Prescott: What I am wondering, Dr. Shaw, is why we can't stay up until 11 every night?

Mrs. Lasker: I feel that way too.

Miss Lindsey: I'm very much concerned about the women's having a say in this. What Mr. Erskine proposes is that the men get two nights of fights while the women only have one night of Studio I. I think it's the principle of the thing, and both men and women should have one night they could pick out.

Mrs. Lasker: Why are you so concerned that the men have two nights while the women just have one?

Miss Lindsey: I suppose it's just part of my illness.

Dr. Shaw: Well, you can always fall back on that one. (There is general laughter in the group.)

Mrs. Lasker: I would like to know how we happened to have this meeting with you, Dr. Shaw?

Dr. Shaw: Well, the doctors had a meeting, and then the nurses had a meeting, and then we came down to have a meeting with you.

Miss Lindsey: I think that's very democratic. I do think though that there ought to be a nurse at this meeting since her duties are concerned.

Miss Prescott: What difference would it make? It's probably been decided ahead of time anyway.

Dr. Shaw: I want to discuss this problem with the patients.

Miss Prescott: You don't mean discuss, Dr. Shaw, you mean explain to us something that has already been decided.

Dr. Shaw (closing the session): Well, we'll leave it at Monday night plus a choice of Wednesday or Friday nights.

At this point Dr. Shaw left the meeting and went off the ward. The patients, however, continued to talk among themselves.

Miss Prescott: It's all a fake and everything is decided ahead of time.

Miss Lindsey: That's not true, I think we really decided something.

Mrs. Lasker: I agree with Helen (Miss Lindsey). . . .

Mrs. Nagle, the nurse on duty on the ward, came into the living room at this point and Mrs. Lasker went over to her.

Mrs. Lasker: Where were you at our meeting?

Mrs. Nagle: What meeting?

Mrs. Lasker: Our meeting about the patients' seeing television late.

Mrs. Nagle: Oh.

Mrs. Lasker: What did they decide up at your meeting when they talked about this?

Mrs. Nagle: What meeting?

Mrs. Lasker: The one the nurses had about television.

Mrs. Nagle: I wasn't present at that meeting.

Mrs. Lasker: Well, you should have been because you're the one who is most concerned. You're the one who is here all the time.

Mrs. Nagle: All I know is that I was ordered yesterday you were to be allowed to see late TV twice a week.

At this all the patients broke into laughter. Mrs. Nagle was bewildered and, sitting down, attempted to talk it out with the patients, but she had little success.

DISCUSSION

The simplest generalization that can be made from the observations that have been presented is that there was a lack of pertinent information available to the staff concerning the events surrounding the television petition. As has been indicated, this lack of information contributed its share to the resultant confusion. Dr. Scott was quite correct when he said in the meeting with the nurses that ". . . we want to know what's behind this request, and this points up our real paucity of knowledge of what goes on on the ward."

Such a state of affairs indicates serious defects in the making and channeling of observations about behavior in the hospital system; the needed information simply was not forthcoming from the nurses and residents. The reasons why this was so are rather complex and involve, first of all, the nature of the relations between the senior physicians, residents, and nurses at this time—a topic which forms a major part of Chapter 5. Secondly, the background and training of the nurses was such that they did not readily transmit the kind of information that was needed, and even when they were able to do so, their contribution was often overlooked because of the relative implicit value attached to various kinds of information in the work of the administrative conference. Information which gave evidence of, or was phrased in, a "psychodynamic" frame of reference was more highly valued than descriptive reporting or observations couched in administrative terms. This was a third reason why adequate information was not available about the television petition. Both in the administrative conference where the petition first came to the notice of the staff, and in the meeting with the nurses, the question was raised almost immediately of, "What is the psychodynamic meaning of this for the patients?" The nurses, because of their training, could not answer the question phrased in this manner, and, being made personally uncomfortable by this, they turned to a criticism of the patients. Thus, the factual contribution the nurses could have made tended to be lost. The residents, who were more able to state their opinions in dynamic terms, did not have the facts about ward interaction to give, since they concentrated their efforts on psychotherapy with individual patients.

None of the above should be taken as belittling the effort to arrive at an understanding of the psychodynamics of the situation, which is an obvious part of the work of the hospital. The point is rather the simple one that it is necessary to obtain sufficient information about what the situation is before going on to the question of what it means—and this would hold true for more administrative matters as well as for those that were more concerned with therapeutic issues. All this is related to the somewhat separate values and attitudes that were held by the various role groups toward life in the hospital and that were incompletely known from one group to the other because of changes that had taken place over the years. These matters are discussed at some length in Chapters 6 through 9.

The question of the values of the various role groups certainly is involved in the confusion often felt by senior physicians or residents between the administrative and therapeutic aspects of their roles. This was true in the observations on the course of the television petition when the chief resident, Dr. Shaw, had the task of communicating an administrative decision, but handled this in such a way as to elicit material more of a therapeutic nature related to the feelings of the patients. This had the effect of leading the patients to believe that they were participating in the making of a decision, which, of course, was not the case.

Such problems raise the procedural issue of the advisability of the separation between administrative and therapeutic responsibilities in the work of a psychiatric hospital. Considerable interest has been expressed in this kind of separation in recent years, and it is usually done by placing the administrative care of all patients on a ward in the hands of one physician, while the other physicians, who are engaged in psychotherapy, are supposed to look upon the conduct of life on the ward as a reality in somewhat the same way that a therapist whose work lay outside the hospital would view the setting of his patient's daily activities. This procedure helps to avoid some difficulties, such as those faced by the chief resident in the situation reported here, but, at the same time, the very process of separation creates its own problems as it increases the likelihood that disagreements will develop between administrator and therapist, both of whom exercise control over the patient (Stanton and Schwartz, 1954). One reason that such disagreements arise is that the administrator usually has less prestige than does the therapist; moreover, the therapist in the name of "emergency" often overrides the decisions and plans of the administrator. As Smith (1955) points out, this is not just a problem for the psychiatric hospital or the general hospital, but is inherent in a situation whenever there are dual lines of authority. Such a situation can arise in military organizations between line and staff control, or it can occur in universities between the faculty members who do the teaching and the administrators who care for the physical upkeep and financial condition of the institution. As such, this is a broad problem which does not admit of any easy solution.

Behind such relatively practical matters as are referred to in the preceding paragraph, there are a number of more theoretical questions about the difference in the sequence of phases through which administrative and therapeutic processes may go. Parsons, Bales, and Shils (1953) have suggested that the same phases are involved in such tasks as reaching administrative decisions as are involved in psychotherapeutic work, but the sequence of phases goes in opposite directions in the two cases. In administrative tasks the sequence moves from the practical statement and implementation of problems, through a period of tension release, and ends with the reaffirmation of social and emotional bonds between members of the group. In psychotherapy the reverse is true, since an initial relation must be established between doctor and patient, which usually then leads to the more open expression of affect by the patient, and finally to the consideration of the meaning of, and appropriate means for implementing, actions. If such is the case, the difficulty in trying to act upon both the administrative and therapeutic aspects of the television petition at the same time, as in the material presented in this chapter, becomes more understandable.

Aside from the possible difference in the sequence of phases in the general nature of administrative and therapeutic processes, there is the further question of whether or not such functions can be handled by the same person in a given position of responsibility. Independently, both Fiedler (1957) and Bales (1956) have discussed this question recently with reference to leadership. Their general position, from much experimental work with small groups, is that adaptive or task functions and expressive or therapeutic functions seem to require different attitudes and roles, which only the exceptional leader can successfully combine. An indication of just how exceptional such leaders are comes from Bales' work,[2] where he found such versatile individuals occurring about 5 per cent of the time, or one person among twenty. Again, this type of research helps in understanding the attempts that have been made to place administrative and therapeutic responsibilities in the hands of different people in the psychiatric hospital.

There does not seem to be any ready answer to the question of whether or not administration and therapy should be separated. There are practical and theoretical reasons both for doing so and for not doing so. Certainly one answer is the need for awareness on the part of the staff, so that they know what they are trying to do and feel comfortable and reasonably assured in doing it. This is particularly important when a situation calls for the exercise of authority either in administrative or therapeutic matters. For example, during the course of the television petition there were many unexpressed tensions related to conflicts with authority, and an avoidance, on the part of all role groups among the

[2] In a verbal communication.

staff, of the necessity to assume responsibility for decisive action. As has been indicated, the reasons for such an avoidance could be traced, in part, to unresolved personal conflicts within the system, as Dr. Scott's underlying feelings of resentment against his superior, Dr. Sutton. Also, however, such an avoidance was related to the effort to shift the policy and procedures of the hospital in the direction of a more psychodynamic orientation. This effort was in line with the recent emphasis that has been placed on changing the psychiatric hospital from an authoritarian to a democratic structure, and from a custodial to a humanistic ideology (Gilbert and Levinson, 1956). Such changes, if serious and realistic, are very much to the good. Often, however, these terms (as also the idea of a "therapeutic community") are invoked with more enthusiasm than knowledge, and are used more in the popular sense they have in American culture than in a technical manner. It sometimes seems as if such desires for change are a specific example of what Riesman (1950) has called the "other directedness" of Americans. This can lead to such extremes as the attitude sometimes held by psychiatrists working in hospital settings that "we are all patients here together" (cited in Rapoport and Rapoport, 1957). Such an attitude can be a useful one, but it can also be an abrogation of the responsibility to assume authoritative control and leadership when these are needed.

The ability to exercise authority would seem to be connected with the freedom to meet and to utilize opposition for creative purposes. The television petition was certainly not viewed in such a way in the events that have been described in this chapter. Similar situations reported from other hospitals, however, have indicated a more creative use of opposition. This is true for the procedures used at Ville-Evrard—a psychiatric hospital in Paris, France—about which Sivadon (1957) says:

> Our service is composed of six pavilions of about 45 patients each. The population of each pavilion meets once each week and is then invited either by certain natural protesters among the patients or upon the more or less insidious suggestion of the personnel, to take cognizance of the imperfections of the service. Motives are scarcely ever lacking—such and such apparatus are not functioning; the meals are served too slowly; there is not enough diversion in the evening, etc. Soon almost the entire group participates in this common protest, and many patients who have up to this point been isolated in their indifference emerge from their mutism. Now human relations have been established. It is only a question of improving upon all the inconveniences of which one is a victim. The premises, the personnel, the doctors, the administration, and society in general bear the brunt of the criticism. Immediately the group

tends to organize. A delegate is elected who is charged with the transmission of the protests to the authorities. Thus six pavilions furnish six delegates who constitute the "Committee of Patients." This committee meets once a week with the doctor and the hostess. In the course of long discussions, which turn into real group therapy, the demands are studied and the whole art of the sociotherapists consists of channelizing the aggressive tendencies thus manifested toward useful activities. The first result obtained is that the doctors, attendants, and nurses, by not seeking to suppress the opposition but by adopting a comprehensive attitude, find themselves included in the group, and the group is extended henceforth to include the whole of the service. An "esprit de corps," the basis for a community atmosphere, is already created; however, it still remains founded upon the common opposition to the environment.

This is a delicate task but one which, by experience, is practically always crowned with success. It promotes the maturation of the protesting attitude into an objective one which is expressed in the need for concrete actualizations. . . .

Perhaps the differences between the way in which the television petition was handled in the American hospital reported on here, and the "maturation of the protesting attitude" developed in the French hospital referred to above, are differences arising out of the cultures within which the two hospitals are set. The French are known for their enjoyment of argument and opposition, whereas Americans would rather arbitrate and conform. This line of thought concerning the cultural context of the psychiatric hospital will be returned to in the final chapter of this book.

In turning to the next chapter, it is useful to ask whether the matter of the television petition was an isolated contretemps, or whether it was itself but a symptom of a more inclusive process. The latter seems to have been true, and the petition can be thought of as simply one instance of the patients' calling attention to themselves. The next chapter is concerned with why the patients felt it necessary at this time to attempt to draw the attention of the staff to themselves.

CHAPTER 5

Occurrence of Collective Disturbances

This chapter represents an attempt to follow the nature of what was going on simultaneously at various levels throughout the entire hospital. It was for this purpose that the term *transactions* was introduced in Chapter 1 to refer to a multiplicity of events taking place over time in a complex field. Thus, the interest here is in the interrelation of behavior within the overt formal and informal structure of the hospital, and within its covert emotional structure.

In a real sense, one of the major aims of this chapter is to point out the reality of the phenomenon that is referred to as the *covert emotional structure* of a hospital. Some of the same data that are used as evidence to support this concept in a clinical or observational manner in this chapter are handled in a quantitative fashion in Chapter 12, where the question is raised of whether indexes could be developed for predicting the direction of shifts in the covert emotional structure. It may be useful for the reader to consider these two chapters as a pair.

The term, covert emotional structure, is not entirely satisfactory, and yet it is hard to find a more adequate one without seeming to attribute anthropomorphic qualities to the hospital structure. For example, as will be seen later in this chapter, there were times when the social structure of the hospital seemed to be characterized more aptly by the term "regressed" than merely by "disorganized." In any case, the phenomenon of the covert emotional structure does not consist simply in the addition of the underlying emotional reactions of separate individuals, and it is not a matter of the sort of emotional contagion that takes over a mob or a crowd. In a hospital, the phenomenon seems to have a structure (it is what is often referred to as a "field"); it is primarily an emotional rather than a rational reaction; and it usually operates out of the specific awareness of the individuals who are participating in it.

One aspect of the covert emotional structure is contained in the reports from psychiatric hospitals in the United States and England, which consistently note the occurrence of mood sweeps in the general atmosphere of the hospital. If these are severe enough, they are known as *collective disturbances*. In a general way, a collective disturbance usually refers to a situation in which the majority of patients on a ward become upset at one time, although as will be seen later the disturbance is probably much wider and includes the staff. Collective disturbances provide a strategic situation for the collaboration of social science and psychiatry, and recently such disturbances have been analyzed by Boyd, Kageles, and Greenblatt (1954), Stanton and Schwartz (1954), Rapoport (1956), Miller (1957), and Caudill (1957).[1]

The focus of this chapter is on a collective disturbance that broke into the open a few weeks after the incident of the television petition had taken place as described in the preceding chapter. Thus, the time span of events in this chapter extends from roughly one month prior to the origination of the television petition on the ward until several months later. The reader will again meet some of the people he has met before.

The collective disturbance analyzed here, as it was seen by the staff at the time it took place, is fairly representative of the way such situations often seem to develop. Without explicit prior recognition or discussion by the staff in the daily administrative sessions that something might happen, certain dramatic events simply occurred which resulted in both the open and closed wards' becoming manifestly disturbed, and a special staff meeting was then called to discuss the matter.

Specifically, all those patients from the open ward who had privileges to go into town left the hospital one evening singly or in pairs, whereas previously they had gone out in groups of four or five. Each pair of patients who left the hospital had a disagreement with one another and returned as separate individuals. All who went out had an unpleasant evening and, depending upon the form taken by their personal problems, returned in an excited, depressed, or drunken condition. The upset state of these patients spread to others on the wards, and this situation persisted for about a week.

[1] The following material in this chapter is adapted from an article by the present author, which appeared under the title, "Social Process in a Collective Disturbance on a Psychiatric Ward," in Greenblatt, M.; Levinson, D. J.; and Williams, R. H. (editors). *The Patient and the Mental Hospital*. Glencoe, Illinois: The Free Press, copyright 1957.

At the conference held by the staff on this situation, the discussion centered around the character disorder patients as leaders, and the schizophrenic and neurotic patients as followers. Three patients—Mr. Erskine, Miss Prescott, and Mrs. Lasker—were singled out as leaders. Suggestions were made, half-humorously, that the passive patients should be encouraged to rebel against the more aggressive ones, and that the staff should play down its attention to the aggressive patients. The head of the hospital, Dr. Scott, responded that he did not want to follow such a punitive policy. A good deal of confusion was expressed, and no one felt able to say what was going on beyond the fact that both the open and closed wards were disturbed. Two recently admitted patients—Mr. Ulrich and Miss Miller—were then suggested as a focus of difficulty in terms of Mr. Ulrich's denial of the hospital situation and his desire to organize the male patients into a sporting fraternity, and Miss Miller's naïve and open sexual provocation, which annoyed the women and which was reacted to by the men partly with humor and partly with fear. The conference ended inconclusively.

After about a week, things became less dramatic on the open ward, although an unsettled state persisted. Within the next two weeks Mr. Ulrich was discharged, Miss Miller was transferred to the closed ward, and a certain degree of social calm was restored.

Without question, the five patients mentioned above occupied a central position, both as individuals and in certain group combinations, on the ward. Since they were prominent,[2] the events on the ward were usually stamped with aspects of their psychopathology. This was by no means always disruptive: Mr. Erskine would throw a temper tantrum or sulk, but he would also (probably for his own security needs but resulting in effective group action) organize a canasta game as a device for warding off the boredom or tension of an evening. In any case, the actions of such patients, individually or in consort, only very rarely coincided with a collective disturbance, and it is intellectually dissatisfying to see in them the sole "cause" of this type of situation.

In order to see the wider social context of the collective disturbance, it is necessary to look at events occurring during the two months prior to, and one month following, the actual disturbance, and to do this with reference to various levels in the hospital—senior physicians, residents,

[2] It is hard to find an adequate word here—aggressive, dominant, leaders, visible. These people were, and yet were not, these things because of the differences in life within the hospital when compared with life in the outside world. Certainly these people "stood out" as individuals in that all other patients reacted toward or against them. They were never neutrally evaluated.

nurses, other personnel (social worker, occupational therapist, etc.), and patients. Upon analysis of the observational data, it seemed that these three months could be divided into a sequence of four types of "balance of forces" between the five main role groups in the hospital, and this sequence is discussed in some detail in the following account. Observations collected over time on five role groups present a complex problem in exposition, and it is hoped that this problem has been handled so that some sense of conviction is retained, even though the data can be given only in summary form.

The sequence of balance of forces that developed in the hospital was related to the state of transition from a diagnostic to a psychodynamic treatment program. In the months preceding the outbreak of the collective disturbance, the senior staff members were engaged in trying to define their own roles, in determining therapeutic policy, and in finding ways to formalize the routines of the hospital so that these would serve to implement therapeutic goals. The residents tended to see therapeutic problems in terms of their individual patients and were opposed to formalized routine. Such disagreement placed the nurses in confusion about their responsibilities and about what were the rules to be followed. In line with the effort at transition, a new activities program, headed by a professional group worker, was started on the wards. This new program was felt as a threat by the occupational therapist and as another area of confusion in routine by the nurses. This unsettled state among the staff was reflected in the patients in a lack of certainty about what were correct and permitted actions. These questions of disagreement among role groups tended to remain covert and were not openly discussed at such expected points as the daily administrative conference. Such disagreements were, however, very often implicit in the discussion of plans for individual patients, who then became the vehicle through which differences of opinion were expressed.

Some two months before the collective disturbance, the observations clearly indicate that the various role groups had attempted to ease the difficulty of the situation by a process of *mutual withdrawal* in which each role group concentrated on the tasks which it felt were most sharply defined for its members and limited its interaction with other role groups to "neutral" activities. This state of mutual withdrawal was still in effect during the weeks preceding the collective disturbance and is the first in the sequence of types of balances between the various role groups.

The second type of balance of forces which occurred was initiated by the outbreak of acute difficulties and may be called the period of *open collective disturbance.* Just prior to the open collective disturbance two key members of the patient group were discharged, and this resulted in a fragmentation of the group structure on the ward. At the same time, two patients who were very upsetting to the patient group were admitted. The patients could not, at this point, re-form adequate companionable groups, and, in various ways, appealed to the staff for greater control over their activities. Because of the state of mutual withdrawal, the patients' attempts at communication did not get through in a meaningful way to the staff, and the open collective disturbance ensued.

Following the outbreak of open disturbance on the ward, the staff were at first bewildered and then were divided in their efforts to help the patients. The nurses and senior physicians tended to work together to help the patients through a greater formalization of routine and a sharpening of the boundaries of the hospital; the resident physicians tried to help the patients by granting greater freedom to individual patients and suppressing information about these additional privileges during the daily administrative meetings. Each staff role group was, in its own way, attempting to act positively, but since the disagreements between staff role groups remained covert, there was considerable confusion among both staff and patients. A situation was created in which the residents identified themselves with the patients, and the nurses with the senior physicians. This forms the third type in the sequence of structural balances—and may be called a *paired role group response* which was taking place in a social field that was seriously split apart.

Such an unstable balance of forces could not persist, and, after several weeks, the discrepancies between the procedures followed by the residents in granting privileges to patients and the general policy of the hospital on this matter were "discovered." This led to several conferences in which the real disagreements between the various staff role groups were openly discussed, and the operation of the hospital returned to a more stable equilibrium. This process of *restitution* comprises the fourth type in the sequence of balance of forces. Evidence from the observational data for each of these types of balances is given below.

MUTUAL WITHDRAWAL

The following observations on the mutual withdrawal of five role groups were all made during the ten-day period preceding the outbreak of the open collective disturbance. Perhaps the best way to present these data would be to indicate what was occurring each day among the five role groups, but this would result in an extremely involved exposition. Hence, the observations are given by role group, but it should be kept in mind that the events, in terms of the order in which they are presented for each group, were occurring at roughly similar points in time.

Withdrawal of the Patients

During these ten days small groups of patients on the open ward continued their attempts to draw the attention of the staff in various ways, such as rather theatrically washing the large glass windows in the living room while complaining about the housekeeping service. Ward conversations were full of references to boredom and tension, criticism that the doctors came around less frequently, a belief that the use of sedation was increasing, and a great interest in the authority hierarchy of the hospital. At the same time the patients intensified their interpersonal and clique relations and assumed greater control over carrying out recreational activities.

In washing the windows the patients indirectly made quite sure the nurse on duty and the residents knew what they were doing. Coupled with other such events, one interpretation of these activities is that the patients were in effect saying: "Look, we want more attention." For example:

Miss Prescott, Mr. Ulrich, Mr. Osgood, Mrs. Lasker, and Miss Peters were sitting around in a rather bored funk. Miss Peters said that the thing she will remember about this place is the endless hours she sat around and did nothing. Mrs. Lasker said that she would like to know whom to speak to about the dirty windows in the living room. She said that she told the nurse the windows were a disgrace and that she washed every piece of furniture in the room this morning. Shortly thereafter Mrs. Lasker said: "Okay, let's wash the windows now if the hospital isn't going to wash them." She went and got a basin of water and rags, and got the group in the living room started on the job. They pulled the tables over to stand upon. Miss Peters said: "This is a lot better than occupational therapy. You know that in a state hospital they let you work." Mrs. Lasker said: "Don't mention that word." Mr. Erskine and Mr. Isherwood came over from the men's side and joined in the washing. Shortly thereafter Mrs. Foster and Miss Murdock came in and watched the proceedings. The job was finished in about an hour. Later in the evening Mrs. Lasker said: "I told Dr. Rolfe (her therapist) about what we did this afternoon and about the dirt in the hospital. He told me on the sly to tell the head of the hospital about it, and I am going to do it."

As indications of the general state of boredom and tension on the ward, observations from the following three days are pertinent:

(6:00 to 11:00 p.m. on the open ward) Miss Peters stormed down the hall and went into her room and slammed the door. She was angry at Mr.

Erskine and said: "No, I won't play canasta and that's final." Miss Prescott was very angry at Mr. Erskine and Mrs. Lasker for disturbing Miss Peters. Mr. Osgood was sitting in the women's living room in the middle of this sea of trouble and said: "I wish I could leave for half an hour and come back and find people in the same mood." Mrs. Lasker came into the living room, and Mr. Osgood said: "Everybody is fighting but me and I have nobody to fight with." Mrs. Lasker said: "Well, I will fight with you. . . ."

(Next day, 3:00 to 6:00 p.m. on the open ward) Miss Peters and Miss Prescott came into the men's living room and wanted to know if a canasta game was going to be played. Mr. Erskine set one up. Mr. Isherwood came into the living room, and Mr. Erskine said: "How are you, my boy?" Miss Prescott called Mr. Erskine down by saying: "My boy, don't be so patronizing." The canasta game went on for a bit, and then Miss Prescott said: "They are getting awfully generous with the sedation around here. Several of the women had their sedation increased." Mr. Ashton suggested: "Let's start an anti-goofball drive." Mr. Erskine said: "I'm on the other team there. Mr. Emerson wrote me a poem, 'The King on the Paraldehyde Throne.' " Mr. Ashton answered: "Yes, and Emerson went to a state hospital after that." He turned to the social anthropologist and asked: "Do they check up on people when they go to state hospitals?" Miss Prescott, answering for the anthropologist: "No, they just let them go." Mr. Ashton said: "I wouldn't sell them that short." Miss Prescott replied: "I would." Mr. Ashton said: "Maybe you are right." Mr. Erskine added: "I found out that my tailor's daughter was at a state hospital." (He laughed at this.) Miss Peters asked: "What's so funny about that?" Mr. Erskine replied: "It's not funny; it's tragic."

(Next evening, 7:00 to 10:00 p.m. on the open ward) Miss Farrell, Mrs. Lasker, Mr. Osgood, and Mrs. Lange were laughing as the social anthropologist came on the ward. Mr. Osgood asked: "Do you think that animals ever get bored?" The anthropologist asked what precipitated this, and Miss Farrell read a bit from a book by Bertrand Russell which she was reading, to the effect that babies should be taught how to sustain boredom because so much of life today was made up of boredom. This led Mr. Osgood to say that he thought that animals had these sorts of feelings and that his dog laughed itself to death. He went on to describe an accident in which the dog was in the car and hit its head against the windshield, and then for all he could see died twenty minutes later after laughing itself to death.

The patients at this time also indicated a particular interest in the hierarchy of the hospital along with complaints that the doctors were cutting down on the amount of time they gave to patients. For example, later the same evening as in the excerpt last given:

Dr. Sutton walked past the living room. There was much comment on this, and Mr. Isherwood said: "We never see him around here. Dr. Shaw you see occasionally. I wish we could know what goes on here, at least who the people are. . . ."

(Next morning) Mrs. Nagle, the nurse on duty, said that she wished she knew where she could get in touch with the doctors, that all the patients were asking for them. On the ward Miss Prescott was yelling her head off for Dr. Shaw, and Mrs. Lasker and Mr. Erskine were asking every few minutes to see Dr. Rolfe. There was a general discussion among the patients in the living room about the fact that the doctors never seemed to be around. Miss Prescott said: "I'm the only one who can't go out this week end. It's difficult to be punished for someone else's sins. The family won't come up, and I can't get out of here because the doctors won't do anything without the okay of the family. Nobody will stand up for me." At this point Mr. Osgood literally stood up for her, and she said: "Thank you, Bill. . . ."

(Later that evening) Mrs. Lasker: I had a delegation visit me today—a big bear, a medium-sized bear, and a little bear. They asked me if I was sick and I fooled them because I said I was. They aren't going to prove me crazy by getting me to say I'm not sick. Who is this guy Sutton anyway?

Miss Lindsey: He's head of all of the hospitals around here, and Dr. Scott is head of just this one. I don't know what happens after that. I think that Miss Noyes is under Dr. Scott.

Miss Fellows: I'm glad someone else can't figure out the hierarchy. I've been trying to do it. I thought that Dr. Sutton was head of the Psychology Department, but now I'm not sure.

Miss Prescott: Well, anyway he owns a piece of it.

Mr. Ashton: Yes, he owns about 51 per cent of the stock. . . .

In the above excerpt it is interesting that Mrs. Lasker makes a joke out of the visit of the psychiatrist-in-chief, the head of the hospital, and the chief resident. At administrative conference the next morning it was noted that there was some discussion in her presence about a possible probate court commitment for her. The residents reacted rather strongly to this saying that this sort of action by the psychiatrist-in-chief disturbed their patients. It is worth noting that Mrs. Lasker did not mention this sort of occurrence to the other patients, but rather made a joke out of the visit, and the use of the patient group as an outlet for anxiety can be seen here.

As part of the withdrawal of the patients, a good many individuals began to intensify their clique activities, and the development of paired relations between men and women increased on the ward. Three such pairs became prominent at this time. One of these pairs consisted of Mr. Osgood and Miss Prescott, both of whom appear in the preceding excerpt. Mr. Osgood was a passive schizophrenic patient whose doctor was attempting to have him reach out for contact. He acted as a balance wheel on the ward through his rather dry humor. Miss Prescott was rather derogatory of the men in the hospital, and had her own boy friend in the outside world. There was pressure on the hospital by Miss Prescott's family not to allow her out of the hospital, as they did not want her to see her boy friend. Miss Prescott's therapist, Dr. Shaw, felt that Miss Prescott could be allowed privileges outside the hospital, but the senior staff felt their hands were tied because of the family pressure, which was backed by the opinion of the referring physician. Dr. Shaw did not feel he could work satisfactorily with his patient under these conditions, and Miss Prescott was full of resentment. This resentment led her to respond to Mr. Osgood's attentions, and these two people consoled each other during a flirtation which began at this time. This flirtation, as did others to be mentioned shortly, caused some apprehension on the part of the nursing staff, who responded with increased vigilance tinged with disapproval. This further decreased the communication between nurses and patients and left the patients in a situation of trying to manage their own complicated relations alone.

The second heterosexual pair which developed at this time was Mr. Erskine and Miss Peters. Mr. Erskine was an immature, dependent person who liked to structure situations so that he was in a secure position. He did this by trying to be the leader in many situations. He turned for support to Miss Peters who, although she tended to depreciate Mr. Erskine, found in him a male who did not threaten her. A third relation that began at this time was between Mr. Isherwood and Miss Farrell. Mr. Isherwood was a talented and intelligent young man with severe periods of depression and feelings of inadequacy. His interests, intellectual and artistic, coincided to a considerable extent with those of Miss Farrell, who was about to be discharged from the hospital. Miss Farrell had come, in her stay of almost two years, to be quite dependent upon the relations she formed in the hospital, which were some of the most meaningful ones to date in her life. As she was fearful of discharge, she welcomed the relation with Mr. Isherwood because it reinforced her ties with the ward.

Some of these aspects of the increasing development of paired relations between men and women on the ward are indicated in the following observations:

(Evening on the open ward) Miss Prescott was very blue and sat with her head sunk in dejection while the Beethoven Sixth was being played on the phonograph. Both Mr. Erskine and Mr. Osgood came in and attempted to cheer her up. Mr. Osgood succeeded in getting her to go over into the other living room. Miss Prescott was not allowed to go out with her boy friend and was feeling double-crossed.

The movie began shortly and Mr. Erskine was holding hands on the couch with Miss Peters. Miss Prescott and Mr. Osgood also held hands throughout the movie. Mrs. Lasker and Mr. Ashton continued their attempt to play-act a rather Noel Cowardish husband-wife relationship—throwing their arms around each other and generally emoting. Miss Farrell went out for the evening with Mr. Isherwood, as neither of them wished to remain on the ward to see the movie.

(The next evening) This evening the patients organized the party on the ward which is described later. At this party the relations which had begun continued to develop. Mr. Osgood and Miss Prescott were very close, as were Mr. Erskine and Miss Peters. These two couples danced for over an hour in the hall where they had more privacy than in the living room. Miss Field changed records on the phonograph for them so that there was a continuous flow of music during this time.

(The next evening) A canasta game began without the usual cutting for partners; just the assumption that Mr. Osgood and Miss Prescott, and Mr. Erskine and Miss Peters, would be partners. During the canasta game Miss Prescott received a phone call from her family and when she returned she said: "Dr. Shaw says that he can't act without my family's permission, and my father says that he can't come up except on Sundays when Dr. Shaw isn't here, and my mother won't come without my father to talk to Dr. Shaw. I'm in the middle, and of course you're not supposed to get neurotic when things are like that." Mr. Erskine and Miss Peters sympathized with Miss Prescott.

In addition to the paired relations, it is interesting that the patients on the open ward sorted themselves into two distinct groups at this time.[3] On the one hand, there was the group, at the core of which were the three heterosexual pairs that have been mentioned, which engaged in card playing, parties, and general conversation as ways of adaptation and defense. On the other hand, there was a somewhat looser group of women patients, five of whom in particular joined together to watch television. The few patients who were not in either of these groups withdrew to their rooms. Also at this time there was a "natural" division of the space on the ward—the card-playing group tended to take over the women's living room and to stay there throughout the evening, whereas the women's group tended to utilize the men's living room where the television set was located.

It may seem as if the division into two groups that occurred at this time was a rather normal sort of thing that might be expected to occur in any case. However, prior to the period of mutual withdrawal, the patients on the open ward acted together much more as a single general group, the sharp division between living rooms was not maintained throughout

[3] This was a duplication of a finding with a previous patient population in the same hospital (see Caudill, *et al.*, 1952).

the evenings, and the more solitary patients withdrew into their rooms less often and more because they wished privacy than because they were anxious and frightened.

As mentioned earlier, another aspect of the patients' behavior during the period of mutual withdrawal was that they began to assume greater control over their activities. In this, they made use of Miss Wright, who was the group activities worker. Miss Wright, however, since her program and job were new, had not developed adequate communication techniques with the rest of the staff, and the details of her actual work remained largely unknown to other staff role groups.

In part as a reaction to the already described feelings of boredom and tension at this time, a number of the patients on the open ward wanted to have a party and approached Miss Wright, who agreed to the plan. The party was largely organized by Mr. Erskine and Mrs. Lasker, as can be seen in the following excerpt from the observations:

> Miss Wright and Mr. Erskine went out during the afternoon to purchase refreshments for the party that evening. Later, Miss Wright, after having discussed it with the open ward patients, invited the locked ward patients down to the party that evening. Miss Farrell and Mrs. Lasker took over the making of the refreshments in the kitchen. Miss Wright started the party off by playing guessing games in which one person went out of the room, the group thought of a situation, and then the person came back and by asking questions attempted to find out what the situation was. There was a tendency for the open ward patients to give the easy questions in this game to the locked ward patients. After the game, there were dancing and refreshments. During the dancing both Mr. Osgood and Mr. Erskine made a conscious attempt to dance at least once with all the women. Similarly, Mrs. Lasker was active as a hostess in being sure that everyone was included in the activities. After the locked ward patients returned to their own ward, many of the open ward patients continued dancing, pairing off into the couples that have been mentioned earlier. At the close of the evening there was a general discussion with Miss Wright about the party, during which Miss Farrell remarked that she wished they could plan this sort of thing more often because it was fun. Mrs. Lasker, Miss Prescott, Miss Lindsey, and Miss Farrell agreed that the men should be complimented on their participation in dancing with all the female patients present.
>
> Earlier in the evening, Dr. Reynolds, who was on duty, walked through the ward but did not stop at the party. Miss Lindsey ran after her, on a bet from Mrs. Lasker, and asked Dr. Reynolds whether she could buy a split-pint of champagne for Mrs. Lasker. Dr. Reynolds said no, as reported by Miss Lindsey when she returned.

At the administrative conference the next morning, Miss Wright, the group activities worker, was not present, and there was no mention of the party in Dr. Reynolds' report of the preceding evening's activity. Dr. Reynolds said:

> It was relatively quiet yesterday. Miss Prescott, Mrs. Lasker, and Miss Lindsey were bitching around in the morning. A number of people were upset at lunch. . . . Mr. Osgood was trying to be helpful but wasn't very effective, and that is about all. Although, in the late evening Mrs. Lange asked if she could bring in champagne for Mrs. Lasker. (This was a mistaken identification on Dr. Reynolds' part, as the patient who actually asked her this question was Miss Lindsey. This would seem to be part of the phenomenon of withdrawal on the part of the resident staff, as a number of such mistakes in reporting occurred at this time.) . . . Everything else was quiet.

Following Dr. Reynolds' report at the conference, other matters were brought up, and there was no discussion of the party in this or later administrative conferences. Miss Wright was not present at the administrative conferences until three days later, at which time she did not give a résumé of the party, but confined her remarks to comments on specific patients that the doctors were discussing in reference to their therapeutic progress.

As indicated in the foregoing material, there was a break in the communication system between the patients and the staff, and the patients increasingly relied on themselves in the planning and carrying out of their recreation. In this process they made use of Miss Wright, since she was the most available staff person on the ward. Miss Wright, however, had not yet established adequate communication with the rest of the staff. Without Miss Wright's being aware of it, she was seen as "doing things with the patients but not telling us what is going on." As will be seen, this led to difficulty in terms of the tension and withdrawal among the nurses and other personnel.

Withdrawal of the Senior Staff

The general situation surrounding the withdrawal of the senior staff is well summarized in an interview with the chief resident, Dr. Shaw, at this time:

> Dr. Shaw said that he had been out of touch with the hospital for the last few weeks. During the same time, Dr. Scott—the head of the hospital—had been away, attending several meetings. Also, the families of several patients had been very much on the neck of Dr. Scott, and indirectly on his, Dr. Shaw's, neck. Dr. Shaw said he felt that he was getting information about the hospital from very second- or third-hand sources. Instead of getting information from being on the ward, or from the residents, he was getting it at the administrative conference and elsewhere, and that much of this information was after the fact.

Dr. Shaw said that he had been surprised during the year that he had not had very much direct contact with the patients, that he had had to force contact. Also during this time he said that he himself had been carrying three patients and had a great increase in charting to do. . . .

Dr. Shaw also said that he thought another problem arose at the point when the procedure at the daily administrative conference was changed some weeks ago: instead of having the resident doctors bring up every small request, they were told that they only needed to bring up things that they felt required a decision. Dr. Shaw said that now if somebody was worried about something, he just didn't bring it up at all.

Dr. Shaw said another difficulty was that the nurses did not speak up in the daily conference. He felt the nurses saw the patients differently and got different information on them. However, when the nurses spoke up, the doctor felt he had to explain away the difference by telling the nurse: "I just can't understand how you can see this in my patient. . . ." Dr. Shaw went on to say that the nurses didn't feel that they had the status to stand up to the doctor, and that the doctors and nurses both got very uncomfortable, so nobody said anything in the administrative conference. Dr. Shaw said he should have brought this up and made an issue of it, but that he felt uncomfortable, and hence hadn't done it. . . .

As indicated in the interview with Dr. Shaw, a good many difficulties in communication were developing at this time. One of these, stemming partly from the residents' interpretation of the change in procedure at the daily administrative conference, was that the residents began to make decisions on their cases without communicating these to the senior staff, and the chief resident was unsure of what course to follow when this happened. This resulted in such lapses in communication as the senior staff's not knowing that patients had been moved from one ward to another until some days later. Equally, the various senior staff members were not in communication with each other about such matters as the impending discharge from the hospital of certain patients. For example:

(At an administrative conference on Saturday)

Dr. Ryan: As Miss Peters is on the open ward, that leaves some room free on the women's locked ward.

Dr. Shaw: Miss Peters has been on the open ward since Monday? Really?

Dr. Ryan: Have you been down on the open ward since Monday? (i.e., during the past five days).

Dr. Shaw: I was just curious. I wondered if that was she I had to bounce out of Mr. Erskine's room the other day.

Dr. Ryan: Probably. . . .

(In a conversation in the hall immediately after the administrative conference)

Dr. Simmons: I think we'll transfer Mr. Innes on Monday.

Dr. Shaw: What?

Dr. Simmons: Didn't Dr. Scott tell you we were going to move Innes?

Dr. Shaw: No, but that's all right. Where is he going?

Dr. Simmons: To another hospital. . . . (Dr. Simmons went on to describe the details of the transfer. He then turned to Dr. Reynolds, who had acted as administrative psychiatrist for Mr. Innes.) Will you dictate up the first two weeks on him?

Dr. Reynolds: Who, Mr. Owens?

Dr. Simmons: No, Mr. Innes.

Some weeks earlier, the policy to be followed in allowing patients privileges to go into town had been a subject for considerable discussion in the administrative conferences. The residents had wanted to individualize the policy, and the senior staff had wanted to routinize it. Out of the discussion, the senior staff finally conceded so many points in its suggested program that very little change in policy resulted. It was at this time that the senior staff also decided to permit the residents to take greater responsibility for decisions concerning their patients rather than bringing small problems to administrative conference each morning. As Dr. Shaw said, this often resulted in the residents' not bringing up even important problems, and, after this policy had been in effect for some four or five weeks, it was during the ten-day period on which observations are being reported here that the senior staff became overtly concerned over the difficulty in communication, but did not take any action beyond bringing the matter to the attention of the residents. For example:

(At administrative conference)

Dr. Scott: I want to emphasize the lack of communication here. We are not using this session correctly, such as for telling about the movement of patients from one floor to another. We have to pay more attention here to this as a communications group, and we also need to get to know all of the patients, and take time to talk to them. There is some feeling, I sense, that patients don't relate to any doctor but their own. . . .

Under the policy of allowing the residents to take greater responsibility, much happened in the hospital of which the senior staff were unaware. Yet, in the nature of the case, the senior staff had to retain ultimate authority in their hands, and the data indicate that the residents sensed they were being given authority which was more apparent than real.

Withdrawal of the Residents

Finding themselves in the above situation, the residents began to concentrate their attention solely on their own patients and to withdraw their interest from the patients of other physicians. This developed into a general lack of interest and a desire to do one's work with as little conflict as possible. At this point the residents often expressed the belief among themselves that the patient load was too heavy and began to mistake the identity of patients on the wards—as in the previously cited instance when Dr. Reynolds mistook Miss Lindsey for Mrs. Lange. The general problems attendant upon such a withdrawal among the residents can be seen in the following excerpts from discussions between the residents while the writer was having supper with them during this ten-day period:

(Supper with the residents) Dr. Ramsay said that he had cleaned out all the patients he was really emotionally involved with, and now he just didn't care. Dr. Rolfe mentioned that many of the patients were showing considerable concern over people's leaving "uncured." He said that they had mentioned to him that Mr. Eliot had left, still with the problem of drinking, and Miss Lyons had been sent to a state hospital. . . .

(At supper with the residents a few days later) Dr. Reynolds and Dr. Rivers were talking about their withdrawal and relating it to their own personal problems. Dr. Rivers said that she felt her withdrawal was caused by the fact that she was never on call, as her program of work was such that this part of her residency was not required of her. . . . However, she said, maybe it was more general, because Dr. Ramsay had said that he was trying to get free of any sort of real involvement in work with his patients, and that Dr. Rolfe had told her that he had never worked in a place with such tension. Dr. Reynolds said that her only interest was in her own patients and that she had taken this position because she felt that the fight was too much in the hospital, and had withdrawn from it. . . . She said that she tended to avoid the women's locked ward because she felt the women patients there liked to have a woman to talk to, and that she did not want to get involved with the other doctors' patients; so, she would sneak on the ward and duck into Miss Packard's room (her own patient) and then try to sneak out without seeing anyone. She said she also avoided the women on the open wards because she felt these women were very hostile to her.

Both Dr. Reynolds and Dr. Rivers felt that Dr. Scott had lost some of his interest and was rather depressed over the whole problem, as he felt very much under pressure from such other senior doctors as Dr. Sutton and Dr. Saunders, since he had to take orders from them. Particularly they sensed that Dr. Scott felt the pressure of disagreement between himself and Dr. Saunders, as for example when Dr. Ryan presented the case of Miss Forrest, and there was considerable disagreement between the two senior men.

Dr. Reynolds and Dr. Rivers went on to say that they felt Dr. Scott had given up when he had, in effect, told the residents that they could do what they wanted about the routine of privileges in the hospital. They felt that the residents were not really as much in conflict with him as he had thought. This, however, left Dr. Shaw without knowing what authority he really had as chief resident.

Dr. Rivers went on to say she felt that back of all this was the unclearness of the hospital about whether it was a private or a teaching institution. She said that the residents were told that it was a teaching institution, which would mean relatively few and highly selected cases for study; but on the other hand, they were also told very strongly by Dr. Scott, who was under pressure from Dr. Sutton, that they must take every patient they could possibly admit and somehow get through the day with their case load. . . .

The withdrawal of the residents seems quite clear from these observations, and it is interesting that the concern with the hierarchy of the hospital among the residents at this time was paralleled by a similar interest on the part of the patients, as previously mentioned.

Withdrawal of the Nurses

During the same ten-day period the observations indicate that the nurses attempted to formalize their routine and showed a good deal of general discontent with the way things were going in the hospital. For example, the following exchange between the residents and the nurses took place at the administrative conference:

Miss Noyes: Can we move Miss Field to the locked ward?

Dr. Rolfe: Yes.

Mrs. Netter: We can use Miss Field's room on the open ward if she is to be moved to the locked ward.

Dr. Scott: You mean, move Ann Forrest to the open ward?

Dr. Shaw: Or Mrs. Matthews. How is she?

Dr. Ryan: She needs a lot of medication. How do the nurses feel about moving her to the open ward?

Miss Nugent: We are very suspicious.

Miss Noyes: We feel when she leaves the hospital she gets some sort of narcotic outside.

Dr. Ryan: I hope that her improvement does have something to do with her going out, but not to get bromides. I have a feeling that she does not get bromides when she is out, and you have the feeling that she does. . . .

(Next day at administrative conference)

Miss Noyes: There is a problem of Mrs. Matthews and the doctor's order which has been written for her to go out unaccompanied from the locked ward. I don't understand this.

Dr. Ryan: Mrs. Matthews really is a patient who should be on the open ward. The only reason she is on the locked ward is because of the nighttime medication for her headaches. . . . She has agreed to stay here and is accepting psychotherapy. I feel that our relation is such that it is good to let her have contact and go out unaccompanied. This was my own idea. Actually, she wants to go out with someone else. However, I did not want to tie up personnel. . . .

Miss Nugent: The real problem on the locked ward is that if the patient goes out unaccompanied, the patient can bring back things which may be bad for the other patients. We had a terrible time with this with other patients. Mrs. Faxon used to go downtown and she'd bring back a compact and toilet water, and such glass being around provides an additional risk. This is a policy matter. Can Mrs. Matthews cooperate, or will she struggle to sneak something in?

Dr. Shaw: We can't settle this here.

Miss Winston (the occupational therapist): I don't think any of the locked ward patients should go out unaccompanied, and there are difficulties even when they are accompanied. Yesterday Mrs. Boswell got hold of some matches and was kidding around saying she would have fun hiding these from the nurse. . . .

After a few such disagreements as the one above, the nurses fell silent at the administrative conferences. For example, on the day after the exchange just cited took place, the atmosphere at the conference was as follows:

Dr. Reynolds: . . . Mr. Osgood has been having a series of ten-minute interviews. He verbalizes his discouragement. At other times he won't talk at all, but on the ward he is much more outgoing. There is a split here in the environment between what's going on in therapy and what's going on on the ward. I am planning to let this take its own course. . . .

Dr. Shaw: Do the nurses have anything to say on these patients?

(There is silence, and nothing is said.)

Dr. Shaw (continuing): Well, Miss Wright, do you have anything to say on the patients? . . .

An example of the withdrawal of the nurses and their greater concern over the formalization of routine can be seen in a failure in communication between the nurses and the head of the hospital, which led to moving the entire men's locked ward—since there were only three patients on it at the time—to the open ward. This had the effect of turning the open ward into a locked ward owing to the increased security precautions that were necessary, and served the implicit function of bringing the activities of the open ward patients more under the direct control of the nurses. This move came about because of a misunderstanding between Miss Nugent, the director of nurses, and Dr. Scott, the head of the hospital. Dr. Scott, in giving permission, believed that the more disturbed male patients would be moved to the open ward only during the afternoon while the locked ward was being cleaned and painted, and that these patients would return to the locked ward each night. What happened was that these more disturbed male patients lived on the open ward for a week. Without prior notification, the situation simply broke upon the open ward patients and the nurse on duty late one afternoon:

(On the open ward) Unlike the usual procedure, an attendant, rather than a nurse, brought the supper trays to the living room. Mr. Anderson and Mr. Eggan had been moved to the open ward from the locked ward. The regular open ward patients were Mr. Ashton, Mr. Erskine, Mr. Isherwood, Mr. Osgood, and Mr. Edwards. There was silence at meal time for ten minutes, and then:

Mr. Erskine: Look, guys, a joy-boy! (This was Mr. Erskine's term for an attendant.)

Mr. Ashton: It looks like he's going to ham up the act.

At this point, Mr. Eggan walked into the room, hallucinating. There was a dead silence among the patients, and then Mr. Ashton discovered that he had taken Mr. Eggan's tray off the supper cart. (The trays had individual name cards on them.)

Mr. Ashton: Gee it's swell that Ted (Mr. Eggan) is here. I didn't know he was here, but I had his tray. (At this point he offered the tray to Mr. Eggan.) I haven't touched it yet, you take it. I'll go get another one.

Mr. Eggan somewhat somnambulistically took the tray and sat down across from Mr. Erskine and stared at him. There was silence. After a while Mr. Erskine spoke.

Mr. Erskine: And that nice Mr. Innes is still upstairs (i.e., on the locked ward).

Mr. Anderson: No, he left today.

Mr. Erskine: Does that mean that the joy-boys will be down here all the time?

Mr. Ashton: Oh, they'll be up and down.

Mr. Edwards: There's nobody up there now?

Mr. Erskine: No, but it does make it nice to have the joy-boys staring at us.

Mr. Ashton: How well I remember the old days, how we used to outwit Killer Netter with cigarettes. . . .

Mr. Erskine and Mr. Ashton, who had been patients at the same time on the locked ward some months ago, continued conversation about the old days in the hospital. Equally, they reverted to their old pattern of behavior on the locked ward, of riding the "joy-boys." Mr. Ashton continued to offer Mr. Eggan food: for example, he offered him a sandwich, which Mr. Eggan took and ate the center out of, after which he crossed his arms and sat and stared at Mr. Ashton. . . .

Miss Norris, the nurse on duty this evening, said she didn't know what was happening. She had no information about the fact that the locked ward seemed to have been moved to the open ward, and she was quite upset.

One of the interesting things that accompanied the movement of the locked ward patients was the "mass regression" of the open ward patients. All the patients on the open ward had previously come to breakfast shaven and dressed, but, in the days that followed, they came out unshaven and in their pajamas. The level of conversation became more primitive and indicative of anxiety on the part of all the patients; the ward became more littered with cigarette butts on the floor; and there were more demands made of the ward personnel for service.

Despite the obviousness of this move, it was not mentioned in administrative conference until the second day after it had occurred:

Dr. Shaw: It was an interesting problem in communication the other day, this move of the locked ward patients to the open ward was quite dramatic, but it wasn't brought up here.

Dr. Rolfe (a bit defensively): Everybody knew about it.

Dr. Reynolds: We all knew about it within an hour.

Dr. Shaw: Well, I must have gotten my wires crossed. . . .

Dr. Scott: . . . About the ward move, my idea was that the patients should join the open ward group in the day, and go back to the locked ward at night, not being really transferred at all. Somehow, however, it didn't work that way, and the patients got transferred. Now we see that if Mr. Eggan has to be transferred back, we should not think of this as a regression in his behavior, since he in fact hasn't really been moved in the first place.

Withdrawal of the Other Personnel

As already indicated, the new group activities worker, Miss Wright, tended to be isolated from the other staff role groups because she had not yet established techniques for communicating about her work. The occupational therapist, Miss Winston, felt at this time that the activities program was interfering with her routine, and she was supported in this by the director of nurses. For example, the following criticism of Miss Wright and her work took place at the administrative conference:

Miss Winston (the occupational therapist): I don't think these activities groups are working out too well. I didn't want to bring it up because Miss Wright is not here this morning. However, with the lower census I could do a lot more with patients if we weren't so rigid about these groups. Also with the doctors' appointments, some people don't get down at all.

Dr. Shaw: We want to discuss these groups. Group Two is supposed to be the high activity group, and it really turns out to be the low activity group. I'll have to talk about this to Miss Wright.

Dr. Scott: I think I will try to get a meeting together of the nurses, Dr. Sears, Dr. Shaw, Miss Wright, and myself. This program should be flexible, and it doesn't seem that it is.

Miss Winston: I wanted to invite the entire patient group down to the occupational therapy shop this morning without having to think in these group terms. I wanted to say we are just going to work on pottery this morning. However, I wanted to bring this up with Miss Wright, but she just isn't here this morning.

Dr. Scott: The function of activities is to keep people doing things.

Miss Nugent: One wouldn't run into trouble by not conforming to these groups on the mornings that Miss Wright isn't here; also, she is not going to be here tomorrow morning either.

Dr. Shaw: On Friday Miss Wright will have a chance to present some of the activities situations.

Miss Nugent: No, she doesn't come in tomorrow either. . . .

A few days later, a meeting between Miss Winston, Miss Wright, and Dr. Sears—who was the senior staff member directly responsible for the activities program—took place in Dr. Sears' office. This was a stormy session in which Dr. Sears said he had heard that the sicker patients were not being reached by the ancillary therapeutic programs. Miss Winston and Miss Wright reacted by saying that they felt such patients were being reached and that the senior staff did not come on the wards enough to know the situation. There was some discussion of the funds available for the occupational therapy and activities programs, and at the end of the session Miss Winston and Miss Wright did not feel that very much had been clarified.

In summary of the situation which confronted the five role groups during the ten-day period under discussion, it seemed that each of the role groups had reacted to the stress of the unsettled state of the hospital in a similar manner by restricting its participation and erecting sharper boundaries between itself and the other groups: (1) the senior staff had given up its insistence on certain administrative matters and had withdrawn from the daily routine of decision making; (2) the residents had restricted their focus to their own patients and reduced their interest in the general work of the hospital; (3) the nurses had decreased their communication at the administrative conferences and had increased the formalization of their routines; (4) the group activities worker had remained isolated from the other staff role groups; and (5) the patients had increased their intra-group relations and assumed a greater degree of independence in the planning of their daily activities. While each group seemed to be conscious of what it was doing, and there was discussion about it between group members, there seemed to be a lack of awareness (or reluctance to communicate) on the part of any one group that much the same thing was occurring in all the groups throughout the hospital system. What appeared to have happened was that an adjustive process of defense against the stresses of change and reorganization in the hospital policy was taking place *within* each group, and looked at from the point of view of each separate group, stress was *reduced* by the defenses used; but, looked at from the point of view of the hospital system as a whole, stress was *increased,* because all groups were still part of the hospital.

Such a state of mutual withdrawal might be roughly diagrammed as in Figure 5–1, where the solid line indicates that cognitive communication had been disrupted, while the dotted line indicates that affective communication was still going on, although the members of various groups were not aware of precisely why they seemed to be sharing certain feelings. Since such a diagram is crude at best, the role category of other personnel has been disregarded because it formed more a residual than a unified group.

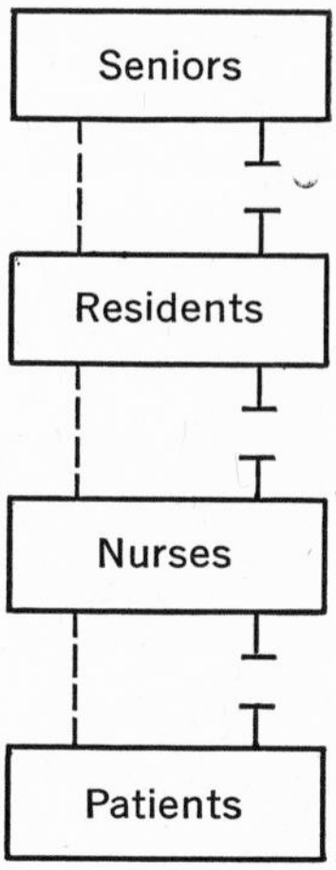

FIGURE 5–1

OPEN COLLECTIVE DISTURBANCE

It was during the period of mutual withdrawal just sketched that the open collective disturbance occurred. In the analysis being made here, it is felt that the state of mutual withdrawal contributed to the development of the open collective disturbance because of the disruption in communication between the various role groups in the hospital. Certain events on the ward grossly upset the equilibrium among the patients, and they were unable to communicate adequately their anxiety about these events to the staff. The main upsetting events seemed to be the following. (1) Two new patients were admitted to the open ward—Mr. Ulrich and Miss Miller, whose behavior was very disruptive for the other patients. (2) Two old patients were discharged from the open ward—Mr. Onofrio and Miss Lindsey, who were key persons in the structure of the ward. (3) The discharge of these two key patients greatly lessened the ability of the remaining patients to plan their activities, and they immediately—the day following the discharge—requested first Miss Wright, the group activities worker, and secondly the anthropologist, who was on the ward at the time, to organize an activity for them. Miss Wright refused to do so on the grounds that she would first have to obtain approval at the administrative conference, and the anthropologist refused because he felt it was outside his research role. Various patients then attempted to contact their individual therapists, and those patients who did receive individual approval then left the hospital for the evening. (4) As indicated earlier, the patients, who had previously gone out in groups of four or five, left the hospital on this particular evening in pairs or as isolated individuals, and all returned in an upset state which, in succeeding days, spread throughout the ward. At this point the staff discussed the ward situation in a conference which stressed the disturbing qualities of three patients as individuals. During this difficult week, and the next, the patients continued their attempts to communicate with the staff and were partially able to do so in the second week through an unplanned group discussion with Dr. Ryan on the ward. This latter event, however, more properly belongs in the period of paired role group response which followed the open collective disturbance.

It is useful to give some of the details from the observations concerning these upsetting events, starting with the admission to the open ward of the two new patients. Mr. Ulrich, an impulsive adolescent man who strongly denied the fact of his hospitalization, and Miss Miller, a sexually provocative young woman, were both admitted a few days prior to the beginning of the open collective disturbance. Mr. Ulrich immediately began to challenge Mr. Erskine's "organizing" role among the patients. Mr. Erskine turned for support to Mr. Edwards, a rather isolated schizophrenic young man who heretofore had not participated in groups on the ward. This is too complicated a sub-aspect of the situation to be gone into here, and the following excerpt is merely to indicate Mr. Ulrich's disturbing qualities, which were manifested from the moment of his arrival on the ward. Upon admission Mr. Ulrich spent a good part of the morning bragging about his athletic prowess to the patients in the living room and asking what there was to do around the hospital. At lunch, Mr. Erskine brought up his favorite topic of seeing fights on television, and Mr. Ulrich attempted to move in on this ground of Mr. Erskine's. The conversation went as follows:

Mr. Erskine: Well, Harold (Mr. Edwards), have you thought it over yet?

Mr. Edwards: Do you want to see the Matthews fight?

Mr. Erskine: It's up to you, my boy.

Mr. Edwards: I'd rather see the Matthews fight.

Mr. Erskine: Well, we'll have to ask the others in the group. . . .

Mr. Ulrich: We ought to take up a fight pool on the ward.

Mr. Erskine: Which fight do you want to see?

Mr. Ulrich: The Marco and Sadler fight is best.

Mr. Erskine (disappointedly): Do you think so? Let's see what Bill (Mr. Osgood) thinks.

Mr. Osgood: I'll go along with the crowd.

Mr. Ulrich: Sadler is an awful peppy fighter.

Mr. Erskine: He is fighting over his weight. I'd put my vote on the Matthews fight.

Mr. Ulrich: How are we going to get tickets for this thing?

Mr. Erskine: We see it here on television. . . . Let me explain the situation. We can see either one fight on Wednesday or Friday nights. . . .

Mr. Ulrich: Hell, we could see the damn things every night. Why don't we just take the set and put it in one of the bedrooms?

Mr. Erskine: That's not quite the problem.

Mr. Ulrich: Well, at Southdown Hospital (another hospital to which Mr. Ulrich had been) the patients pay a dollar a day and they can see television right in their own room. I think we ought to have that sort of thing around here. . . .

Miss Miller was also a disturbing influence, as is indicated in the following excerpt from the observations made during her second day on the ward:

Mr. Ulrich and Miss Prescott were playing as partners against Mr. Erskine and Miss Miller in canasta. Miss Prescott and Mrs. Lasker were riding Mr. Erskine very hard about the rules of canasta, and Miss Miller was yelling, "shit, shit, shit," and saying that she hoped that Dr. Ramsay would hear her. Miss Miller then asked a question of Miss Prescott:

Miss Miller: Does your doctor ask you about your sex life?

Miss Prescott: Yes.

Miss Miller (turning to Mr. Ulrich): He'll ask if you sleep with your girl.

Miss Prescott (to Mr. Ulrich): There's a guy who is new here. He is still alive and not just existing.

The canasta game continued through the afternoon, and periodically Miss Miller would yell, "shit, shit, shit," for about five minutes, and finally Miss Prescott said: "Oh, for Christ's sake, stop the act." And Miss Miller did so.

(Later at supper in the men's living room) Miss Miller came over and threw her arms around Mr. Erskine. He heard her coming, and was about to try to go to his room. She said: "Joe, dear, did you get me a Hershey bar?" There was general laughter among the men, and Mr. Erskine tried to ignore Miss Miller and get to his room. Miss Miller said to Mr. Anderson: "Let's play cards." Mr. Anderson said: "Not right now," and Miss Miller went away down the hall.

As indicated earlier, it was also just at this time that two key patients, Mr. Onofrio and Miss Lindsey, were about to be discharged. The evening before their discharge, the other patients on the open ward decided to give them a going-away party. Both Mr. Onofrio and Miss Lindsey had been working at part-time jobs outside the hospital for the preceding few weeks and returning to the ward after work. The party came about in the following manner:

(On the ward) . . . About 3 p.m. Mr. Onofrio came into the living room and told the patients he had found a room in town. The patients congratulated him on his being able to leave. Mr. Onofrio then left the ward to do an errand in town.

Mrs. Lasker said she thought they ought to have a going-away party for Miss Lindsey and Mr. Onofrio. This was seconded by Mr. Erskine, Mr. Osgood, and Miss Prescott. Mr. Osgood went to ask Mrs. Nagle, the nurse, if the patients could go out and get refreshments for a party. Mrs. Nagle said that they could go out if they could get someone official to go with them. Mr. Erskine then went to see if he could find Miss Wright in her office on the ward, and, finding her, said: "Sweetie, you know that Miss Lindsey and Mr. Onofrio are leaving, and we would like to give a party for them, if you could go out with us to get the goodies." Miss Wright said that she would be glad to go out with them. The patients in the living room decided to make a collection from the other patients, asking everyone on the ward, so that no one would feel left out. Mrs. Lasker then went to collect donations from the women patients, while Mr. Erskine collected from the men.

The party, held that evening, was a most successful one, but can only be summarized in the briefest terms here. Of the total twenty-seven patients in the hospital at the time, twenty-three participated in the party. The attendants, who came down with the patients from the locked wards, entered into the spirit of the party and enjoyed it while also being generally helpful. The same was true for the nurse on the open ward, Mrs. Nagle, who later said she thought it was the best party the patients had ever held. Miss Wright, the group activities worker, was not present as this was not one of her nights to work in the hospital, although she had carried the load of helping to organize the party during the afternoon. Dr. Ramsay, who was on call that night, walked briefly through the ward at 10:00 p.m. as the party ended, but did not otherwise come on the ward. Dr. Scott came on the ward to draw Miss Lindsey aside for a few minutes' talk, but left immediately thereafter. Thus, the burden of communicating something of this very complex event fell on the nursing staff. However, Mrs. Nagle, despite her enthusiasm, did not transmit the details of the party, so that almost nothing of its effect reached the staff level. The evening ended with Mr. Onofrio and Miss Lindsey, both of whom were visibly affected by the situation, singing "thank you" to the group. Various of the patients then individually said their good-byes to Mr. Onofrio and Miss Lindsey. After this Mrs. Nagle brought the party to a close, saying she didn't want to, but bedtime had arrived. The patients quietly went to their rooms.

The next morning at administrative conference there was a minimum of communication about the party, and only the following was reported:

Dr. Ramsay (who had been on duty the preceding evening): The only possible untoward event last night was that Mrs. Lasswell was irate. Otherwise there was a large and extremely good party on the open ward.

Dr. Reynolds: What sort of party?

Dr. Ramsay: Well, they danced and had cheese and salami.
Mrs. Nolan: This was a farewell party for Mr. Onofrio and Miss Lindsey.
Dr. Shaw: Well, okay, that's all for today.

On the morning following the party, Mr. Onofrio and Miss Lindsey were discharged and left the hospital. The atmosphere on the ward that day was one of gloom, coupled with tension and a shortness of tempers. For example, during the male patients' mealtimes:

(At breakfast, Thursday morning, the day after the going-away party)
Mr. Erskine (to the group): The Yankees are not going to broadcast or put their games on television next year.
Mr. Ashton (very angrily and very loudly): That's a lot of crap!
Mr. Erskine (somewhat taken aback): Okay, okay, have it your way, but it's in the headlines here.
Mr. Osgood (in a somewhat mediating fashion): The headlines on baseball are the last things you want to take seriously. . . .

(At supper that evening) The patients were eating in silence. Mr. Erskine was not eating because he had a dinner date. The attendant went over to Mr. Erskine's room and knocked on the door saying: "Supper is ready."
Mr. Erskine (very angrily): That's the second time you've called. For Christ's sake, leave me alone. In about two minutes I'm going to sic Walt Ashton on you if you aren't good.
Mr. Ulrich (yelling out to the group): Joe must have a date because he's shaving.
There was no response to this, and Mr. Ulrich muttered to himself and went back to eating in silence. . . .

A group outing in town, composed of those patients having regular going-out privileges, had been planned by the patients for this evening, but the discharge of Mr. Onofrio and Miss Lindsey had broken up these plans. The remaining patients who wanted to go out together decided, therefore, to ask Miss Wright if she would arrange an activity for them that evening. She said that she could not, as it would first have to go through the administrative conference. The patients then asked the anthropologist if he would organize an activity, and he said that he could not do so. This left the patients who wanted to go out together at loose ends, as they could not arrive at any focus for their plans as a group.

At this point, various patients tried to make separate plans for the evening. Mrs. Lasker decided to go out to dinner with Miss Peters because, as Mrs. Lasker expressed it: "I don't think I would get in as much trouble if I felt I were responsible for someone." Miss Peters called her therapist, Dr. Ryan, for permission to go out, but he did not want her to leave the hospital. Miss Peters then retired to her room in a huff and remained there all evening. The result was that Mrs. Lasker went out by herself, ended up at a bar, and came back drunk. Miss Prescott had initially intended to go out with Mrs. Lasker, but not being sure that she wanted to go along with Miss Peters, she decided to go to the movies with Mr. Osgood—an engagement she later said she would have preferred not to make. As it was, Miss Prescott and Mr. Osgood had a disagreement in town and came back separately to the hospital. Mr. Erskine asked Miss Farrell to go to dinner with him, where they were to be joined later by Mr. Ashton, and the three of them were to go to the home of a previous patient for a visit. This did not work out, as Mr. Ashton did not arrive for the dinner date, and the visit to the previous patient did not turn out well. Mr. Erskine returned to the hospital in an acute anxiety state, and Miss Farrell came back a little later in a mildly depressed condition.

Additional examples, beyond those given above, might be cited, but the point is that all the patients who went out on this particular evening came back having had an unpleasant time, and their upset states spread to the other patients on the ward, most of whom were already jittery. This was reported at the administrative conference the next morning as follows:

Dr. Ramsay: Last night Miss Peters was very upset about the projected going out. Mrs. Lasker was upset, but went out. Mr. Ulrich went out and drank, and came back about 10:00 p.m., and was very ill and vomited several times. . . . The whole open ward crew seemed to be extremely upset last night.

Miss Nicholas: All the patients seemed to be lost on the open ward. I met Miss Murdock downtown, and she certainly seemed that way. . . .

Interviews on the ward with the patients during the week of the open collective disturbance indicated that they were upset by the discharge of Mr. Onofrio and Miss Lindsey, and particularly had missed the stabilizing influence of the plans they had made with these patients. This, coupled with the upsetting effect of the presence of Mr. Ulrich and Miss Miller, seemed sufficient to keep the ward in a tense state for some days.

In regard to the discharge of the two key patients, Mrs. Lasker, for example, said: "I felt bad that Helen (Miss Lindsey) was leaving . . . and I think most of us dread going out alone. . . . When Helen left I felt a real sense of loss. This was a real friendship I had built up with her. . . ." Equally, Mr. Isherwood said: "Nick's (Mr. Onofrio) leaving sort of left me hanging around on the ward alone, and that upset me a good deal. I was very close to him. . . ." Also, Miss Prescott said: ". . . I didn't want to go out alone with him (Mr. Osgood), as I knew what would happen. I tried to get a group going, but no group formed, and Bill (Mr.

Osgood) was also getting into his newly found aggression at the time. He said: 'Dammit, you said you would go out with me, and now you'll go where I want you to.' . . ."

In the following days, Mr. Ulrich increased his attempts at ascendancy over Mr. Erskine, Mr. Ashton was frequently sick at his stomach and vomiting, and so on with the other patients, but one example of the state of the open ward at this time will have to suffice:

(On the open ward after supper a canasta game was in progress) Miss Prescott and Mr. Osgood were playing partners in canasta against Mr. Erskine and Miss Miller. Mr. Ulrich had the phonograph on very loud, and was dancing as if he had a partner, and clowning around. The four canasta players were not paying any attention to him.

Mr. Ulrich (to the anthropologist): How about taking a group out dancing on Friday night?

Miss Prescott: You'll have to learn that this is not a night club, but an institution.

Mr. Ulrich: Well, we're not all looney. I'm only 75 per cent looney, anyway.

Miss Miller: Shit and bullshit, and Dr. Ramsay says bullshit to me.

Mr. Osgood (raising his eyebrows): Just a nice quiet evening at home.

Miss Miller: With Joe (Mr. Erskine) and his big fat face.

Mr. Osgood got up and went out of the living room.

Miss Miller threw down the remaining cards she had in her hand.

Mr. Erskine got apoplectic with rage, his face got very red, and he began to stutter, "Why, why, why, you, you, you," and beat with his hand on the table.

Miss Miller (shouting at him): Oh, shit on you, fuck you, piss on you, shit, shit, shit.

Mr. Erskine was sweating now, and the perspiration was standing out on his face. Miss Prescott took a candy box lid off of the table and fanned him with it.

Miss Miller got up and went over to Mr. Ulrich and said: "Let's dance," and Mr. Ulrich and Miss Miller danced for the next fifteen minutes.

Mr. Erskine went to find the nurse and asked if he might have some hot milk. . . .

The upset state of the open ward seemed also to have spread to the women's locked ward, as was indicated in the administrative conference the next morning:

Dr. Reynolds (who was on call the preceding evening): Well, last night the women's locked ward was unrelieved gloom. Nothing specific, but Mrs. Lange was upset. Mrs. Foster wanted to sign out, and Mrs. Litchfield was bad. Everyone at one time or another, nothing very specific. I had the feeling that there was sort of a group panic on the ward.

Dr. Shaw: How was Mrs. Monroe?

Dr. Reynolds: She is a little better.

Miss Newcomb: Last night she was the only bright spot on the locked ward.

Dr. Scott: And also the only bright spot on the open ward. Mrs. Monroe and Mrs. Foster said that the open ward was too noisy when they were down there.

Dr. Reynolds: Also too competitive.

Dr. Shaw: I think we might explore this, and there is going to be a meeting this afternoon, and we might discuss the situation on the open ward as an interacting group.

Dr. Ryan: I wanted to talk about Mrs. Matthews.

Dr. Scott: Couldn't we talk about both problems?

Dr. Shaw: I think it would be more profitable to discuss the open ward.

At the meeting to discuss the collective disturbance, as has been indicated earlier, attention was focused on Mr. Erskine, Miss Prescott, and Mrs. Lasker as possible sources of the disturbance. Only a little was said about Mr. Ulrich and Miss Miller, and even less about the wider context of events that has been sketched in the foregoing pages. There was a good deal of bewilderment about what was happening and about what remedial action to take.

In summary, the situation at the close of the open collective disturbance might be indicated by a crude diagram (Figure 5–2) in which the various role groups were still in a state of mutual withdrawal, and there was still a disruption of communication. During the open collective disturbance the patients were unable to maintain a state of relative equilibrium in the face of events on the ward, and the integration of the patient group was shattered.

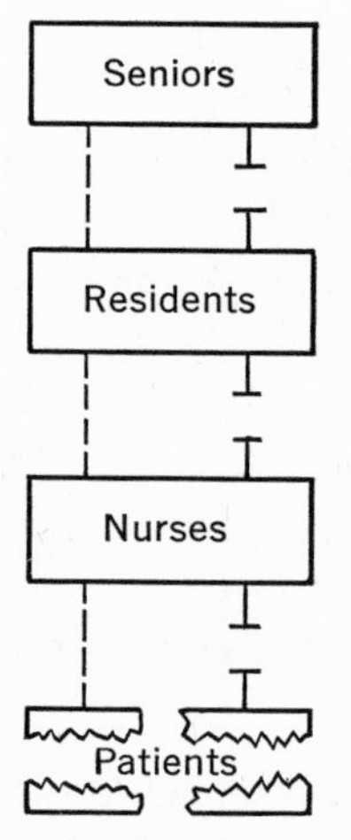

FIGURE 5–2

PAIRED ROLE GROUPS

All the staff role groups wanted to alleviate the situation created by the open collective disturbance. In trying to help, however, the residents followed one course of action while the nurses followed another.

The residents tried to help by granting greater individual freedom to patients and avoiding the mention of this at the administrative conference. This led to an identification with the patients, as a part of which, for example, the residents began jokingly to call their own quarters Ward Five, while referring to Miss Lindsey's apartment—where several parties were held by the patients—as Ward Zero. These terms were an extension of the regular numbers for the wards such as One, Two, and so on.

The nursing staff, on their part, felt that something was going on, but not being in possession of the facts, were somewhat bewildered. After a number of upsetting episodes, they attempted to help by suggesting a greater formalization of routine and appealed to the senior staff to put such a policy into effect.

The patients on the ward alternated between being gloomy and depressed, and being rather frantically gay (at times somewhat hysterically so) in the planning of activities outside the hospital. They continued their attempts to develop communication with the staff, as, for example, in a long discussion on the ward with Dr. Ryan, but when Dr. Ryan reported this discussion in the administrative conference, it was ignored. Many of the patients turned to the use of Miss Lindsey and her apartment in town (which she had rented after her discharge) and carried out a series of parties there. Mr. Ulrich and Miss Miller continued to be a focus of tension for the other patients on the ward until, about a week after the outbreak of the open collective disturbance, Mr. Ulrich was discharged, and Miss Miller was transferred to the women's locked ward.

Altogether, the above state of affairs, which is here called the period of the paired role groups, lasted for two weeks—the residents and patients being paired on the one hand, and the nurses and seniors on the other. During this time, cognitive communication was somewhat better between the role groups which were paired with each other, but the two sets of pairs were not in communication on a cognitive basis—indeed, there was active resistance to this type of communication, as when the residents withheld information from the administrative conferences. Affective communication, however, in the sense of emotional discharge, continued to spread throughout all role groups in the hospital system as it had done during the preceding periods of mutual withdrawal and open collective disturbance. Nevertheless, to the extent that cognitive communication was to some degree re-established, no matter in how strained a fashion,[4] between the particular role groups which were paired, the balance of forces represented in this type of response would seem to be a stage in the movement toward a restitution of an effective integration between cognitive and affective communication.

[4] The phrase, "no matter in how regressed a fashion," comes to mind as perhaps more accurately conveying the nature of such a communication network except, as mentioned at the beginning of this chapter, for its unfortunate anthropomorphic connotations.

The kinds of processes that occurred during the period of the paired role groups have been sketched above, and may be seen in operation in the observations that were made at the time. On the open ward, the beginning of the first of a series of three parties at Miss Lindsey's apartment, and the lack of communication about this party at the administrative conference, can be seen in the following:

(On the ward during the evening of the day of the staff conference on the state of the open ward) This evening there was considerable activity with reference to the planning of Miss Lindsey's party on the part of a number of the patients. Miss Wright had a square-dancing and charade activity on the ward this evening, and after 9 o'clock there was much secrecy and kidding back and forth between Miss Farrell, Mr. Isherwood, and Mrs. Lasker over the party at Miss Lindsey's apartment tomorrow night. Miss Lindsey came in to visit tonight and immediately took Mr. Erskine aside and talked with him.

Other than this, things were very dull and gloomy. At supper almost no conversation took place. Each of the patients found his tray, ate silently, and then went to his room.

(At breakfast with the residents the next morning) This morning at breakfast the residents decided that it was just as well not to mention Miss Lindsey's party at the administrative conference, but Dr. Ryan was not present at breakfast when this decision was made, and he brought the matter up at the conference.

(At the staff conference)

Dr. Ryan: . . . A second thing, Miss Peters wants to go to a group activity which is being held at Miss Lindsey's apartment, and Mr. Erskine, Mr. Isherwood, Mrs. Lasker, and Mr. Osgood are going. These seem to be people who get together on the ward.

Miss Nugent: I don't know about that.

Dr. Ryan: It is a problem for her to go. She fits into the group on the ward, but if there is to be drinking. . . .

Mrs. Nolan: Miss Lindsey came in to visit last night, and there were many secrets flying around.

Dr. Shaw: All we can do is handle this when it comes up in therapy. As far as Miss Peters goes, no, I don't think she should go, as it is not healthy for patients to find their social life with former patients in any case.

Dr. Reynolds: But that's life, I guess, in an unknown town. . . .

(Later the same day, at lunch with the residents) The other residents told Dr. Ryan that he certainly had let the cat out of the bag this morning. Dr. Ryan said somewhat defensively: "Why doesn't somebody tell me these things? We have to have our lines of communication clear." The residents went on to discuss the fact that they thought things would go much better for the patients therapeutically if they simply went ahead and made decisions themselves without bringing them up for general discussion at the administrative conferences.

The patients, on their part, were still attempting to get the lines of communication about their activities clear in their minds, and succeeded the following evening in drawing Dr. Ryan, who was on rounds, into a long discussion about this. However, when Dr. Ryan attempted to bring up the matter of this discussion at the administrative conference the next morning, he was cut off. In the following excerpt, the situation begins with the male patients' talking at supper about activities prior to Dr. Ryan's entrance into the living room:

Mr. Ulrich: From here on in we've got to get group activities really going. Miss Wright is not so enthusiastic, and she said we couldn't go to the hockey game, she said we should go skating on Sunday.

Mr. Erskine: I think you are unreasonable.

Mr. Ulrich: She can't face it.

Mr. Osgood: Let's face it. There's a system of authority here, and we're at the bottom, and Miss Wright is a step above us.

Mr. Ulrich: Who's above her?

Mr. Osgood: About six officers.

Mr. Ashton: She's done a hell of a lot of good around here.

Mr. Ulrich: If you're talking about going to concerts, yes, but skating, no.

Mr. Ashton: That's selling her short. She's done more about getting people out of here than anyone since the cornerstone was laid.

Mr. Erskine: You know darned well, Walt, that she's a failure. She gets done what she wants to get done.

Mr. Ashton: Dammit, I'll talk to one guy at a time, not both of you.

Mr. Osgood (directing his remarks to Mr. Ulrich): They want to have group activities inside and not outside of the hospital.

Mr. Ashton (speaking to Mr. Erskine): If, Joe, later you can explain the day-to-day planning of this skating thing maybe I can understand it, just now it sounds like so much horseshit to me.

Mr. Ulrich: I explained it to her.

Mr. Ashton: By God, let's get her in here. You're trying her out of court. . . .

Mr. Erskine: I am surprised Dr. Shaw doesn't have a meeting and explain the policy. We had one on television, and now we know.

Mr. Osgood: Yes, but just apply what happened at that television meeting to this. They already make the decisions ahead of time, and you're just finding out how often you can go, not doing any deciding about it. . . .

Mr. Ashton (who is very red in the face, begins to shout at this point): It's the doctors! It's the doctors!

(As Mr. Ashton was shouting this, Dr. Ryan came into the living room, and Mr. Erskine addressed him.)

Mr. Erskine: Dr. Ryan, will you spend a few minutes with us? We'd like to talk over why we were turned down on skating. The doctors always say they want us to exercise.

Dr. Ryan: Tell me about the skating rink. Have you ever been there?

Mr. Ulrich: It was too crowded last Sunday when we were there, because they let all the little kids in on Sunday afternoon, but they don't let kids in on Friday night.

Dr. Ryan: I was aware that it was crowded, but you say that it is not crowded on Friday?

Mr. Erskine: It is less so.

Dr. Ryan: This presents several problems, our own unfamiliarity with the situation; and once people get there, they tend to go off in a hundred different directions. But the skating activity was presented in such a way that I felt that nobody really knew what it was about, and it was not investigated thoroughly.

Mr. Ulrich: That's what I mean, it's not presented right.

Mr. Erskine: Can't the patients and the doctors get together so that there isn't so much bickering?

Dr. Ryan: Yes, we realize that and are trying to do something about it. Let me tell you my own reaction. First of all, a doctor has to decide whether his patients can go out and take it, whether it will be disturbing or comfortable to them. Secondly, he has to think whether the thing has been thought out sufficiently ahead of time.

Mr. Ulrich: That's okay, I can understand that.

Dr. Ryan: If we could plan two weeks ahead of time.

Mr. Erskine: Suppose we wanted to go to a basketball game. What should we do?

Dr. Ryan: Pick out a game and approach Miss Wright.

Mr. Ulrich: I'm just a newcomer, but I think someone from this group should go into those meetings. (Mr. Ulrich means a patient should attend the daily staff administrative conference.) If it's Joe (Mr. Erskine), or whoever else might go in.

Mr. Erskine: I don't want to go to the locked ward again, don't send me in to those meetings.

Mr. Ashton: I question that sending a person to those meetings would do any good. What could a person do? I think that what really happened was that nobody on the staff was familiar with the skating arena. . . .

Mr. Erskine: Okay, let's not talk about it any more. Dr. Ryan now knows how we feel. We want to work this out.

Dr. Ryan: We need a routine channel of communication for these things.

Mr. Ashton: You are good to cut it off at this point. We have stated our case to Dr. Ryan, he knows how we feel about it, now let's stop talking about it and see what happens.

(At this point Dr. Ryan left, and the group broke up.)

Later the same evening, after supper and the discussion with Dr. Ryan, the first of the parties at Miss Lindsey's apartment took place. Nine of the patients from the open ward went to the party. At the administrative conference the next morning, the matter of the party was de-emphasized by Dr. Reynolds, who had been on duty. Following this, Dr. Ryan tried to bring his discussion with the patients to the attention of the staff, but he was unsuccessful in this as can be seen in the following excerpt:

Dr. Reynolds: Mr. Eggan was rather disturbed last night. . . . Beyond that, all the open ward people went to the party and had a good time.

Mrs. Nolan: Miss Peters went without permission, and Miss Miller and Miss Forrest didn't get to go.

Dr. Ryan: That's not right. Miss Forrest did go. . . . (After this the matter was dropped, and the group went on to other discussion.). . .

Dr. Ryan (later in the conference): I had a long discussion on the open ward with Mr. Osgood, Mr. Erskine, Mr. Isherwood, Mr. Ulrich, and Mr. Ashton. They were concerned with their ability to participate effectively in the activities program. They spoke very seriously, and I thought it was a good discussion. They wanted a channel of communication to us. They used the iceskating party as an example. . . . The whole group wanted to know how they might set up their requests so that the staff wouldn't refuse them. I told them my ideas about the skating party and the basketball games. They were willing to plan two weeks in advance for two activities. . . .

Dr. Shaw: They already have the Friday meeting with Miss Wright.

Dr. Ryan: But they wondered why it always bogged down, and they wanted a doctor there, either you or another doctor.

Miss Wright: There is an interesting thing here. I told Mr. Ulrich that most of the people on his list could go skating alone on Sunday.

(After this, the matter was dropped and received no further discussion in subsequent conferences.)

During the following week end a rather unfortunate series of incidents occurred. Both Mr. Ulrich and Miss Miller openly refused to abide by Dr. Ramsay's orders, and were placed on the locked ward. Mr. Ulrich smashed his hand into a door and fractured one of the small bones on the way to the locked ward, and Miss Miller insisted she was going to take a walk with Miss Prescott. Mr. Ulrich returned to the open ward the next day and was discharged during the following week, while Miss Miller remained on the locked ward. These events raised the anxieties of the open ward patients, and this situation was handled very well by Mrs. Nash, the nurse on duty, who spent the evening with the patients in the living room—laughing and talking with them. It is important for a theoretical point mentioned at the end of this chapter, that it was Mrs. Nash, whom the patients had always enjoyed, who was on duty on this particular evening, rather than another nurse toward whom the patients had less positive ties.

Such events as those just cited had the effect of bringing home rather sharply to the nursing staff that something should be done, and in the next administrative conference they suggested a tightening of ward routine. This suggestion was, however, resisted by the residents as can be seen below:

Dr. Ryan: Well, all of us had an "opportunity" to work with disturbed patients. . . . (Also) Miss Prescott wanted to go out at 10 o'clock, and of course she is allowed to stay out until 11 on Saturday nights. It seemed logical that if she wanted to take a walk between 10 and 11, she could, but the nurse, of course, has to come and answer the door to let her in after hours.

Mrs. Netter: They are not careful in ringing the bell; they just keep their finger on it.

Miss Nugent: I think we should clarify this matter of rules, both for ourselves and for the patients. In discussing the three-step plan for privileges, there was no limit on the number of times one could go in and out, and at what time. It used to be that they couldn't go out after 9 o'clock. I'm sure I don't know what a person can do between 10 and 10:30, unless they are making some sort of gesture of defiance against the hospital.

Dr. Reynolds: Well, they might want to go out and get a cup of coffee, or just take a little walk in the evening before going to bed.

Miss Nugent: Well, I don't think so.

Mrs. Nolan: It means the doorbell is ringing all the time.

Dr. Shaw: One of the purposes in staying out late is to go to things that last a late time. My own feeling is that no one should go out after 9 o'clock.

Dr. Ryan: Why don't we leave it up to the individual doctor?

Dr. Reynolds: We ought to explain this to the patient group.

Dr. Rolfe: I think so too. This should be handled in a group session, and there is no sense in using therapeutic time for this.

Miss Nugent: I think Dr. Scott will bring up these things; all of these things need to be discussed.

Dr. Reynolds: It depends on whether it's really a problem for the individual. But if you just had an urge to go out for a cup of coffee, I don't see anything wrong in that, and the patients probably don't think of the doorbell's ringing as being a disturbing factor.

Mrs. Nolan: I have talked a great deal to Mr. Earle about this. He rings the bell a great deal. (This is Dr. Reynolds' patient.)

Dr. Shaw: We can miss or take these opportunities when the patients express their defiance and rebellion. And the therapists can take it up or not. . . . Going out at 9 to 9:30 seems to be a reasonable time limit to me.

In general, the alignment of the role groups at this time seems clear from the discussion at the administrative conference. The residents, in stressing the planning for individual patients, were opposed to the nurses and seniors, who emphasized routine. Two other matters of importance can be seen in the material just given: (1) the expression of disagreement indirectly through the medium of an individual patient, as when Mrs. Nolan spoke of Mr. Earle, who was Dr. Reynolds' patient (see also Chapter 1); and (2) the concentration on the "defiance and rebellion" within the patient group, without bringing out the possibility that similar feelings were present among the residents and nurses.

The above situation, with its attendant difficulties, continued to exist for the next ten days. During this time, the structure of the four main role groups in the hospital might be roughly diagrammed (Figure 5–3) by indicating with solid lines the fact that the residents and patients had re-established a degree of cognitive communication, as had the nurses and seniors, but that there was little such communication between the two pairs of role groups. As in previous diagrams, the dotted lines are a crude attempt to represent the free flow of affective communication throughout the system, which went unchecked by any effective cognitive communication concerning the disagreements over policy in the hospital.

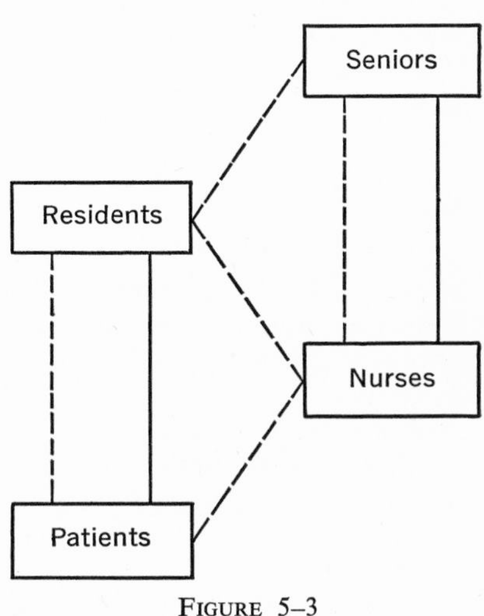

FIGURE 5–3

On the ward, there were two further cycles in which there was first an atmosphere of depression, followed by a period of frantic gaiety during which a party was planned at Miss Lindsey's apartment. These events did not form a topic of discussion at the administrative conferences. On the night of the third party, Dr. Shaw, the chief resident, checked the order book and discovered that a number of patients, who, he felt, should not have left the hospital, had been given permission to go out. He raised this question the following morning, and this led to a restitution of communication among the staff role groups:

(At the administrative conference)

Dr. Shaw: One thing came up last night that I was rather surprised about, and that we didn't discuss here. This was the matter of the party. . . . I had to make some changes. Miss Field was expecting to go, and as I have said again and again, insulin patients don't go out of the hospital without hospital personnel. Also, Miss Peters was upset, and should not have gone out, and Miss Forrest is depressed.

Mrs. Wells (the social worker): What party?

Dr. Shaw: Miss Lindsey's.

Dr. Rolfe: I am sorry I made a mistake about Miss Field. I was sure myself that Mrs. Lasker would have taken care of the matter adequately, but if it's a legal problem. . . .

Dr. Reynolds: I have administrative charge of Miss Peters while Dr. Ryan is away, but I didn't know about this party. That is, I knew it was arranged. As far as my other patients go, where they are on Thursday is their own problem. I don't probe into what they are going to do. . . .

RESTITUTION

During the next week many of the underlying issues which had been causing difficulty were discussed openly. One of the first of these was the desire expressed by the residents to explore what they felt was a restrictive policy concerning patient privileges, and the positive tenor of the administrative conference in which this was done, along with a shift in the content and manner of discussion, can be seen in the following:

Dr. Shaw: . . . I sense that there is some feeling that we are too restrictive, too conservative, but it doesn't seem to get discussed here. If there is a difference of opinion, it should come out.

Dr. Rolfe: I think that with going out we are really very restrictive. Take the experience of the past week. The trouble is, we make our decision on psychodynamic reasons, but we have nothing more than really just a few ideas about this. You take the case of Miss Fellows. Her psychodynamics are that she hates her father, yet in the last week or so we have let her go home, and she gets along very well. Or you take the case of Mrs. Foster. Her psychosis can be considered as a fight with her husband, yet when she goes home, everything goes fine. This shows that the psychodynamics, perhaps, aren't the best basis on which to plan for patients' going out. . . .

Dr. Reynolds: The important point is to judge on the basis of the individual and the situation. It's good, I feel, for the patients to tolerate a little tension in going out, if they have a constructive activity to engage in. If you wait until you are sure they are not tense, you may wait forever.

Dr. Shaw: It is true that you have to run some anxiety-producing risks in terms of the patient, but the other side is important too—that when you have a patient who is excited and who withdraws, one of the functions of the hospital is to help him avoid these experiences and to help him work toward the handling of such experiences. . . .

Dr. Reynolds: Another way of answering, however, is to show the patient that you are not so frightened about his going out.

Dr. Shaw: It's a mistake to say that you're frightened of the patient's reaction, so you don't let him go out.

Dr. Reynolds: Well, what is your position, then?

Dr. Shaw: You put it on the basis that it's my anxiety. In this way it's the doctor who is analyzing his own anxiety, and that's a thing we have to watch. . . . It is true that it is normal to go out, but it is also true that the patients are here because of their pathology, and we have to assess what it means to them to go out.

Dr. Rolfe: It's very important to know how they act when they go out and what effect the experience has for them when they come back. But more than this, I feel there is a tremendous pressure on the doctor who wants to be liberal. If the hierarchy is against people's going out, the doctor who is liberal is under terrific pressure, and the willingness to risk going out has to go much higher up. I think that you and Dr. Scott are not in favor of such a situation, and I remember Mr. Ashton's wanting to go to a party, and the tremendous pressure which was placed on you by the referring physician and the family not to let him go. If it's true that these outside pressures on you are more frequent than I know of, then I can understand your reluctance to let people go out.

Dr. Shaw: We should discuss this whole problem some more and really know. Also the patients' ability to bring it back. There is a feeling of many people here that in psychotherapy the present is important, and it is almost impossible to leave it out. However, the present is often much more painful than what happened way back in their lives, and it is this which makes the present much more valuable to psychotherapy.

Dr. Reynolds: However, patients will only talk about the present and do this freely if they feel it is not going to be used as a basis of further restriction and punishment, and I think there is a very general feeling among the patients of insecurity. They feel when they talk to their therapists, this really means that they are telling so many people, that perhaps they had better not tell the therapist. They feel: "My therapist will tell another one, and it will get back to the hospital." And also, the patient will feel that he has been a traitor to other patients. This came up in relation to Miss Lindsey's first party. This was talked about in therapy, and the patients I know were very concerned about how the information got out.

Dr. Shaw: It got out through the patients' own communications with the nurses, and with each other. . . .

As can be seen, the issue was joined, and in subsequent conferences a great many further topics were discussed. These included: (1) the difficulties the resident staff had in presenting their cases to the senior staff; (2) the senior staff's supervision of the therapy done by the residents; (3) the whole area of the administrative management of patients and its effect upon therapeutic progress; (4) the financial situation of the patient and the meaning of this both therapeutically and administratively; and (5) the practical and emotional needs of ward personnel and residents which had to be satisfied in order for them to function effectively in the hospital.

During this period of restitution an equilibrium was reached in the balance between cognitive and affective communication among the various role groups, and, in line with preceding diagrams, this might be indicated as in Figure 5–4.

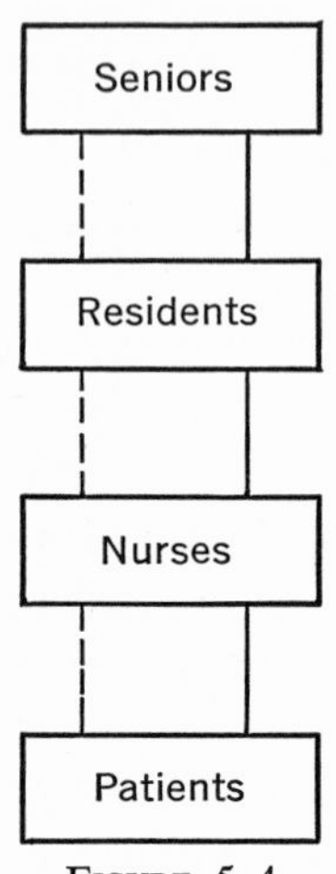

FIGURE 5–4

Although detailed observational data of the kind presented here are lacking, some five months later the hospital was able to avert successfully an acute outbreak of open collective disturbance, caused in part by the presence of a difficult alcoholic patient on the ward, by responding to the patients' pressure for increased organized activity, and with the wider social context of the situation more specifically in mind.

DISCUSSION

The aim of this chapter has been to show that, in the case of one collective disturbance, a fuller understanding could be gained when attention was focused not only on what occurred among the patients on the ward, but also on what occurred at other levels of the hospital. In presenting the data, there have been many points at which it would have been easy, and perhaps profitable, to turn aside for a discussion of practical and theoretical details, but the major emphasis has been placed here on the general point that a hospital really is a social system, and that this has truly meaningful implications in addition to being a topic of serious intellectual interest.

If this is so, it is necessary first to determine the structure and component parts of the overt formal and informal and covert emotional systems in the hospital, and secondly to follow the processes of balance between these parts over time, particularly as this involves shifts in the network of communication. During all four phases of the collective disturbance outlined in this chapter, affective communication between the various role groups was maintained, but the lines of cognitive communication were at first broken, then re-formed rather strangely in the period of the paired role group response, and only finally re-established during the period of restitution. Thus, the covert emotional structure of the hospital was operative throughout the three-months' cycle that included the acute period of the open collective disturbance, but the spread of emotions in the system was not supported by the effective operation of the overt social structure, which was fractured and twisted in many ways before it returned to normalcy.

This chapter has been written largely in terms of five role groups, and thus the emphasis has been on the structure and process of role group relations. For other problems, however, it is more necessary to keep track of specific individuals as personalities occupying positions in the structure over time. For example, it was important to know the nature of the general balance in the hospital at the time of the paired role groups, but in addition (not in lieu of), it was also necessary to know that Mrs. Nash, in whom the patients had confidence, was the nurse on duty during a particularly upsetting evening. Further, it is also probably necessary for some problems to keep track of *combinations* of specific individuals who occupy various positions in the system. Other data than those presented here from the study suggest that agitation on the ward was less severe on those evenings when certain combinations of nurses and physicians were on duty. This point was raised in Chapter 1 in connection with the discussion of the hypothetical example of Miss Jones and the fire engine. As indicated in Chapter 1, the various permutations of such a problem, involving combinations of specific individuals in hierarchical role arrangements, go beyond what is usually meant by the study of interaction, and are better characterized by a term such as transaction. Practically speaking, additional attention might be given to the scheduling of combinations of nurses and doctors on duty with reference to their congeniality and usefulness as a therapeutic team; equally, research might be done about the effects of particular combinations of nurses and doctors on various diagnostic or social groupings of patients.

The state of affairs sketched in this chapter raises the question of what might be done to avert a collective disturbance, and perhaps the answer is that one would not wish to do so. The process referred to here as a collective disturbance is not necessarily bad, and, in fact, much good can come of it. A hospital (or any other organization for work) which did not have some rhythm in its activities would not be a good hospital, it would be a dead one. The opposite is also obviously true—the ups and downs in everyday life can reach too great proportions for adequate functioning. In between a state of extreme oscillation and one of dead calm there is much to be learned from such processes and many ways in which they can be put to use for truly therapeutic ends.

Rapoport (1956) has expressed the same point of view in his discussion of similar processes taking place at Belmont Hospital in England. He indicates that "these tension states need not be seen as antitherapeutic and therefore categorically to be avoided. On the contrary, they may have therapeutic value." He proposes the term "sociotherapy" for the activities associated with the didactic, beneficial resolution of these tension states. Concerning this he says: "The resolution of a hidden staff conflict might alleviate a patient's disturbance and thus be beneficial, but it would only become sociotherapeutic if it were done to the accompaniment of an analysis of the patterned personal significance of the development and alleviation of discordant relationships for those concerned. The criterion of *didactic* accompaniment to tension-reduction is conceived of as important in enhancing the possibility that persisting change in capacity to sustain harmonious relations will occur."

The conclusion would appear to be that rather than attempting to do away with the processes that make up a collective disturbance (at bottom an impossible task because of the nature of both staff and patients as human beings), what is needed is the development of methods for studying the covert emotional structure in its relation to the overt social structure with the goal of first coming to some understanding and then perhaps bringing about changes in both. Such study is needed, as to date there has been too much enthusiasm for, and too little understanding of, what goes into the concept of a therapeutic community.

If the type of material presented in this chapter (and in Chapter 12) has seemed to have a use in the daily work of a psychiatric hospital, certain practical questions arise, such as who should gather these data. The task could properly belong to the nurse, but this would mean that her training and duties on the ward would undergo considerable change. It is also possible that a program of research and actual clinical responsibility in this area could be under the direction of a "clinical anthropologist" or, more broadly, a "clinical social scientist."

A second practical question concerns where and how such material as appears in this chapter should be communicated in order for it to become part of the information on which the daily work of the hospital is based. A possible suggestion, using the routine of the hospital discussed here as a model, would be for the person charged with the responsibility for keeping track of the hospital system as a whole to make his report at the administrative conference once a week, or more often if necessary, in a manner analogous to that of the residents reporting upon the progress of their patients in psychotherapy.

A third question, of both practical and theoretical importance, is whether or not the gathering of material from various levels is an invasion of privacy which is perhaps necessary for the maintenance of the system. This is particularly a question for patients in psychotherapeutic treatment in a hospital where ward life, at best, does not afford much privacy. In this study, however, the patients did not seem to resent the presence of the anthropologist, and it is felt that such material could be gathered, communicated, and acted upon, for therapeutic gain. The questions raised in the above paragraphs are discussed at greater length in Chapter 14.

It is hoped that the preceding chapters have demonstrated with sufficient convincingness that there are important social processes that go on largely out of awareness in the work of a psychiatric hospital. In the next section of the book, attention is shifted from the observational data to interviews which were carried out with staff and patients in order to learn something further concerning their perceptions of the hospital and their attitudes toward life in it.

Section III

PERCEPTIONS OF THE HOSPITAL

Use of the Picture Interview

CHAPTER 6

Development of the Picture Interview

The preceding three chapters on interrelations have attempted to show some of the processes that came into focus when events occurring over time were seen within a wider context than was usually accorded them in the daily work of the hospital. In line with the conceptual position taken in the first chapter, the material has been presented so as to highlight the systematic interplay—or "transactions"—between the internal psychological reactions of individuals, interpersonal events, and shifts in the equilibrium of the over-all social structure of the hospital.

In a more categorical sense, the preceding chapters have discussed processes arising in the various areas of hospital life centered on therapy, administration, and human relations—the latter being how people got along with each other from day to day within and between role groups. Thus, the doctor-patient relationship was the center of attention in Chapter 3 and administrative decisions in Chapter 4, while the analysis of the collective disturbance in Chapter 5 involved all areas of hospital life, including human relations. These three chapters have also been concerned with what might be thought of as a fourth area of life: the interaction of staff and patients with the hospital-in-general, where the hospital has been thought of as an entity—either as a physical or a social structure.

In the present section, the attempt is made to gain additional understanding of the events of hospital life by approaching them somewhat differently than through the sort of contextual analysis utilized so far. Some of the processes that have been described may be further understood by testing the assumption that the hospital meant quite different things to doctors, nurses, and patients as these groups interacted within the four areas of life which have been separated out for discussion: the hospital-in-general, therapy, administration, and human relations. For example, residents, patients, and nurses might hold very different ideas concerning what was involved in psychotherapy, and hence the communication of these groups might be distorted in this area. Similarly, a nurse might define her role differently from the way in which a resident would define a nurse's role, and this could become a source of confusion in daily work. In general, the idea to be explored here is that the perceptions of any individual, or the shared attitudes in a role group, are highly colored by an underlying set of both cognitive and affective assumptions about what is "reality."

In order to gather material on the similarities and differences in attitudes and role perceptions of the various groups, an interviewing program was carried out by means of a series of pictures of hospital life which were drawn specifically for this research. The development of these pictures is described in more detail shortly. At this point it is appropriate to indicate why it was felt important to carry out interviews at all, rather than rely entirely upon observation.

The interviewing program was needed for at least two reasons: (1) to serve as a check on observations; and (2) to gain information on problems which could not be solved from observation alone. In the latter case, for example, the observations indicated that nurses on the open ward spent very little time with patients, whereas nurses on the locked ward spent considerably more time in this manner. While it is possible to make some inferences about why nurses did not spend very much time with patients on the open ward, about all that can be said with complete assurance from the observations is that they did not, indeed, do so. There was a need, therefore, to ask nurses and patients to talk about their relations on the wards. There was a third, and further, reason for the interviewing program: (3) in certain areas of hospital life it was not at all clear what the significant questions to ask were, and a series of unstructured interviews might reveal some of these questions. This third reason leads directly to a discussion of the particular way in which the interviewing was carried out.

Neither a highly formalized schedule nor a set of explicit questions was used, because although the *areas* in which information was desired were clear enough, the *specific questions* to ask in these areas were less clear, and it was necessary to avoid delimiting a person's response by structuring questions too narrowly. On the other hand, the objective was not to obtain completely free interviews, as it was planned to subject the material gathered to a systematic content analysis in order to find what were areas of agreement and disagreement between role groups on specific problems.

For these various reasons, it was decided to use pictures as "visual questions." The belief was that such pictures would structure a situation sufficiently within an area of interest, but would not predetermine the way in which a person responded to as great an extent as would a schedule. This method of interviewing was quite close in overt form to that used in such psychological projective techniques as the Thematic Apperception Test (Murray, 1943). Indeed, this method of interviewing grew out of the writer's fairly extensive use of the TAT in several cultures (Caudill, 1949, 1952). He had found that, just after having taken a Thematic Apperception Test, a person often would spontaneously, and with little apparent anxiety, provide important material that would have taken longer to obtain through ordinary interviewing. Acting on this clue, the series of hospital pictures was used more as a method of gathering general interview material than as a method designed to elicit "psychological test" data. The use of this method resulted in a fairly flexible, but still "focused" (Merton, *et al.,* 1956) interview situation. This is not to say that the same material could not have been obtained by ordinary interviewing; however, the use of the method resulted in material which was more readily comparable from one interview to the next.

If this picture interview method is to be considered by other workers, it is also probably of importance that the writer liked to interview in this way and found it enjoyable. In part, these feelings also grew out of his experience with the TAT, where he noted that the picture often served as a "convenient fiction" in the interpersonal situation between interviewer and interviewee. For example, in the hospital, if the interviewer used a direct question to ask a nurse how she conceived of psychotherapy, or directly asked a resident doctor about the nature of his relation to his senior staff supervisor, such questions might well raise the defensiveness of a nurse or resident who felt personally vulnerable in such an area, and little material would be forthcoming. If, however, the interviewer presented a picture to the nurse or resident, and in talking about the situation in the picture they found themselves getting into emotional material, they would usually feel a need to continue and to explain what they meant. On the other hand, they could always retreat into the rationalization that they were only talking about a picture—it might be of another hospital, not be concerned with real life, and so forth. Such a "convenient fiction" was, therefore, useful in keeping the interview from becoming stalled on one emotionally loaded topic, and in moving the interview along from topic to topic by presenting the interviewee with another picture.

As for the development of the pictures themselves, it was decided to have an artist make simple line drawings of the desired scenes and then have these photostated.[1] As interest was on both intra- and inter-role group relations in the four areas of life in the hospital, the number of possible topics for pictures was very large. Some compromise with this large number of topics had to be made in practical terms. The artist and the writer worked together on the wards, with the artist sketching pictures from a list of topics prepared by the writer. These sketches were then revised and prepared as finished pictures. Altogether, twenty-two pictures were drawn and photostated. Eighteen of these were used in interviews with patients, while fifteen were used in interviewing hospital personnel. Of the fifteen pictures on which all persons were interviewed, the material from twelve pictures was analyzed and forms the basis of the presentation in the following chapters.

The pictures were drawn so that the manifest content of about half of them showed intra-role group activity in the hospital, while the other half showed several role groups in interaction. Among the pictures of intra-role group activity, some dealt with persons who were essentially on a similar status level, as two patients talking together in a private room on the open ward. Other pictures showed intra-group status differences, as a resident doctor talking over his case load with a senior supervising physician. The pictures on interaction between role groups were concerned with such topics as the doctor and patient in psychotherapy, and the nurse-patient relationship in administrative matters.

A second way of categorizing the subject matter of the pictures was by the area of life that would most likely be conveyed by the manifest content of the picture. Thus, such a picture as a patient standing before the door of a locked ward would be likely to provide material on how the various role groups saw the patient in interaction with the physical structure of the hospital. Similarly, a picture of a patient on the steps of the hospital—either entering or leaving—would probably elicit material centering around a general evaluation of the hospital experience of the patient. Stimulus in the area of therapy came from such pictures as a doctor and a patient in an interview situation, or a nurse and a patient talking together in the patient's room. The administrative area was the

[1] The author is indebted to Mr. Paul Lambert, the artist, who came to the hospital for several extended visits in order to make these drawings.

focus of attention in pictures of a patient signing the book which recorded absence from the ward, or a staff administrative conference. The area of human relations included such pictures as a social gathering of patients on the open ward.

A pilot study, to be described later, indicated the need for some revision of the pictures, but, as the research budget did not permit this, a selection from the original pictures was used in the final study. There were several reasons why it would have been useful to revise some of the pictures. (1) Matters of factual inaccuracy had crept in—for example, the picture of the administrative conference contained too many figures which could be interpreted as nurses, and not enough as doctors. In the final study, however, most of the staff and patients identified this as the daily administrative conference; if they did not do so at first, they were later asked to please treat it as such. (2) It was found that pictures which were somewhat pleasanter than a general evaluation of the reality of the hospital warranted often elicited more material than pictures which reflected actual conditions in the hospital. For example, Picture 9, showing a nurse and patient chatting in the patient's room, was very productive at all role levels; the interviewees would usually start by saying, "This is the way it should be," and then go on to move back and forth between actual conditions and those they felt were more desirable. If the present series of pictures were to be redrawn, or another series constructed, it probably would be useful to have a greater number of pictures portraying ideal rather than actual conditions.

The pictures were numbered in a standard sequence in which they were presented during the interview. The rationale for the sequence was: (1) the earliest pictures should be familiar scenes, which would most likely be comprehensible to all role groups; (2) the pictures more likely to arouse anxiety should be presented later; and (3) there seemed to be some sense, in order to elicit fuller material, in having two pictures on the same topic (e.g., nurse-patient relations) follow one another.

The twelve pictures which were finally used in the analysis, classified by the area of life about which it was hoped they would produce material, are indicated in the following list, and can be seen in the accompanying illustrations. The numbers refer to the sequence of presentation in the interview.

HOSPITAL-IN-GENERAL (as a physical or social structure)

1. A patient looking through the doors of the locked ward
4. A patient at the front door of the hospital (either entering or leaving)
5. A patient in seclusion

THERAPY

2. A psychotherapeutic session
9. A nurse talking with a patient
10. A resident psychiatrist in discussion with a senior supervising psychiatrist

ADMINISTRATION

3. Signing the book upon leaving or returning to the hospital
11. The daily morning administrative conference attended by seniors, residents, nurses, and other personnel
17. The night nurse making rounds on the ward

HUMAN RELATIONS

6. The men's locked ward
12. Evening on the open ward
14. Two patients talking together

Initially, a pilot study using twenty of the pictures was carried out with five resident doctors, five student nurses, and five patients. This pilot study was done nine months prior to the beginning of the actual research interviewing program, and none of the subjects used for the pilot study were any longer connected with the hospital. These pilot study subjects were asked not to talk over the type of interview with their colleagues. So far as it was possible to tell, all the regular research subjects later came to the situation without prior knowledge of the method of interviewing.

From the results of the pilot study decisions were made concerning the best way to instruct subjects about the interview, the most productive pictures to use, and the sequence of presentation. In the pilot study the subjects were told a standard title for each picture as it was handed to them. This procedure was later abandoned, and in the actual research the interviewee was simply presented with the picture and asked to begin talking about the area of life that the picture represented to him. If he started by talking within the area of life portrayed in the manifest content of the picture, the interviewer said nothing. If, however, the interviewee interpreted the picture to be in an area other than that in which information was desired, the interviewer let the interviewee continue and recorded the material until there was a pause. During the pause the interviewer indicated that perhaps this was a picture with which the interviewee was not familiar; the interviewer then suggested the area of life within which the picture might fall and asked the interviewee if he would talk in this particular area even though he might not be personally familiar with it. For example, Picture 10, showing a resident doctor and his senior supervising physician, was sometimes interpreted by patients

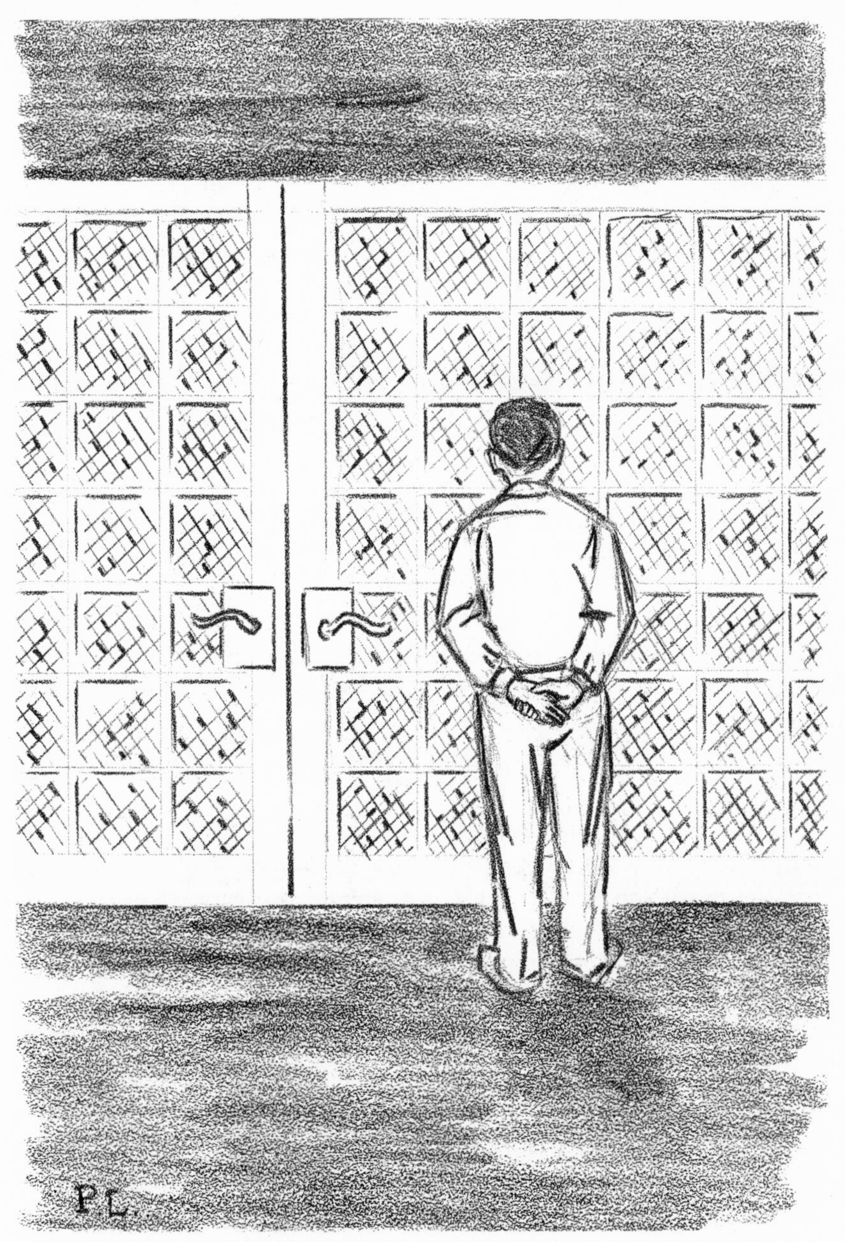

PICTURE 1. A patient looking through the doors of the locked ward

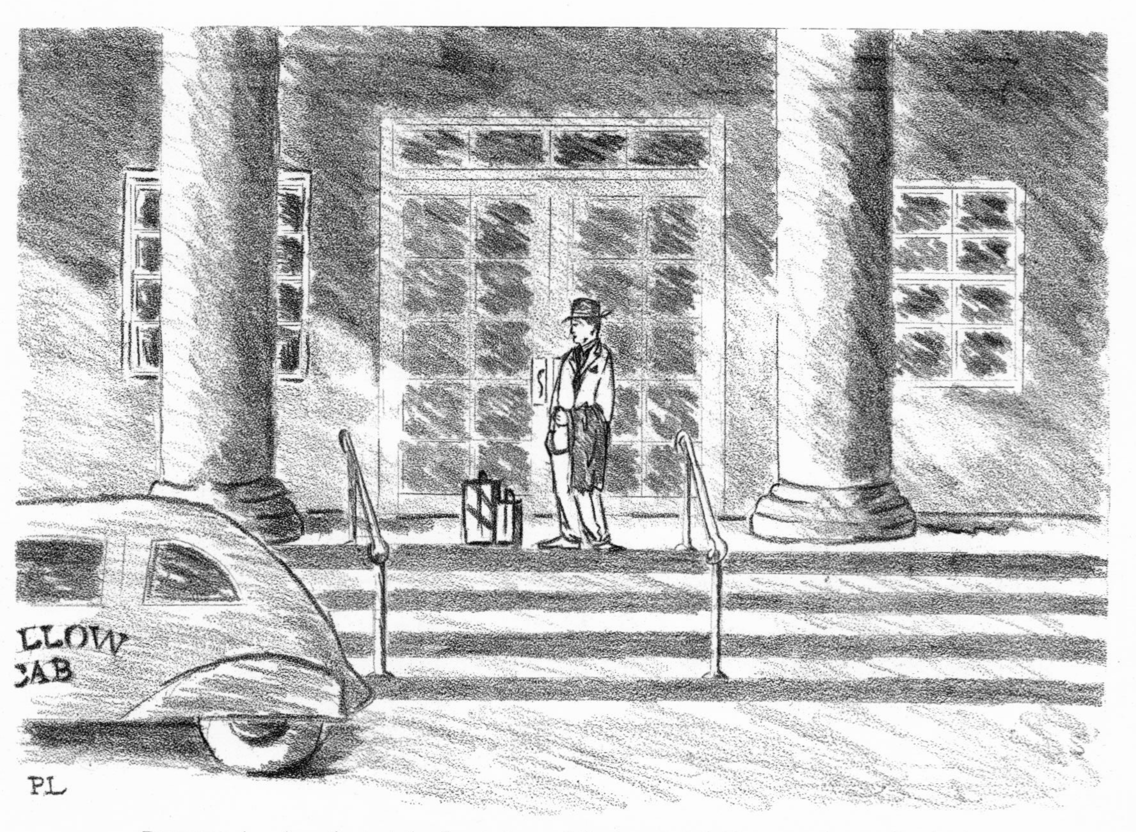

Picture 4. A patient at the front door of the hospital (either entering or leaving)

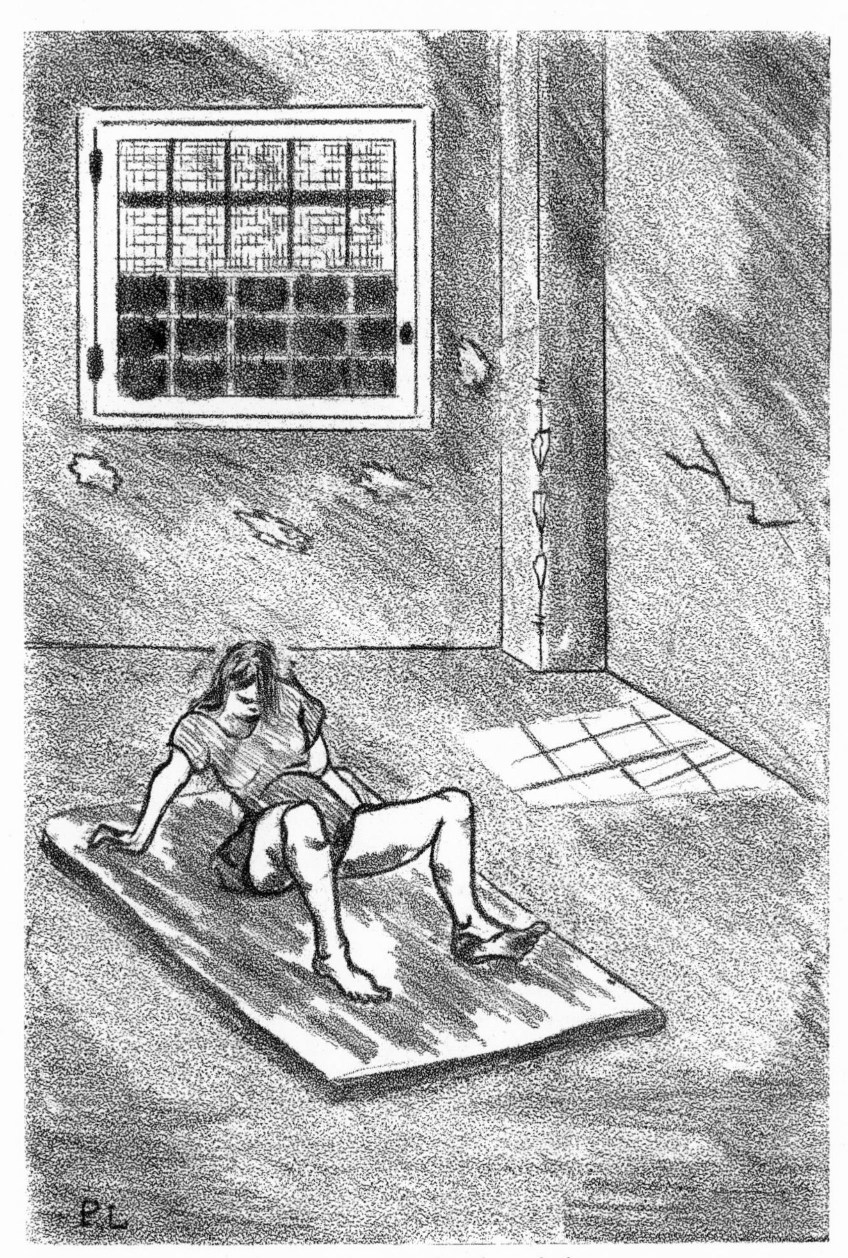

Picture 5. A patient in seclusion

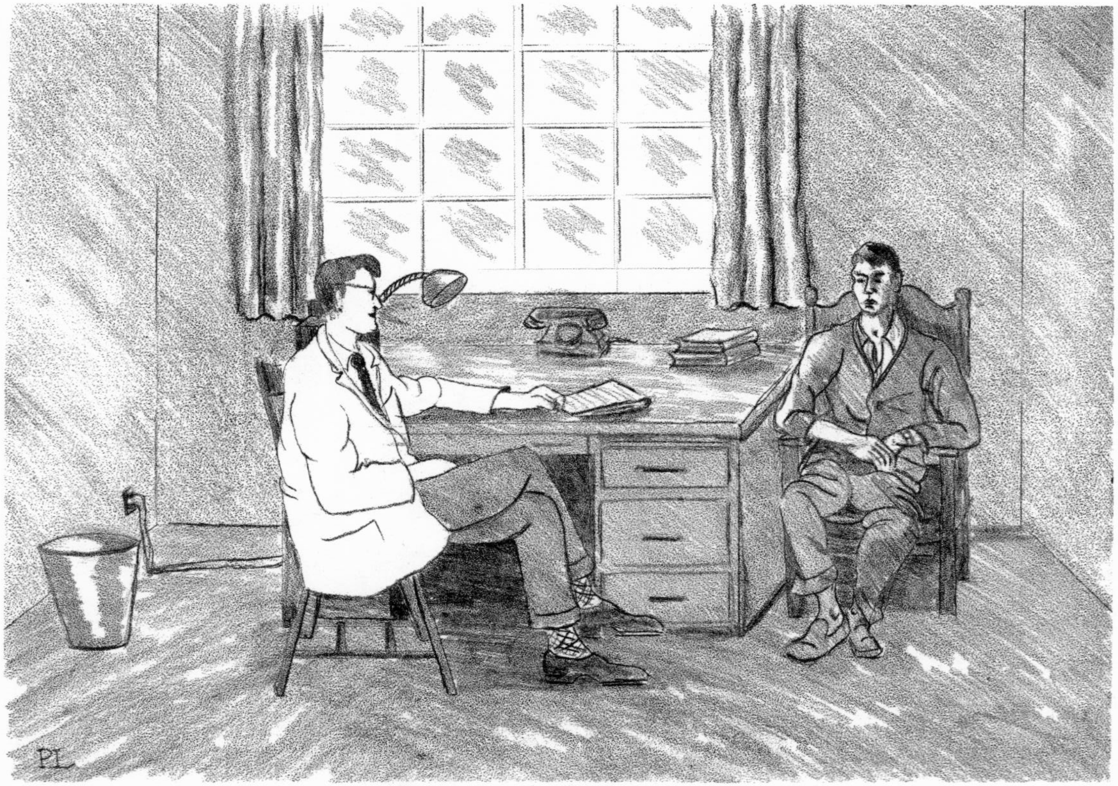

PICTURE 2. A psychotherapeutic session

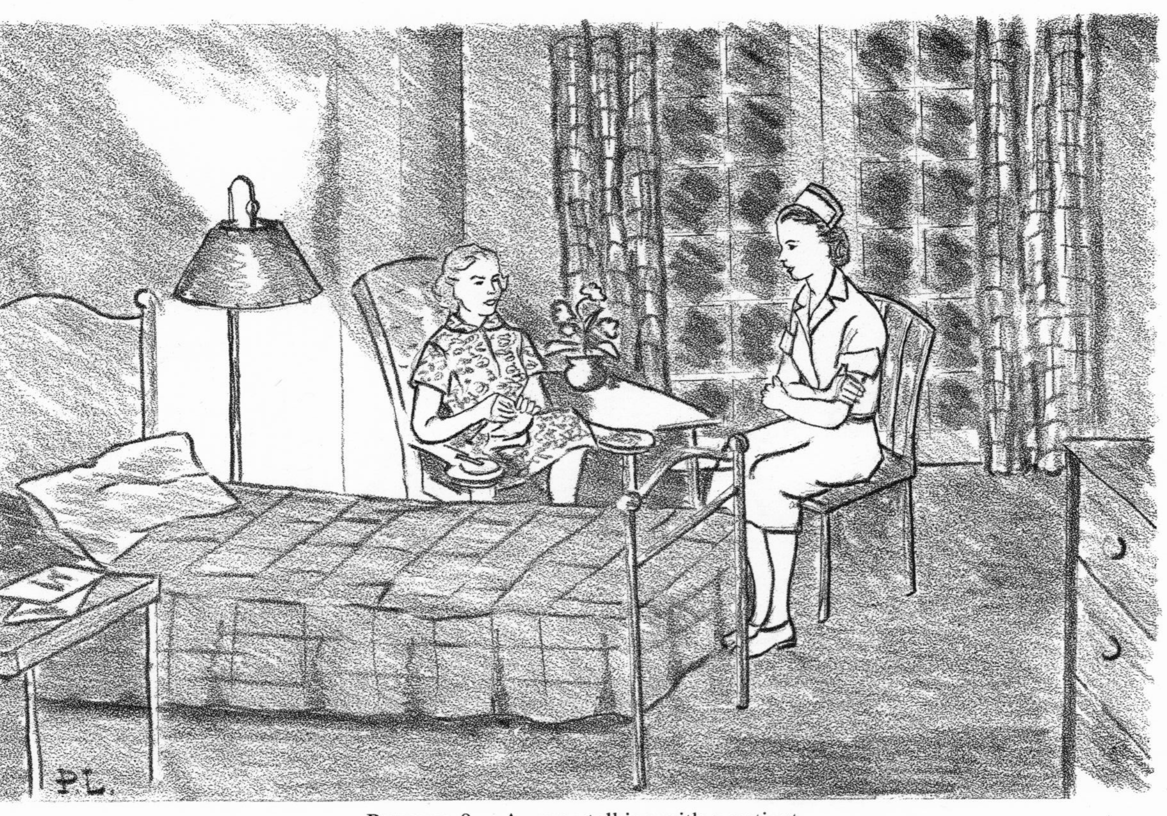

PICTURE 9. A nurse talking with a patient

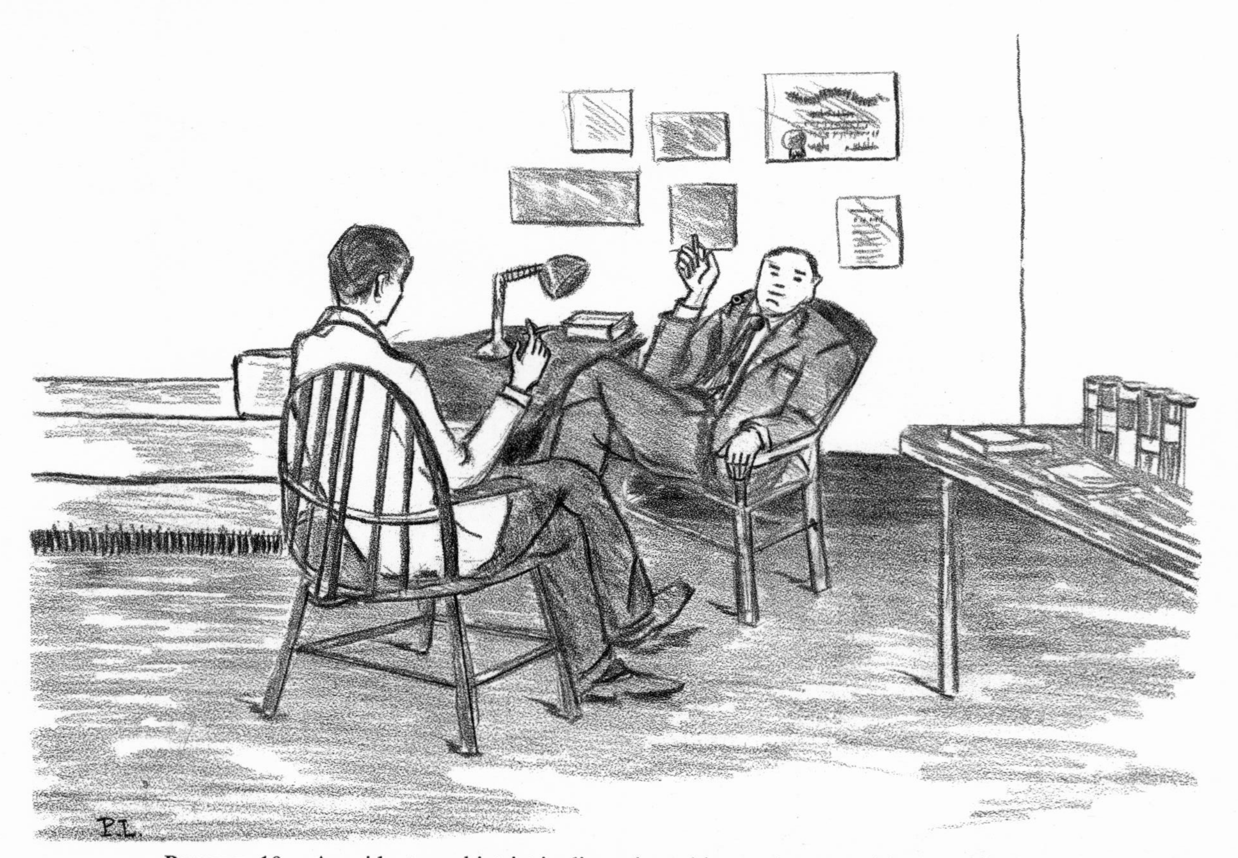

PICTURE 10. A resident psychiatrist in discussion with a senior supervising psychiatrist

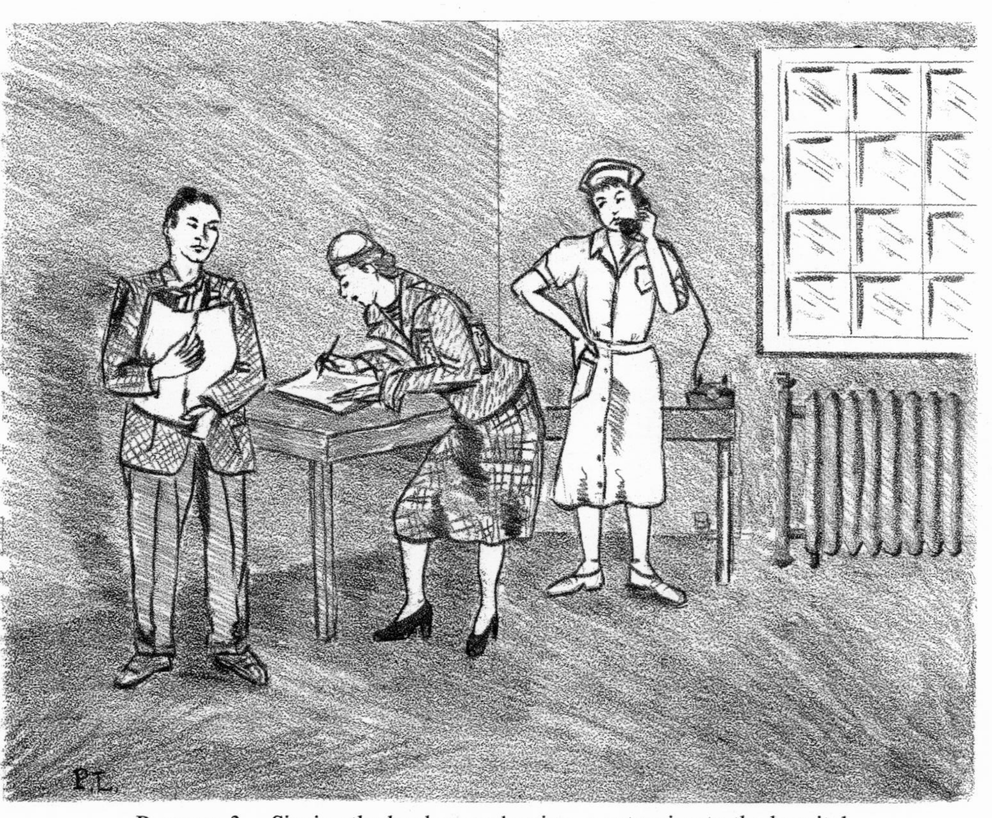

PICTURE 3. Signing the book upon leaving or returning to the hospital

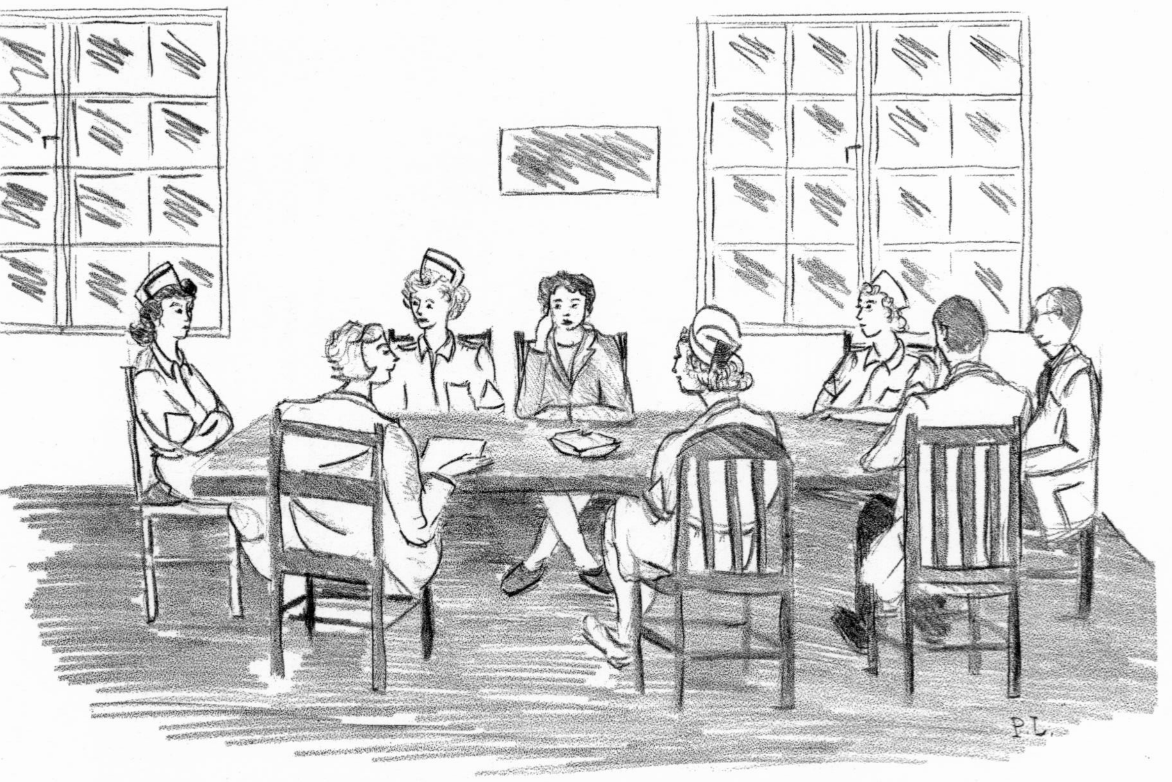

PICTURE 11. The daily morning administrative conference

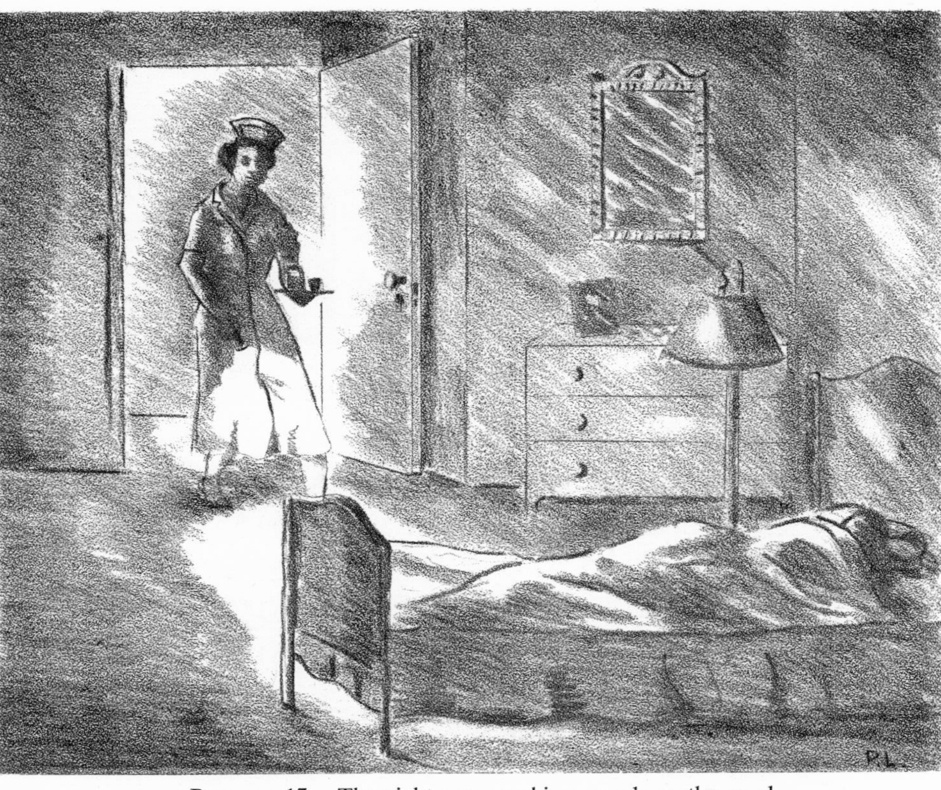

PICTURE 17. The night nurse making rounds on the ward

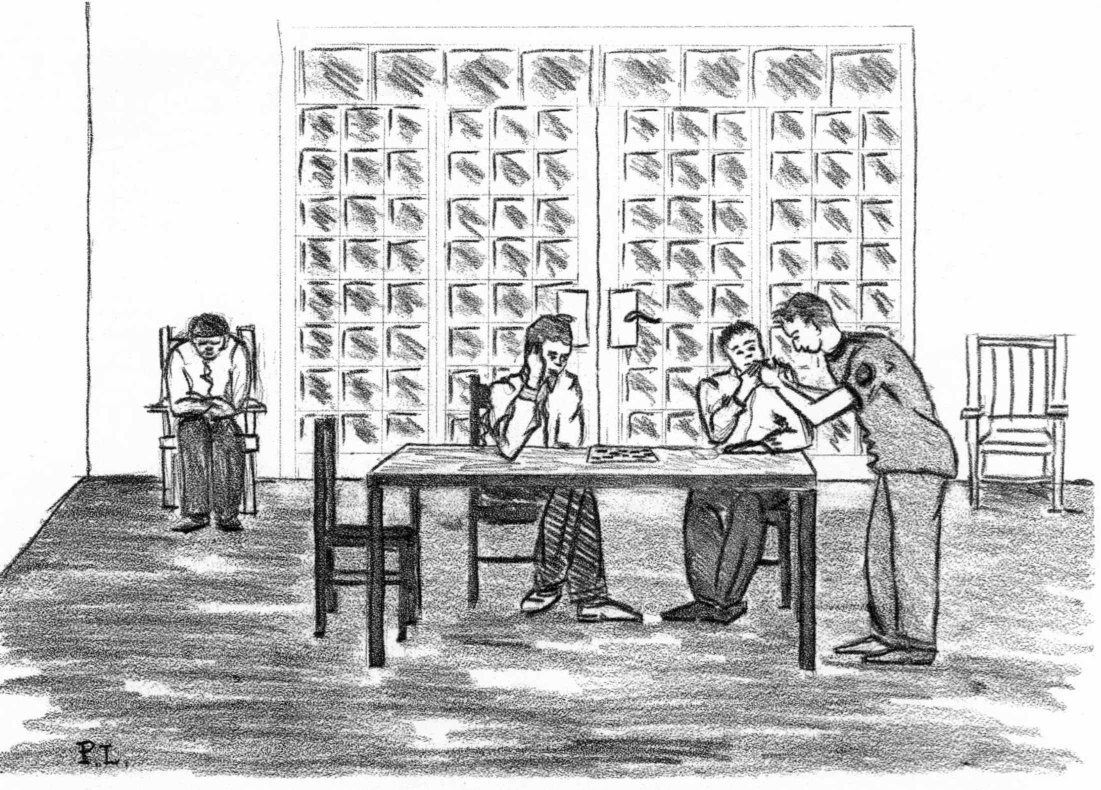

Picture 6. The men's locked ward

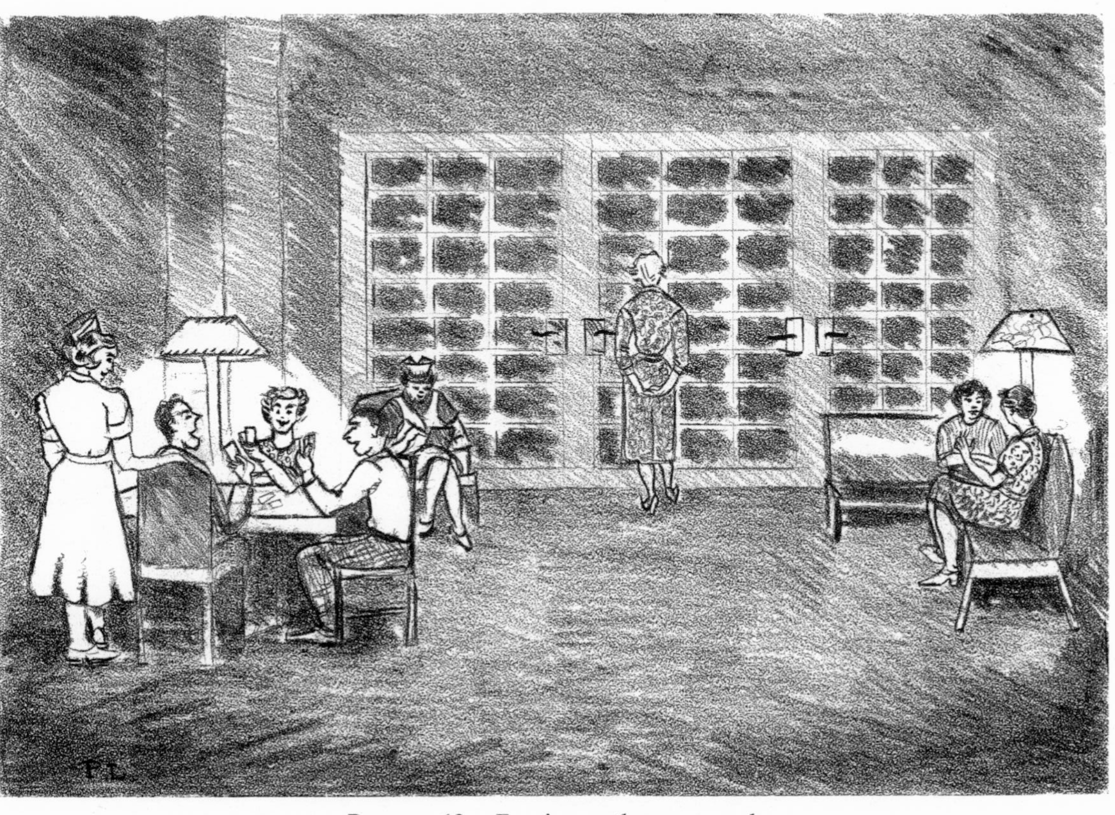

PICTURE 12. Evening on the open ward

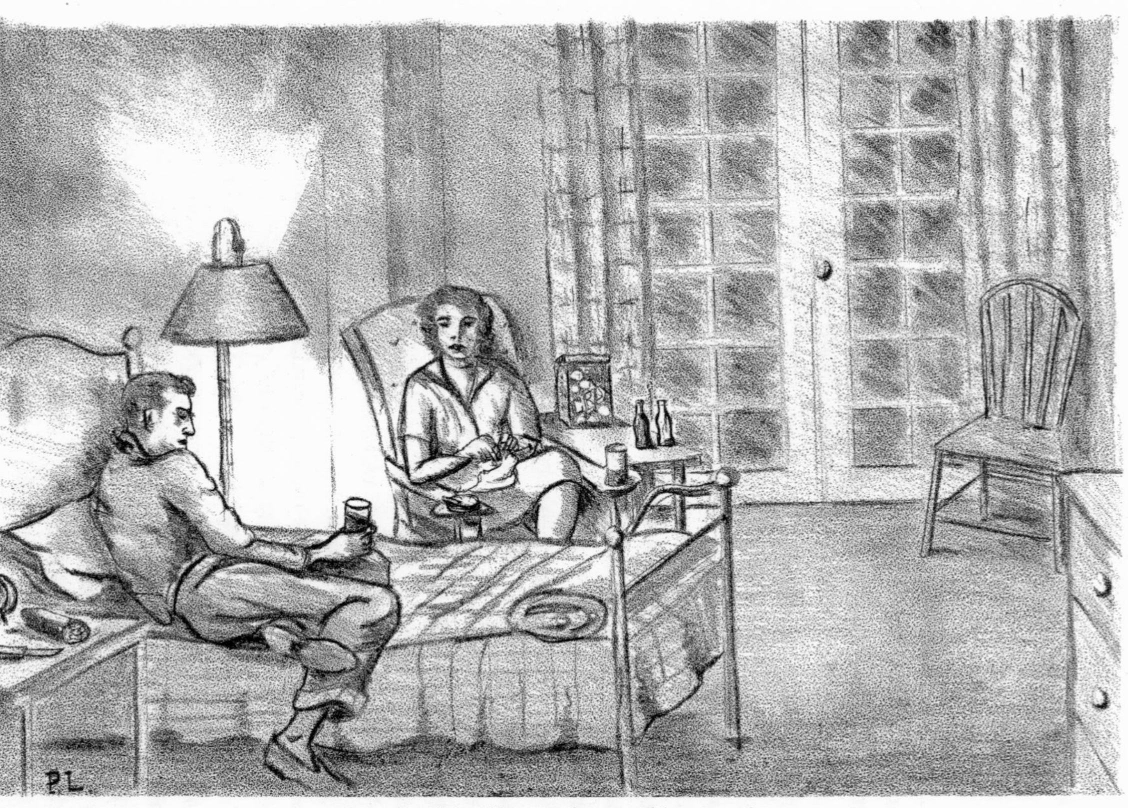

PICTURE 14. Two patients talking together

and nurses as a picture of a patient and a doctor in a psychotherapeutic session. No senior doctor or resident so "misidentified" this picture. After the patient or nurse had told a story about psychotherapy, it was suggested that he might not be familiar with the area of life which the picture attempted to portray, and he was asked to consider it to be a resident physician talking with a senior man.

The research interviewing program was started after three of the four months of intensive observation had been completed. The interviewing program continued over a period of six months. Thus, by the time the interviews began, there had been a chance to become well acquainted with the hospital personnel and patients. The writer, a social anthropologist, did all the interviews. When necessary he would first clear with the proper authority, such as the nursing supervisor and the patient's therapist, and then make an appointment with the interviewee. All the interviews were carried out with only the two persons present in a private office, and without any pressure of time. Almost all the interviews required at least two sessions of several hours each, and the total time required to complete a full picture interview ranged in length from three to ten hours. All persons were assured that the material they gave would be held in confidence and would be used only for research purposes. As will be seen later, the quality of the material indicated that the subjects believed this assurance of confidence, and they had already had proof of it in contacts with the writer during the preceding three months of research work.

The following instructions were given each interviewee, although the exact wording was not invariably used. The attempt was made to standardize as far as possible the emotional situation between the interviewer and the interviewee, rather than to standardize the nature of the instructions given. That is, the goal with all persons was to bring about a fairly free and easy talking relation. In essence, the following instructions were given:

In this research, I am interested in learning how patients, doctors, and nurses feel about certain everyday life occurrences in a mental hospital. I have drawn up a series of pictures of typical happenings in order to have a number of situations to talk about. Some of these situations may be more familiar to you than others. A wide variety of pictures has been included because I am asking all the doctors, nurses, and patients to talk about them.

You may have had some experience with telling stories about pictures as part of a psychological test. This is not like that. I am interested in what you, as one of the [doctors, nurses, patients] feel is important in the common occurrences that make up everyday living around the hospital.

Everything you say will be held in confidence. The interview material you tell will be used only for research purposes.

I will hand you a series of pictures, one by one; and, as I want to write down [or sound record] what you tell me about them, I may ask you to slow down a bit if we get to going too fast. On each picture, even if you are not too familiar with it, I would like you to try to include three things in your material about what is happening: First, try to tell me what you think the situation is—that is, just a simple description of where you think the action is taking place, who the various people are and why they are there. Second, try to tell me what the situation means to the people involved—that is, what are the feelings, emotions, and personal thoughts of the various people, and what are their relations with one another? Third, try to tell me what final actions the various people will take in order to end the immediate situation shown in the picture. That is, what will be the outcome? How will the various people evaluate the situation? What personal thoughts will they go away with?

Feel free to use any of the personal experiences you have had in the hospital yourself, and to be as specific or as general as you would like.

Mechanically, the collection of the interview material was similar to the procedure followed with the Thematic Apperception Test: either the interviewer wrote down the verbatim statement of the interviewee, or the material was recorded by having the subject dictate his material into sound-recording equipment. This latter method was used with the doctors, who were familiar with it through their dictation of case records. Three of the five interviews with residents, and five of the six interviews with senior doctors, were sound recorded in this manner. The remainder of the interviews with doctors, and all the interviews with the patients and nurses were written down by the interviewer.

As indicated, the hospital was a small one, and ideally it would have been advantageous to interview all personnel and patients in it. However, even if this had been done, the number of persons interviewed in any one role group would have been too small to be a statistically adequate sample. Even including all personnel and patients in the hospital, the number was still small. It was expected, however, that such an interviewing program would lead to some knowledge about how the entire hospital was put together and how it ran. The final sample included all senior doctors, all resident doctors, all nurses except one, and all patients on the open wards at the time of the research. Numerically, this means interview material was obtained from six senior doctors, five resident doctors, ten nurses, and eighteen patients. For the sake of simplicity, these figures will not be repeated each time a role group is mentioned in the remainder of this chapter, but the reader should be aware that these are the numbers of individuals included in the sample.

Some further characteristics of the role groups interviewed are useful. Of the ten nurses, five worked on the open wards and five on the locked wards. The eighteen patients were divided into eight males and ten females. Six of the eight males, and eight of the ten females, had spent at least a month on the locked wards before being transferred to the open wards. Thus, fourteen of the eighteen patients had had experience on both the locked and open wards, while four had had experience only on the open wards. All the patients had been in the hospital at least a month before being interviewed, and most of them for much longer periods of time, ranging up to a year-and-a-half. By diagnosis, eleven of the eighteen patients were classified as having one of the various psychoses (seven males and four females); six were classified as having severe neuroses or character disorders (one male, five females); and one female patient had organic impairment. Of the eleven patients with psychoses, nine were schizophrenic and two were manic-depressive. All the patients at the time of interview were in relatively good contact with the world around them.

As can be seen from the sample stories quoted shortly, and from the substantial amount of interview material given in Chapters 8 and 9, there was a great deal of ego-involvement with the subject matter of the pictures on the part of all the interviewees. That is, the interview was not a casual, nonaffective experience for any person—each person worked hard at the intellectual aspects of the task and openly expressed his conscious feelings in the various areas covered by the pictures. So far as the interviewer could tell, both hospital personnel and patients cooperated with him to the very best of their ability.

After the interview material had been obtained, the next task was to devise a method of analyzing the content. The primary purpose in making a quantitative content analysis (see Chapter 7) was to present certain general aspects of the interview material. It is strongly felt that the more qualitative nuances of the data (see Chapters 8 and 9) are just as important as the patterns discernible from the quantitative analysis. In scoring the interviews, the material was separated into *topics* dealing with *interactions* in the hospital in four mutually exclusive (for purposes of analysis) *areas of life*. It is necessary to define these various terms.

A *topic* was the basic unit for counting. In order to be counted, a topic had to meet criteria of length, area, and interaction. (1) *Length:*

a topic had to be, arbitrarily, five or more lines of typescript. (2) *Area:* a topic had to be a discussion about one of the four areas of life within the hospital. These areas, defined more fully below, were the hospital-in-general as a physical or social structure, therapy, administration, and human relations. The important point here is that the discussion had to center on what went on inside the hospital rather than outside it. Thus, topics that dealt with the patient's family, the referring physician, the environment of the community surrounding the hospital, and so forth, were excluded and were not counted. This arbitrary distinction was in line with the purpose stated in Chapter 2 of exploring intensively what went on within the hospital itself. (3) *Interaction:* a topic had to be explicitly concerned with the relations between an individual and his physical or social environment. Thus, topics were counted that dealt with the interaction between two or more individuals within a role group, or the interaction between two or more individuals in different role groups. Interaction with the physical or social environment included discussions where an individual was explicitly considered to be responding intellectually or emotionally to the quality of his external environment. For example: "This patient feels comfortable and secure on the locked ward because he knows he is protected from people on the outside by being in the hospital." Similarly: "The nurse is fed up with all the red tape in this place, and she knows it's no use trying to get a definite decision on her question, so she is frustrated." The topics which were not concerned with interaction, but were concerned with what might be called "self-action," were excluded. The term "self-action" was applied to topics in which an individual was considered to be influenced solely by certain qualities inherent in him, or responding solely to cues arising from within himself. For example: "This patient is hallucinating because he is schizophrenic." Or: "The resident here is very unsure of himself, and I would guess that this is related to problems in his own background that he has not worked out as yet." Such topics were excluded because, while they were of considerable interest, they were not in line with the immediate goal of trying to understand how interaction, explicitly recognized as such, was evaluated by the various role groups in the hospital. In summary, then, the first task in scoring was to separate the interview material into topics which were concerned with interaction going on in one of the four areas of life within the hospital.

After it had been decided what a topic was, the next task was to decide the *area of hospital life* within which it fell. For scoring purposes, the four areas of life were made mutually exclusive, and could be divided into: (1) problems of interaction with the *hospital-in-general,* considered either as a physical space or as a social structure; (2) problems of getting well—that is, *therapy;* (3) problems of getting routine done—that is, *administration;* (4) problems of getting along with others—that is, everyday *human relations.* A topic was scored in the area of the *hospital-in-general* if it concerned an individual who was in interaction with the physical or social structure of the hospital. Examples of this have been given under the discussion of what a topic was. A topic was scored in the area of *therapy* if it indicated a conscious and specific attempt on the part of an individual to participate with, influence, or evaluate another person with reference to the therapeutic implications of getting well. A topic was scored as *administration* if it concerned the day-to-day aspects of the routine work of the hospital on any of its levels, and if the emphasis was on getting work done (rather than on helping people or getting along with people). A topic was scored as *human relations* if it involved rather general day-to-day problems and feelings which were phrased in terms of getting along with one another in the hospital (without any particular regard to therapy or routine). Thus topics of human relations involved matters of human dignity, self-respect, and mutual liking, without reference to any immediate and specific task or goal.

A third kind of decision that had to be made was concerned with the *type of interaction* under discussion in a topic. That is, was the interaction between the hospital-in-general and the patient, between the resident and patient, between nurse and patient, and so forth?

A fourth decision to be made concerned an evaluation of the interviewee's feeling of *optimism* or *pessimism* about the matter under discussion in the topic. It must be emphasized that this was not a measure of how the person doing the scoring felt about the topic, but rather whether the interviewee himself expressed optimism or pessimism about the topic he was discussing. Stories which were neutral in their emotional tone were scored as optimistic, so that every topic was scored as either optimistic or pessimistic.

In summary of the over-all scoring system, every topic was scored with reference to four points: (1) whether it was a topic or not—one main criterion being five or more lines of typescript; (2) the area in which the topic fell—whether it was hospital-in-general, therapy, administration, or human relations; (3) the type of interaction going on—between the hospital-in-general and individuals in any of the four role groups, between two or more individuals from different role groups, or between two or more individuals in the same role group; and (4) the emotional tone of the topic—whether it was optimistic or pessimistic. One final aspect of the scoring system needs to be mentioned: a topic could be scored only once in the interview material to a particular picture. For example, if a topic was scored as "administration, nurse with patient, optimistic," then this score could not be repeated on that particular picture. Thus, once a topic had been scored, all material of the same nature, even though spatially separated in the interview material, was placed under the initial scoring. The same topic could, of course, be scored again in the material given to another picture.

Sample stories and their scoring may be seen in the following examples, and will serve to illustrate the foregoing explanation. It will be noted that the interview material to a single picture may contain only one topic, or it may contain several topics. Equally, parts of a topic may be separated by material belonging to a different topic. All the interview material given by an individual to a picture is cited in its entirety in the examples.

The first topics to be quoted as illustrations are taken from interview material in the area of the hospital-in-general. The following material was given by a senior physician, Dr. Scott, to Picture 1:

[Topic Score: Area—hospital-in-general; Interaction—hospital with patient; Tone—pessimistic]

Well, it occurs to me that this is before the doors. It could very well be our own hospital, actually. I get an impression of the massiveness and the heavy finality of the meaning of the doors in terms of the restraint on the freedom of the patient, who, I would presume, is the person standing in front of it. It occurs to me first of all that the individual is on the inside, wondering about the barrier that is presented to him in the form of the psychiatric hospital, with its doors as a symbol of pretty definite restraint on freedom. The patient stands, there's not too much evidence of tension in the way his posture is; he seems to me to be more mildly reflective and probably not too stressed by the idea of being in the hospital, but certainly some mild depressive emotion is evidenced by his posture about his situation. My own projection here is one of mal-depressive wondering and some kind of evidence of futility being expressed, and my feeling is that this circumstance for the patient is not going to change quickly. This seems to represent again the slow tempo of the hospital, generally the fact that he is going to be here for some time, and that tomorrow is not going to bring the immediate magical change which maybe all of us might hope for. So, I would see this kind of—in other words, I think this is a very good picture of the general slow tempo, the mild depressive apathy, of the hospital atmosphere itself.

A second illustration comes from the material given by a resident physician, Dr. Reynolds, to Picture 9, and includes a topic in the area of therapy as well as one in the area of the hospital-in-general.

[Topic Score: Area—therapy; Interaction—nurse with patient; Tone—pessimistic]

This patient is on the open ward and the nurse is stopping by for one of her periodic visits with the patient. The nurse seems to be a little bit uneasy in this situation; she seems to be sitting in a way that suggests that she is planning to get up as soon as it is reasonable to do so. She is anxious to do her best to help the patient out and to make a relation with her, but she has so many other things to do on the ward that it is really difficult to find the time to settle down and to have any kind of a relaxed, uninterrupted visit with the patient. The patient feels the desire to be pleasant and agreeable on the part of the nurse, but she also feels the lack of spontaneity, and in spite of both of their best intentions to enjoy each other, there is a feeling of tension between them. The patient is grateful to the nurse for having come in to see her; she is rather glad when she leaves. (The anthropologist asked: "Tell me a little bit more about the feelings of the two people.") The feeling of the patient toward the nurse would depend a good deal on what the problem of the patient was; if she saw the nurse as a kind of a frustrating mother figure, she might have considerable hostility to the nurse. On the other hand, if she were anxious to, if she were anxious to make the appearance of a good social adjustment in order to get more privileges, and be able to demonstrate that she is handling herself more adequately, she may have a considerable need and desire to make a satisfactory relation to the nurse. For the most part, she has very little opportunity to come to know the nurse as a person, and often sees her only as an authority figure or someone who is there, more or less to wait on her.

[Topic Score: Area—hospital-in-general; Interaction—hospital with nurse; Tone—pessimistic]

This seems to be related to the system in which the nurse has so many clerical and administrative and general duties around the ward that her ability to make relations with the patients is curtailed. It may also have a great deal to do with the personality of the nurse. To some nurses, this whole role in which they are cast is very frustrating, and they would like to have a great deal more time to be with the patients and to make relations with them. To others, the uniform and the role of the nurse is a protection against their own feelings of insecurity, and this might be a somewhat threatening situation, threatening to their security if the patient was seeing them as a person. These nurses cling to the role in which the system casts them, even though they may feel at times that it prevents them from doing things they would like.

[This material goes with the initial topic in the area of therapy and is not scored separately]

The nurse in this particular situation is trying very hard to be pleasant. She wants to do something for the patient. The patient has been showing some anxiety lately, and the nurse is anxious to be friendly with her, and to demonstrate her willingness to help, but she feels uncomfortable, and the patient senses this and is really unable to bring out her feelings that she would like to talk over with the nurse. After a brief conversation, the nurse is called away rather abruptly and terminates her interview with the patient. The patient is left with the vague feeling of frustration, and yet has a good feeling toward the nurse for having tried.

The next example falls in the area of therapy, and was given by a patient, Mr. Earle, to Picture 2:

[Topic Score: Area—therapy; Interaction—resident with patient; Tone—optimistic]

This is the familiar situation of the doctor's office, certainly. Might be "Long Tom" Ruthers, who has a particular meaning to me—was my doctor for seven months. Looks to me like just now the fellow is discouraged. His clothes unkempt, hair uncombed, shirt out of his sweater. Most fellows find themselves this way some days when the going is particularly hard. The doctor seems definitely to encourage the fellow to come out with the whole story—he has a benign look, is comfortable, is not perturbed about—which is encouraging to the patient. I've put on an expression that way when I think of mistakes sometimes. The doctor is gaining insight, sees the patient is in one of his moods. The patient leaves with the idea that the doctor is very encouraging as far as wanting to hear the whole story and not being prejudiced one way or the other. As for the doctor, I think he has got the idea that he feels sorry for this fellow, that he had to go through something rough, and he leaves with the determination to help him see the various angles. The doctor is not writing, just listening intently. It's an important incident, but there's not too much to write down. The guy walks back to the ward—hears card playing going on, goes to his room, gets out her picture. He might do what we saw in the first picture, a situation that stays with a person for a long time, but in the end he works well with his doctor and is helped.

The following examples occur mainly in the area of administration, although the material also includes topics in other areas. A senior physician, Dr. Sloan, said on Picture 17:

[Topic Score: Area—therapy; Interaction—nurse with patient; Tone—optimistic]

Well, this could be one of a couple of situations. It may be a nurse coming in at a certain hour of the night to see if the patient is asleep. I think it's somewhere about 11 or 11:15, perhaps later, that they walk around, flash a flashlight at the patient. She is carrying some liquid in her hand which may or may not be for this particular patient. So, if we assume that it is for this patient, it isn't necessarily her rounds, but she is using a flashlight so she wouldn't have to put on the light in the room. The patient may be calling for some, have asked for some milk or some other drink, and the nurse is bringing it to the patient, or it may be some medication that the nurse is giving to the patient. The patient looks to be fairly quiet, lying down, the bedclothes aren't too disturbed, so perhaps the patient isn't too agitated. The nurse will give the patient the medication or milk or other drink, perhaps say a few words, and then will leave, at which point the patient will settle down and sleep the rest of the night.

[Topic Score: Area—administration; Interaction—nurse with patient; Tone—optimistic]

(The anthropologist queried: "The nurse says a few words?") Well, of course, the relation between the nurse and the patient may be a relation that could be no relation, merely a nurse acting as a carrier of something to give the patient, or it may be a very close one, depending on what went on before. To the patient, however, she may be an extremely important figure—what the emotional reaction of the patient toward the nurse is, we can only guess. In some instances it may be resentment and anger, and hatred, even though the nurse is bringing the patient something, and at other times it may be one of great gratitude and comfort. I would say that this relation here is a very close one. I ask myself, why do I say that? Well, one clue only, and that is that the patient is lying apparently quietly in bed waiting for the nurse, so that apparently there is no agitation involved. A feeling of confidence that the nurse will come, will bring this, and the patient then is being composed and relatively calm knowing that. I would say that the feeling is a good feeling on the part of the patient and also on the part of the nurse for the patient. The nurse will try to be soothing and comforting to the patient.

A further example in the area of administration, as well as one on human relations, was given by a patient, Mrs. Matthews, on Picture 11:

[Topic Score: Area—administration; Interaction—nurse with patient; Tone—pessimistic]

This looks as though it might be nurses, doctors, and social workers having a conference. Do they have combined conferences? I'd like to be a fly on the wall there. Well, you don't have to quote me verbatim—looks as though a couple of real sourpuss nurses are here who had a hard night on the ward and have a few gripes about the patients. Could be Mrs. North complaining about my window's being open all the time—freezing her out of the place. Now if she were a real good—well, let me revise that, she is a good nurse, it just wouldn't do her any good to bring up the point, such as the complaint about having the window open. I resent that, so she comes along and closes the window, and I have to get up and open it. Of course, she knows we are allowed to have the windows open, and she can't introduce that at the meeting and have it changed, even though she freezes. Of course, all this is supposition. None of us has the vaguest idea. Lots of things you wish they would talk about—doesn't seem they will report a petty little incident, yet maybe they do report all these things. If they have this sort of staff meeting every morning, doesn't seem as if enough important things come up unless they really are observing, but you feel as if they were spying on you—like they are eavesdropping to find out, let's say, "natural" reactions, because most patients act differently toward the nurses.

[Topic Score: Area—human relations; Interaction—nurse with patient; Tone —pessimistic]

I think that as a general rule the patients act toward the nurses just the way the nurses act toward the patients. If they are nice, the patients respond nice, and if they aren't, they sort of build up a resentment. Many times these feelings are imaginary—not imaginary, but unfounded. On the locked ward Mrs. Nixon—for weeks I didn't actually know who she was—didn't come near me, didn't speak. All the other nurses came in and introduced themselves. I resented it. She never came near me. Even when I was outside her office she'd walk right by. So I decided one day I'd find out what the story was. So I asked her, and she said she was very busy and generally just spoke to the patients as a group, and unless she had some specific reason to go into a patient's room, she didn't go. She said she had no personal feeling against me, and was very glad I brought it up. And I was too. It's ridiculous to go on having a feeling of antagonism without knowing why. Wait a minute, she said she was on a vacation, but after all, I was still a new patient to her. To me, it wouldn't have hurt her to say hello, but I couldn't endure the fact that she ignored me. Wouldn't have taken more than two or three seconds to say hello. It makes you feel more at ease.

The material just quoted contained a topic in the area of human relations. Another topic in this area may be seen in the interview with a nurse, Miss Neal, on Picture 9:

[Topic Score: Area—human relations; Interaction—nurse with patient; Tone —optimistic]

I think this is a patient on open ward. It's on a week end when most of the group have gone out or have visitors, so the nurse has stopped in for a chat. The patient was very eager to talk with the nurse, she's lonesome. Probably has no family or friends living near enough by to visit. The patient probably enjoyed having someone to talk to about her children. The nurse always enjoys talking with this particular patient. The patient is always friendly, and the nurse is feeling sorry for her because she has no visitors and is left in practically by herself today. The patient is talking about her home and her children, their activities. She is showing pictures of them taken since she has come to the hospital and showing the changes in them. The nurse asks questions and may tell of a niece she has or a nephew, and describes similar antics of his. The patient is anticipating a visit with her family the following week end, and the nurse is helping her to make plans for this—where she will go, what she'll wear, places to eat. The patient was so enthused about it that the nurse was also enthused, and it was almost as much fun for her as it was for the patient. It's in the middle of the afternoon, and only a few patients are on the ward, and so she asks the patient if she wouldn't like to join her in the kitchen—she has asked her several times before—and help get refreshments out. She joins her in a snack, and by that time it is time for report.

After the method of scoring illustrated in the foregoing examples had been decided on, a check was run on reliability between scorers. Earlier, a graduate student in sociology was trained in the scoring method.[2] Facility in scoring was developed by analyzing interview material from the pilot study. Following this, an actual research interview was selected at random from each of the four role groups. The anthropologist and the graduate assistant independently scored the material in these four interviews on the twelve pictures selected for analysis. The anthropologist arrived at a total of 91 topics on the four interviews, while the assistant arrived at a total of 82 topics. Both scorers divided the material into the same 82 topics—the additional topics scored by the anthropologist were owing to his having made a somewhat finer breakdown of the material at certain points. On these same 82 topics the two scorers agreed completely in their scores for 75 of the topics. If any part of the scoring of a topic was dissimilar, then that entire topic was said to be a disagreement. Thus, if the scoring of emotional tone was dissimilar on a topic but there was agreement as to area and type of interaction, the entire topic was still considered to be a disagreement between the two scorers. Counting the additional 9 topics scored by the anthropologist as disagreements, the two scorers were in complete agreement on 75 of the 91 topics, or an over-all agreement between scorers of 82.4 per cent. As this seemed to be a satisfactory agreement, the entire body of the interview material on the twelve pictures was then analyzed.

The next three chapters present some of the results of the analysis of the interviews. Chapter 7 is a discussion of the more quantitative overall characteristics of the attitudes and role perceptions held by the four role groups toward areas of life in the hospital and types of interaction in the hospital. In Chapter 8 these two aspects are put together in a detailed qualitative presentation of how the interaction of patients and staff with the hospital-in-general was perceived. Chapter 9 is a qualitative analysis of various types of interaction in the areas of therapy, administration, and human relations. The discussion of the picture interview material is brought to a close at the end of Chapter 9 with the suggestion of a hypothesis concerning relations between role groups in the hospital.

[2] This student was Miss Dorrian Apple, and her sustained interest and help in the analysis of the interview material is gratefully acknowledged.

CHAPTER 7

Patterning of Attitudes among Staff and Patients

As indicated in the preceding chapter, the picture interview material came from six senior physicians, five resident physicians, ten nurses, and eighteen patients. Although this represented all the staff in the particular role groups, and about half the patients in the hospital, the sample is still small. The quantitative analysis in this chapter is not, therefore, presented in any attempt to create an illusion of statistical validity, but rather in the effort to state with as much precision as possible certain characteristics of the interview material which can be put into numerical form.

AREAS OF LIFE IN THE HOSPITAL

Altogether, the 39 persons in the sample were scored on 723 topics. The distribution of these topics by role group and area of life can be seen in Table 7–1. This table shows that the manifest content of the pictures did its work, and a fairly good spread of topics was obtained from each role group in each area of life. Looking at the percentage columns for the various role groups, it can be seen that the seniors and residents tended proportionately to talk more than the other role groups about the hospital-in-general. The nurses concentrated more on administration and therapy. The patients spread their topics rather evenly throughout all four areas. The residents were somewhat low, when compared with the other groups, in the proportion of their topics devoted to therapy. This might be thought rather odd since the residents did most of the formal therapy, but, as will be seen later, this low proportion of topics was owing to the concentration of the residents' topics on matters that concerned only the resident and patient, or the resident and senior physician. In general, the residents did not give topics of a therapeutic nature in

TABLE 7–1. Number and percentage of topics, by role group and area of life

Area of life	Seniors (N=6) Number	Seniors (N=6) Per cent	Residents (N=5) Number	Residents (N=5) Per cent	Nurses (N=10) Number	Nurses (N=10) Per cent	Patients (N=18) Number	Patients (N=18) Per cent
Hospital-in-general	44	36.7	49	41.2	37	19.6	84	28.5
Therapy	25	20.8	20	16.8	55	29.1	65	22.0
Administration	25	20.8	31	26.0	61	32.3	74	25.1
Human relations	26	21.7	19	16.0	36	19.0	72	24.4
All areas	120	100.0	119	100.0	189	100.0	295	100.0

discussing the relation between nurse and patient, or between patient and patient. The other three role groups, however, did discuss these relations in therapeutic terms.

Reading across the table by area, it can be seen that the patients had the highest proportion of all role groups in human relations, the nurses were highest in administration and therapy, and the residents in the hospital-in-general. All the preceding points reflect the differential emphases given various areas of life in the hospital by the several role groups.

It is important to stress that within no role group was a greatly disproportionate share of topics contributed by any one person, nor did any person fail to give at least one topic in each area of life, and usually gave several. Within the various role groups, the average number and range of topics per person in all areas may be seen in Table 7–2. The data in Table 7–2 also include the average number per person and the range of topics for each area of life.

As indicated in the preceding chapter, the topics were scored according to whether they were predominantly optimistic or pessimistic in emotional tone. Of the total 723 topics, 350 were optimistic and 373 were pessimistic. No person had a completely optimistic or pessimistic inter-

TABLE 7–2. Average number and range of topics per person, by role group and area of life

Area of life	Seniors (N=6) Average	Seniors (N=6) Range	Residents (N=5) Average	Residents (N=5) Range	Nurses (N=10) Average	Nurses (N=10) Range	Patients (N=18) Average	Patients (N=18) Range
Hospital-in-general	7.3	2–15	9.8	5–14	3.7	1–13	4.7	2–11
Therapy	4.2	2–10	4.0	1–6	5.5	3–9	3.6	2–6
Administration	4.2	3–5	6.2	4–9	6.1	4–9	4.1	1–6
Human relations	4.3	3–6	3.8	3–5	3.6	1–5	4.0	2–6
All areas	20.0	14–27	23.8	15–29	18.9	15–26	16.4	11–25

view. Of the total 39 persons, 19 had 50 per cent or more optimistic topics, while 20 had more than 50 per cent pessimistic topics. Separating the 39 persons into role groups: the patients had the most optimistic ratio with 11 of the 18 patients having 50 per cent or more optimistic topics in their interviews; the senior physicians came next with 3 of the 6 seniors having an optimistic balance; the nurses were less optimistic with only 4 of the 10 nurses showing a preponderance of optimism; while the residents came last, since only 1 of the 5 residents was optimistic in his interview. These various aspects are summarized in Table 7–3.

The reading of the number of optimistic or pessimistic topics shown in Table 7–3 should be quite easy to follow. For example, the 6 senior physicians gave a total of 120 topics (59 optimistic, 61 pessimistic). Of these total topics for seniors, 44 (7 optimistic, 37 pessimistic) occurred in the area of the hospital-in-general, and so forth.

The number of persons judged to be optimistic or pessimistic in Table 7–3 needs a word of explanation. As will have been apparent from a careful reading of the foregoing text, the following convention was used: if a tie occurred in the number of optimistic and pessimistic topics in an interview, the balance of the total interview was judged to be optimistic. That is, if a person had an equal number of optimistic and pessimistic topics in his interview, the interview would be considered as optimistic. In fact, there were no ties in the total topic count per person concerning the balance of emotional tone.

TABLE 7–3. Number of persons and topics showing optimism or pessimism, by role group and area of life

	Seniors (N=6)		Residents (N=5)		Nurses (N=10)		Patients (N=18)	
Area of life	Persons	Topics	Persons	Topics	Persons	Topics	Persons	Topics
Hospital-in-general								
Optimism	2	7	0	9	5	16	8	29
Pessimism	4	37	5	40	5	21	10	55
Therapy								
Optimism	4	15	5	14	7	35	13	37
Pessimism	2	10	0	6	3	20	5	28
Administration								
Optimism	5	16	1	9	4	27	13	44
Pessimism	1	9	4	22	6	34	5	30
Human relations								
Optimism	5	21	3	11	3	12	13	48
Pessimism	1	5	2	8	7	24	5	24
All areas								
Optimism	3	59	1	43	4	90	11	158
Pessimism	3	61	4	76	6	99	7	137

TABLE 7–4. Number of persons and topics showing optimism or pessimism in total of all areas of life, by role group, with percentage optimistic

	Seniors (N=6)		Residents (N=5)		Nurses (N=10)		Patients (N=18)	
	Persons	Topics	Persons	Topics	Persons	Topics	Persons	Topics
Number optimistic	3	59	1	43	4	90	11	158
Number pessimistic	3	61	4	76	6	99	7	137
Percentage optimistic	50.0	49.2	20.0	36.1	40.0	47.6	61.1	53.6

The same convention was also used in determining the balance of emotional tone on a person's interview *within* a particular area of life. For example, if a person gave 4 topics about therapy, 3 of which were optimistic and 1 pessimistic, his interview was considered to be optimistic in the area of therapy. If, however, this person's 4 topics about therapy had been split into 2 optimistic and 2 pessimistic, his interview would still have been considered as optimistic in the area of therapy following the rule for ties. In fact, ties occurred in the balance of emotional tone within areas of life only 8 times out of a possible 156 chances (39 persons times 4 areas).

The remainder of this section will be concerned with the implications of some of the points raised by Table 7–3. For convenience in discussion, the data in Table 7–3 will be presented in a series of supplementary tables. Thus, Table 7–4 represents only the data for all areas, while Tables 7–5 through 7–8 indicate the figures for each area of life separately.

In general from Table 7–4 it can be said that considering total topic response, there was not a great deal of difference between the four role groups regarding their over-all optimism about the hospital. The patients, seniors, and nurses were, however, somewhat more optimistic than were the residents.

Since it will not be a matter of direct concern in the remainder of this chapter, it is useful at this point to mention an interesting difference between male and female patients that is not apparent from Table 7–4 because a breakdown by sex is not made. The males were more optimistic than the females. In terms of total topics, male patients had 69.1 per cent optimistic as compared with 42.4 per cent for the females. This difference was not due to the interview of any single patient, as 7 of the 8 male patients, compared with 4 of the 10 female patients, had 50 per cent or more optimistic topics in their interviews.

Anticipating the differences by area of life a bit, as this male-female distinction will not be mentioned again, it is noteworthy that the greater degree of over-all optimism on the part of the male patients tended to hold up in three of the four areas of life. That is, with reference to the hospital-in-general, 50.0 per cent of the topics given by male patients were optimistic, while only 24.0 per cent of the topics given by female patients were optimistic. The corresponding figures by persons were: 5 of the 8 males had 50.0 per cent or more optimistic topics on their interviews, whereas this was true for only 3 of the 10 female patients. Similarly, in the areas of therapy and human relations, the male percentages for topics were 76.0 and 92.0 per cent optimistic, as opposed to 45.0 and 53.2 per cent optimistic for the females. By persons within these areas: all 8 of the male patients were optimistic on both therapy and human relations, compared with 5 of the 10 female patients. Male and female patients were closer in their agreement about administration as an area of life. The topic count for males was 66.7 per cent optimistic and for females 51.4 per cent optimistic. The corresponding figures by persons for the administrative area of life were: 6 of 8 male and 7 of 10 female patients were optimistic.

It is difficult to say what these differences between male and female patients may mean. They certainly reflected a general opinion in the hospital, where it was frequently remarked by patients and personnel on both the open and locked wards that the men's wards were quieter and caused less trouble than the women's wards. Equally, the research observations indicated that on both open and locked wards the women were more noisy, insistent in their demands, and irritable. Such a sex difference has, of course, long been noted on psychiatric wards in our culture, where it is usual to find female patients in a more excited and turbulent state. A good deal of this probably has little to do with "psychiatric illness" *per se* and more to do with the relatively greater deprivation experienced by female patients, especially on locked wards, when they cannot easily obtain everyday necessities such as lipstick, bobby pins, mirrors, access to a hairdresser, and so forth. There is also probably a relation with the somewhat more "emotional" role played by women in our culture. A third factor that undoubtedly enters in here is that the male patients were interacting with female nurses, as opposed to the female patients interacting with female nurses in the day-to-day life on the wards. Female nurses are perhaps prone to judge female patients somewhat more harshly regarding their behavior than they judge male patients. This would result in greater friction between nurses and female patients than between nurses and male patients. An extended discussion of any of these

TABLE 7–5. Number of persons and topics showing optimism or pessimism about hospital-in-general, by role group, with percentage optimistic

	Seniors (N=6)		Residents (N=5)		Nurses (N=10)		Patients (N=18)	
	Persons	Topics	Persons	Topics	Persons	Topics	Persons	Topics
Number optimistic	2	7	0	9	5	16	8	29
Number pessimistic	4	37	5	40	5	21	10	55
Percentage optimistic	33.3	15.9	0	18.4	50.0	43.2	44.4	34.5

points would, however, move too far afield from the main line of development in this chapter.

Turning to an analysis of the various areas of life, the hospital-in-general will be discussed first. As can be seen in Table 7–5, all role groups agreed in their pessimism about the hospital-in-general. This pessimistic outlook on the hospital included the physical structure, the emotional climate, and the general social organization. The details of this outlook may be found in the next chapter. As in previous instances, the distribution by topics in Table 7–5 was not owing to the concentration of pessimistic topics in any particular individual's record, as is indicated by a comparison of the distribution by persons and topics. The nurses present the most equivocal group in that by topic count they were pessimistic, but by person count were optimistic (by extending the logic of the rule set up earlier in which ties are counted as optimistic).

The differences shown in degree of pessimism—the nurses and patients being less pessimistic than the seniors and residents—might be caused by the fact that neither the seniors nor the residents really had very much investment in the hospital-in-general and could be more openly critical. The residents were only on the inpatient service for a period of a year, and were more concerned with their relations to individual patients than they were with the nature of the hospital-in-general. The seniors, on their part, devoted only a fraction of their time and interest to the hospital-in-general, and spent much more of their time in other activities. This was not the case for the nurses or patients. The nurses' entire occupational life was bound up with the hospital-in-general, and it was from this source that they received their financial security. Equally, the patients' life was bound up with the hospital-in-general for the time that they were living within it, and it was from the hospital-in-general that they received treatment as well as from their doctors.

A second reason for the greater degree of pessimism among residents and seniors might lie in the fact that both these groups were per-

TABLE 7–6. Number of persons and topics showing optimism or pessimism about therapy, by role group, with percentage optimistic

	Seniors (N=6)		Residents (N=5)		Nurses (N=10)		Patients (N=18)	
	Persons	Topics	Persons	Topics	Persons	Topics	Persons	Topics
Number optimistic	4	15	5	14	7	35	13	37
Number pessimistic	2	10	0	6	3	20	5	28
Percentage optimistic	66.7	60.0	100.0	70.0	70.0	63.6	72.2	56.9

haps more acutely aware of discrepancies and difficulties between psychotherapy as a system and the hospital-in-general as a system. This question is related to one of the major points of this book. If, as indicated in Table 7–5, all role groups were agreed about the inadequate nature of the hospital-in-general, the system would seem ripe for change.

The general conclusion to be drawn about the attitudes toward the area of the hospital-in-general is that none of the role groups seemed to derive very much satisfaction from the hospital as a system. One would not predict much day-to-day disagreement on this matter—merely a general frustration felt by the majority of persons in all role groups.

Just as all groups were relatively pessimistic about the hospital-in-general, so all role groups were relatively optimistic about the matter of therapy. This can be seen in Table 7–6. It is interesting that the resident doctors, who were most directly responsible for psychotherapy in the hospital, were the most optimistic about this area of life (100.0 per cent by persons and 70.0 per cent by topics). In general, therapy as an area of life in the hospital was seen rather hopefully.

Unlike the preceding two areas of hospital life where there was relative consensus among the four role groups, the area of administration indicated a divergence of opinion, with the seniors and patients being fairly optimistic and the nurses and residents more pessimistic. These divergences in attitudes may be seen in Table 7–7. It is interesting that those role groups having the most to do with the day-to-day control of

TABLE 7–7. Number of persons and topics showing optimism or pessimism about administration, by role group, with percentage optimistic

	Seniors (N=6)		Residents (N=5)		Nurses (N=10)		Patients (N=18)	
	Persons	Topics	Persons	Topics	Persons	Topics	Persons	Topics
Number optimistic	5	16	1	9	4	27	13	44
Number pessimistic	1	9	4	22	6	34	5	30
Percentage optimistic	83.3	64.0	20.0	29.0	40.0	44.3	72.2	59.5

administration—the residents and nurses—were the least optimistic, while the patients, who lived under the administrative control, did not seem to feel it as too frustrating. Most of the senior physicians, largely removed from these matters except at the policy level, had a rather unrealistic and somewhat "rosy" view of administration, as will be seen in the next two chapters, where these points are given more extended discussion. It is also interesting that the least optimistic group, the residents, who had to juggle the psychotherapeutic and administrative care of their patients, were the least hopeful.

In general, from Table 7–7, administration is an area of life where one would predict day-to-day inter-role *disagreement,* with the result that administrative matters could become a source of misunderstanding, tension, and confusion in the hospital. This is in contrast to the areas of life of the hospital-in-general and therapy, where there was more of a consensus of opinion among the four role groups.

The area of human relations was, like administration, one within which there was a divergence of opinion. As can be seen from Table 7–8, the balance of emotional tone in the topics on human relations was optimistic for seniors, residents, and patients, whereas it was pessimistic for nurses. The seniors, as in administration, had a somewhat unrealistic picture of life in this area and, in fact, had very little daily contact with it. The residents and patients, having more to do with day-to-day human relations, were not so whole-heartedly optimistic as were the seniors, but were far from being as pessimistic as the nurses. As with administrative matters, the prediction would be for disagreement among the role groups, particularly between doctors and nurses, in the area of human relations.

The material on areas of life in the hospital can be summarized by following the procedure of calling a role group optimistic about an area of life when 50 per cent or more of its topics in this area were optimistic, and pessimistic when more than 50 per cent of its topics were so scored. The same rule can be applied to the count by persons. The results of this

TABLE 7–8. Number of persons and topics showing optimism or pessimism about human relations, by role group, with percentage optimistic

	Seniors (N=6)		Residents (N=5)		Nurses (N=10)		Patients (N=18)	
	Persons	Topics	Persons	Topics	Persons	Topics	Persons	Topics
Number optimistic	5	21	3	11	3	12	13	48
Number pessimistic	1	5	2	8	7	24	5	24
Percentage optimistic	83.3	80.8	60.0	57.9	30.0	33.3	72.2	66.7

TABLE 7–9. Tendency toward optimism or pessimism in areas of life, by role group

Area of life	Seniors	Residents	Nurses	Patients
Hospital-in-general	Pessimism	Pessimism	?	Pessimism
Therapy	Optimism	Optimism	Optimism	Optimism
Administration	Optimism	Pessimism	Pessimism	Optimism
Human relations	Optimism	Optimism	Pessimism	Optimism

procedure may be found in Table 7–9. If the counts by both topics and persons were in the same direction, an entry was made in the table. If, however, the counts by topics and persons were in opposite directions, a question mark was entered in the table. As can be seen, the seniors and patients were alike in the *pattern* of their predominant attitudes and were the two most optimistic groups—being so about all areas of life except the hospital-in-general. The residents were next most optimistic, being so about therapy and human relations, but pessimistic about the hospital-in-general and administration. The nurses were the least optimistic of the role groups, being so only about therapy, while they were pessimistic concerning administration and human relations. A question mark was entered for the nurses in the area of the hospital-in-general as the two counts were in opposite directions in this area (see Table 7–5).

With regard to the intriguing similarity in pattern between the seniors and patients, it is interesting that neither of these groups had day-to-day responsibility for the operation of the hospital, and hence both groups could more easily be optimistic as they were less in touch with these immediate problems. In addition, it is very likely that this is a specific instance of a general phenomenon in social relations: the tendency for alternate levels in a hierarchical structure to show certain similarities in attitudes and feelings, whether the alternate levels are in a kinship system (Murdock, 1949) or a factory (Roethlisberger and Dickson, 1939). It is a common anthropological observation that there frequently is a pattern of mutual indulgence and affection between alternate generations, such as that between grandparents and grandchildren. In the case of grandparents and grandchildren, neither generation usually has direct responsibility for the other, and the two groups are united in having experienced frustration with the intermediate generation. That is, the grandparents have had to rear the parents, and the children have had to be reared by the parents (Radcliffe-Brown, 1952; but also see Apple, 1956). In an analogous way, the residents and nurses are in an intermediate position between the seniors and patients. The seniors have the problem of responsibility for policy and ultimate decision over the residents and nurses, but do not enter into the day-to-day operation of the hospital, and usually come into contact with the patients only on "visits" to the wards. The residents and nurses exercise direct control over the patients; and indeed much of psychiatric theory supports the notion that patients are in the position of "children" in the hospital. If one were to carry this analogy somewhat farther, it would place the residents and nurses in the roles of "father" and "mother" in the hospital, with the seniors in the role of "grandparents." While these groups do seem often to occupy these roles, unfortunately it is sometimes the case that the residents and nurses do not appear as a very harmonious couple. There is a good deal of appeal to higher authority on the part of both the residents and nurses, and a use (often unconscious) of the patients to defend a personal position. Both the seniors and patients may experience some impatience with the intermediate groups and speculate (rather fancifully because of their infrequent meetings) on how matters would be if they were in more direct contact—a type of speculation not uncommon among grandparents and grandchildren, top management and workers, and high government officials and the average citizen.

Returning to Table 7–9, one would anticipate a fair amount of agreement among the four groups about the hospital-in-general and therapy; equally, one would expect administration and human relations to be areas of greater disagreement. To some extent one would also expect the residents and nurses to share an underlying attitude toward administrative matters that diverged from the attitude held by seniors and patients. Somewhat differently, the seniors, residents, and patients would be more likely to be in accord with each other on matters of human relations than they would be with the nurses. These various combinations did indeed seem to occur, as will be indicated in Chapters 10 through 12 where the actual administrative operation of the hospital is considered in detail.

TYPES OF INTERACTION IN THE HOSPITAL

The over-all characteristics of types of interaction reported in the interviews are given in Table 7–10. As in the analysis by areas of hospital life, the various frequencies in topics in Table 7–10 were not caused by a concentration of a particular type of interaction in any one person's interview, but rather represented a spread from all the interviews, as may be seen in the count by persons. The same procedures were used to determine optimism and pessimism concerning type of interaction as were used in scoring area of life.

TABLE 7–10. Number of persons and topics showing optimism or pessimism, by type of interaction and role group

Type of interaction	Seniors (N=6)		Residents (N=5)		Nurses (N=10)		Patients (N=18)	
	Persons	Topics	Persons	Topics	Persons	Topics	Persons	Topics
Hospital-in-general with patients or staff								
Optimism	2	7	0	9	5	16	8	29
Pessimism	4	37	5	40	5	21	10	55
Staff with staff								
Optimism	4	8	1	2	7	14	15	26
Pessimism	2	6	4	12	3	14	3	10
Staff with patients								
Optimism	5	30	3	23	4	57	11	66
Pessimism	1	16	2	20	6	51	7	60
Patients with patients								
Optimism	6	14	3	9	3	3	17	37
Pessimism	0	2	2	4	7	13	1	12
All types of interaction								
Optimism	3	59	1	43	4	90	11	158
Pessimism	3	61	4	76	6	99	7	137

For logical reasons inherent in the scoring system, the figures for type of interaction in the hospital-in-general are the same as the figures for the hospital-in-general as an area of life (see Table 7–3). The reason for this is simple: in order to be included as a topic in the area of the hospital-in-general, the interview material had to meet a criterion of interaction between the physical or social structure of the hospital and the staff or patients. This logic does not apply at any other point in the scoring system because the other three areas of life are independent of the specific type of interaction occurring in them: that is, interaction between residents and patients may occur in the areas of therapy, administration, and human relations; equally, the area of administration may encompass interaction between seniors and residents, residents and patients, nurses and patients, and so forth.

The topics included in the interaction category of staff-with-staff in Table 7–10 came largely from the interview material given to the picture of the daily administrative conference (Picture 11). Most of the interaction in these topics concerned the day-to-day administrative relations between seniors, residents, and nurses. It is interesting that the patients were the most optimistic here, and this was probably so because they could only infer that interaction among the staff went relatively smoothly.

TABLE 7–11. Tendency toward optimism or pessimism in types of interaction, by role group

Type of interaction	Seniors	Residents	Nurses	Patients
Hospital-in-general with patients or staff	Pessimism	Pessimism	?	Pessimism
Staff with staff	Optimism	Pessimism	Optimism	Optimism
Staff with patients	Optimism	Optimism	?	Optimism
Patients with patients	Optimism	Optimism	Pessimism	Optimism

The nurses, who were in somewhat more direct contact, were also optimistic about staff-with-staff interaction. Part of the reason for this probably was that nurses tended to leave decisions to doctors in this type of interaction and, if the nurses did disagree with the outcome, this disagreement was frequently expressed covertly and indirectly rather than as a part of open discussion (see Chapters 3 through 5, and Chapter 11). The senior physicians, who were somewhat removed from matters of daily administrative interaction and worked on a higher policy level, were also optimistic in the balance of their attitudes. The residents, however, upon whom fell the real responsibility for day-to-day administrative work, were quite pessimistic about staff-with-staff interaction.

Turning to the interaction of staff-with-patients, the seniors, residents, and patients were optimistic in the balance of their attitudes, while the nurses were indeterminate. The category staff-with-patients hides a number of important distinctions in types of interaction, such as resident-with-patient and nurse-with-patient. These finer breakdowns in types of interaction will be considered in Chapter 9.

The seniors seemed to be overly optimistic concerning the relations of patients-with-patients, as they were more optimistic about this type of interaction than were the patients themselves. The residents also were optimistic, but less so than seniors or patients, whereas there was a real disagreement with these three role groups on the part of the nurses: the nurses were quite pessimistic in their view of the interaction of patients with each other.

All the foregoing points can be summarized, as was done in the analysis by areas of life, in terms of a table indicating the tendency toward optimism and pessimism about the various types of interaction. This summary may be seen in Table 7–11. The same similarity in pattern obtained between seniors and patients with reference to their optimism about types of interaction (Table 7–11) as obtained between these two role groups with reference to areas of life (Table 7–9). Both seniors and patients were optimistic concerning all types of interaction except those involving the hospital-in-general.

The residents and nurses were less optimistic than the seniors and patients. However, the residents and nurses differed regarding the various types of interaction they viewed with optimism or pessimism. The residents were pessimistic about staff-with-staff interaction, whereas the nurses were optimistic. Just the reverse was true for patients-with-patients interaction, where the residents were optimistic and the nurses pessimistic.

The lack of determinancy for the nurses in two of the four types of interaction may well reflect the poorly defined role of the nurse in the hospital—often she was not sure what attitude or action she should take in a particular situation. In general, the role of the psychiatric nurse is much in need of clarification in order to bring it into line with recent developments in psychiatry (see Robinson, *et al.,* 1955).

From Table 7–11, one would tentatively predict that there would be agreement among the role groups regarding the inadequacy of the hospital-in-general when either staff or patients tried to interact with it as a physical or social structure. Equally, there would be agreement about the relative adequacy of the interaction between staff and patients. On the other hand, there probably would be more disagreement over matters involving the interaction of staff-with-staff or patients-with-patients.

It seems reasonable to conclude from the material in this chapter that the various patterns of agreement and disagreement among the role groups in areas of life and types of interaction represent underlying differences in perception of the world of the hospital. These underlying differences are probably not readily verbalizable as such, yet such covert differences strongly affect the smoothness with which the day-to-day operation of the hospital is carried out (see Chapters 3 through 5).

The patterning of these underlying perceptions is related to what the anthropologist calls the implicit culture of a group (Kluckhohn, C., 1951). As pointed out in earlier chapters, because of the hierarchical structure and interpersonal formality in a psychiatric hospital, a somewhat different subculture exists for each of the various role groups. In such a situation, the various role groups in the hospital will be likely to meet with difficulties in communicating and working together, just as the peoples of two cultures would have problems in relating to one another if the underlying assumptions of their cultures differed on important matters. These ideas are in line with the work of Mishler (1955) who, in studying two state hospitals by means of schedules and intensive interviews, found that the differences in attitudes expressed by various role groups were much greater than the differences between the two hospitals.

The foregoing discussion has presented some of the more formal characteristics of the interviews rather than the specific content. It is now time to turn to a more detailed and qualitative analysis of the material, and to examine how the various types of interaction are seen within the several areas of hospital life.

CHAPTER 8

The Hospital in General

The content of all the interviews was very rich in both intellectual and emotional expression, and the purpose of this chapter and the next is to try to convey some of the more clinical insight to be gained from the material. This will be done through a discussion of the types of interaction that occurred in the various areas of hospital life. Interaction of the patients and the staff with the hospital-in-general will be discussed first.

INTERACTION OF PATIENTS WITH THE HOSPITAL-IN-GENERAL

As may be seen in Table 8–1, there was somewhat more optimism about the interaction of patients with the hospital-in-general than there was about the interaction of the staff with the hospital-in-general. The optimistic topics about the interaction of patients with the hospital referred mostly to the security the patients felt in a protected setting and to the therapeutic effect of being in the hospital. The pessimistic topics were largely concerned with boredom, dreariness, and the monotonous atmosphere. The majority of both optimistic and pessimistic topics concerning the interaction of patients with the hospital-in-general came from interview material on Pictures 1, 5, and 4.

On Picture 1—the picture of a patient looking through the doors of the locked ward—the distribution of optimistic and pessimistic topics by role group was: seniors—1 optimistic and 4 pessimistic, residents—no optimistic and 5 pessimistic, nurses—2 optimistic and no pessimistic, and patients—8 optimistic and 10 pessimistic. The low number of topics for nurses is interesting, as it coincides with a similarly low number of topics in this area of interaction produced by nurses on Picture 5. This was

TABLE 8–1. Number of persons and topics showing optimism or pessimism about hospital-in-general, by role group and type of interaction

Type of interaction	Seniors (N=6)		Residents (N=5)		Nurses (N=10)		Patients (N=18)	
	Persons	Topics	Persons	Topics	Persons	Topics	Persons	Topics
Patients with hospital-in-general								
Optimism	1	7	1	8	8	16	8	29
Pessimism	5	24	4	24	1	10	10	51
Staff with hospital-in-general								
Optimism	0	0	0	1	0	0	0	0
Pessimism	6	13	5	16	6	11	4	4

owing to the fact that the nurses did not see the patient as being in interaction with his environment in either Pictures 1 or 5, but rather saw the patient's state as due solely to "his illness" without relation to his surroundings.

The only senior doctor, Dr. Shaw, who saw Picture 1 as optimistic, stressed that the patient would shortly come to a sense of direction regarding how he was to proceed:

(Picture 1, Dr. Shaw) I have an impression that this is one of the patients standing on the inside looking out. . . . He's kind of caught by forces, and he stands sort of passively, feeling rather in the power of things that are quite out of his control now. . . . Given a little time, he'll find himself through the group and begin to find that his way out is through activity in the hospital. . . . I think his way out is a combination of his participating with the group, and . . . his treatment, working with the doctor or with the nurses, also gives him a sense of direction as to how he is going to proceed.

The pessimistic topics by the seniors were concerned with the coldness and tediousness of the ward as reflected in the topic by Dr. Scott on Picture 1 cited in Chapter 6 and as indicated in the following topic given by Dr. Sutton:

(Picture 1, Dr. Sutton) . . . This brings to mind this whole business of locked wards; they are necessary and they are a terrible nuisance. If anything, I have a strong tendency against it. . . . Some people say that they close up the locked ward to keep people from the outside from annoying the patients, but I never really believed that. I think it is really some peculiar inherent tendency in psychiatry—still even in modern psychiatry today to keep the patient locked up, not to take chances. . . . The poor fellow, how he looks at that so intently. I can feel with him. I mean, this to me is the horrible part of our business. You should always ask doctors if it is justified to keep them locked up. . . .

The topics of the residents were similar in tone to those of the seniors, but were more specific in referring to issues arising out of the fact of hospitalization. Dr. Reynolds, for example, felt that hospitalization seemed to focus and precipitate the patient's latent dependency needs. Dr. Reynolds also stressed the problem of finances for the patient, in that most families could not afford long-term treatment in a private hospital:

(Picture 1, Dr. Reynolds) . . . If it was a patient on the locked ward, he would be looking toward the outside, but with a feeling of hopelessness at ever getting out. A feeling that he is in there, and he doesn't know quite what the situation is all about, and just from the position in which he is standing, it gives me the feeling of indecision and of conflict and of hopelessness about the situation. The family eventually runs out of money, and he gets transferred to a state hospital. . . . He came into the hospital with some hope that short-term therapy would solve his problem, but the very fact of hospitalization seems to focus and precipitate all the latent dependencies that were at the basis of his problem, and rather than clearing the situation, it accentuated the difficulties to the point where they had to be treated on a long-term basis. (The anthropologist asked about the situation of finances.) It was possible for the family and relatives to raise sufficient capital to keep him in the hospital for a short time, but when they found it was going to run into a long-term treatment problem, they felt unable to handle it on a private basis and had to send him to the state hospital. This raises the whole point of conflict between the kind of treatment the patient needs and the ability to pay for what may turn into long-term treatment. . . .

A further specific point raised by the residents was the tendency for patients to learn to conform and to hide their symptoms in order to facilitate transfer to an open ward. This point was not mentioned by any of the seniors or nurses, but formed an important part of the interview material told by the patients about Pictures 1 and 5. Among the residents, for example, Dr. Rolfe said:

(Picture 1, Dr. Rolfe) . . . The feeling is always what a locked door is like, and I dislike it. A reasonable psychiatrist opens the door, and it will be done a little later. In this situation with a patient, to be resigned in front of the door without banging, he is on the way to conform and behave and slowly work his way out—either to improve or to hide his symptoms. . . . Here we have the basic conception of a hospital, an evil that has to be used as constructively as possible, but it is always better to get out. . . .

As mentioned, the nurses only gave two topics involving interaction between patients and the hospital-in-general on Picture 1. Both these topics emphasized the security and protection provided the patient by the hospital. This was very evident in the interview with Miss Nicholas, who, in addition, showed a creative attitude toward the use of locked wards. She was in charge of the men's locked ward and, when on duty, would usually open the doors while at the same time maintaining close, friendly contact with the patients. In her interview Miss Nicholas said:

(Picture 1, Miss Nicholas) How appropriate. This is one of the patients. This can be Ted standing by the door, which isn't really locked, but being so submissive, he doesn't even try the lock though he sees the staff going in and out. . . . I imagine he must have, in a way, some feeling of enclosure—of this wall's being the limitation of his existence at the present time. Right now I think he is very grateful. The wall not only means he can't go out, but that others can't come in, such as the family. It's a protection to him. . . . (The anthropologist asked Miss Nicholas when she started the open-door policy on her locked ward.) We've had it going off and on for a month. . . . After I had been doing it, Dr. Scott mentioned it to me, and asked me what I thought. I said that I had been doing it for a month, and it was an interesting thing to try, gives them a feeling of not being so completely confined. I hope that the doors between the men's and women's locked wards can be opened so that they can be in each other's living rooms at certain times. A much more realistic situation. Last Sunday we brought the men over to the women's music appreciation group, and it worked out very well; at least on the surface there were no untoward effects.

The interaction and feeling tone evident in Miss Nicholas' material was in direct contrast to the approach taken by most of the nurses to Picture 1. In general, the nurses saw the patient as having little or no awareness of his surroundings. For example, he was "preoccupied with his own thoughts," or he had "very little feeling about anything, just within himself right now." These topics were not scored, since they did not involve interaction (see Chapter 6). A pointed example of this kind of thinking was the response of Miss Nye to Picture 1:

(Picture 1, Miss Nye) . . . He could be paranoid, doesn't realize he's sick enough to be in the hospital, and that this is a form of protection for him. . . . He might perhaps wind up in a state hospital, or be transferred to another hospital on the same order as this one. This certainly is a common occurrence in a place like this. It's part of their illness. . . . Could be hallucinating in a case like that. Voices telling him what to do. You are apt to get a good blow if you try to tell them to disobey their voices, and I understand that it doesn't help to try and do that anyway. Can't give medication when the voices tell them not to take it. . . . Funny, the brain works that way, and yet it's real to them.

A further interesting aspect of the nurses' material on Picture 1 and elsewhere throughout the interviews, although it was not scored separately as a topic in itself, was the number of times that nurses working on the open ward indicated that they really had not had contact with the locked ward for several years and were at a loss concerning what to say about a picture of a locked ward. Those nurses working on the locked ward were equally at a loss when faced with pictures of situations on the open ward. For example:

(Picture 1, Miss Nagle) . . . It looks like the locked ward. I can't speak too well for the locked ward. I haven't been up there for two years. . . .

(Picture 1, Mrs. Nolan) . . . I haven't been on the locked ward in five years to work. . . . I guess the poor thing just stands there until the doctor or nurse comes in and gets him interested enough to leave the door.

(And on Picture 5, Mrs. Nolan said:) . . . It doesn't mean much to me. . . . I've avoided the locked ward, as I am terribly uncomfortable with people as disturbed as that. . . .

(Picture 9, Miss Nicholas) The open ward. This is funny. I have so little feeling what's going on here. . . . I am not really familiar with this at all, I've never worked on the open ward. . . .

This kind of statement, when it appears as frequently as it did, has many implications. It would seem that nurses on the various wards had very little conception of what went on elsewhere, and this was reflected in an interesting gap in the information contained in the routine nursing notes about the behavior of patients. For example, the nurse on the locked ward wrote a note on the behavior of patients during the time they were actually present on her ward, but she did not observe the behavior on the open ward of those locked ward patients who had progressed to the point of being permitted to visit on the open ward for several hours each day. On the other hand, the nurse on the open ward did not feel that charting the behavior of these patients was her responsibility, particularly as the records in which the nursing notes were written were kept on the locked ward. Thus, an important area of information, the behavior of locked ward patients who were visiting on the open ward, was missing from the day-to-day nursing records in the hospital. Such material could be of considerable use in the making of decisions concerning the transfer of patients from the locked to the open wards.

In a wider sense, such statements in the interviews serve to point up the lack of knowledge between individuals and role groups occupying different positions in the social structure of the hospital regarding the spatial arrangements and activities of each other's jobs. This problem is not confined to the nurses and will arise again in connection with other role groups later in this chapter. In terms of the totality of structural positions in the hospital hierarchy, the patients were frequently in real contact with more situations during the course of the day than was any other group. For example, the locked ward patients referred to in the preceding paragraph were likely on a given day, in addition to the regular life on their own ward, to be in contact with: (1) the open ward patients and nurses, (2) the occupational and recreational therapists, (3) the residents through individual psychotherapy, and (4) the senior physicians if they happened to be making rounds. This sort of simple explanation, in terms of contact with a greater number of people on different levels, goes a considerable way toward helping to explain the seemingly mysterious process by which patients often sense, and even concretely know, what is happening in the hospital before such information is disseminated among hospital personnel.

While the seniors and residents saw Picture 1 predominantly as pessimistic, the patients were about equally divided between optimism and pessimism (8 to 10) in that they recognized the security and support provided by the hospital as well as its more confining aspects. The positive feelings among the patients were usually coupled with an underlying ambivalence about the whole problem of hospitalization, as in the following topic:

(Picture 1, Mr. Osgood) In one sense, he feels quite safe where he is—and from my own personal experience—I wish the doctors would get around to the idea that I'm normal and let me move (meaning transfer to the open ward). Let's say: look at it as the locked ward's being "your mother made you stay here because you were bad. Wouldn't go out and play." One of the things that first came into my mind—the size of the doors struck me. I suppose you might say the guy is waiting to be cured and when he does get cured, the doors are going to look pretty big to him, all that space to go out into. Right now the doors are closed and God only knows what the outcome will be.

As indicated earlier, the patients and the residents, in contrast to the seniors and nurses, felt that often a patient had to learn to conform and suppress his symptoms in order to be moved from the locked to the open ward. For example, a patient, Mrs. Lasker, brought up the topic of conformity over and over again in her interview, as is indicated by the following excerpt from her material to Picture 1:

(Picture 1, Mrs. Lasker) It's evidently a patient looking through the doors to the outside and thinking of the spot he's in and how the hell to get out of it. The doors represent barriers. He's standing there wondering what the hell to do about it. . . . Well, sooner or later he realizes he must conform to get out of those closed doors. If he's not completely insane, he works his way to a place where the doors are open and he gets privileges, and sooner or later manages to get out. He'll see that beating his head against the wall won't get him any place, literally or figuratively, and he'll try to adjust at least outwardly, so sooner or later he gets moved. (The anthropologist questioned:

"At least outwardly?") He'd be a damn fool, unless he was really insane, unless he was throwing things around, he has to sort of come out of himself and adjust and that way eventually he'll do what he wants.

On Picture 5, none of the role groups saw the use of the seclusion room as an optimistic situation. The distribution of topics concerning the interaction of patients with the hospital-in-general on this picture by role group was: seniors—1 optimistic and 7 pessimistic, residents—2 optimistic and 3 pessimistic, nurses—1 optimistic and 3 pessimistic, and patients—1 optimistic and 8 pessimistic.

The few scattered optimistic topics in the various role groups stressed the positive function of seclusion as a place where a patient, removed from outside stimuli, could calm down. For example, Dr. Reynolds said: "She probably will only be there for a short time and will become quieter, partly because of removal from the stimulation of other patients, and partly because of the extra attention she will get from some of the nurses and attendants. . . ." Among the nurses, Mrs. Nixon felt that the situation represented security for the patient: "I don't think the nurses feel as strongly as the doctors about patients' being in isolation. Some patients feel more secure out there, some like the attention they receive when they are there. It's more disturbing to the nurses to have a patient in this condition on the ward than in isolation. . . ."

The pessimistic responses of the seniors and residents largely reflected their concern over their inability to find a solution for such a problem.[1] Dr. Shaw, for example, expressed concern that hospital personnel were not able to handle such situations adequately:

(Picture 5, Dr. Shaw) The real impression of personal indignity is enhanced by the fact that we haven't managed really to get the place fixed up: the cracks in the wall, the chipped corners. . . . Here is a place where the hospital administration and the doctors struggle with two things: one is that we very often don't have enough personnel to handle it adequately, and then the personnel don't know what they're doing. That is, they don't have a sense of direction, a sense of real understanding of what's going on with the patient and with the treatment. Therefore, much too much trial and error goes on. First, an attempt to get very close and be personally reassuring and relieving, and then a sense of frustration and uncertainty, and perhaps withdrawal and even isolation on the part of the patient follows after. . . .

As did many of the staff, Miss Nicholas recognized the anxiety-producing aspects of isolation, but she also went on to indicate how she had been able, in part, to overcome this problem by showing the seclu-

[1] This study was carried out prior to the extensive use of such tranquilizing drugs as chlorpromazine, reserpine, etc.

sion rooms to the patients early in their stay, and routinely making use of empty seclusion rooms for ordinary housekeeping purposes, or as places where a patient could be comfortably alone (as opposed to isolated) if he so desired. Again, as in her material to Picture 1, Miss Nicholas was indicating how the existing facilities of the hospital could be used creatively:

(Picture 5, Miss Nicholas) . . . Think she's probably pretty well frightened by the room. Plaster is off of the walls, some markings on the wall, and she doesn't understand, but she feels they are put there because she is in the room. . . . And she is all alone, which makes her even more frightened. But having people with her makes her frightened too. . . . That's the point we often feel guilty about, that we shouldn't leave them alone. Yet, . . . we may be answering our own needs in staying with them. . . . To have a person in there with them most of the time may make them more anxious. They should be enclosed and allowed to act out. If they scream and yell, I'd be in favor of letting them do it for a while instead of sedating them. . . . It's a good idea to bring patients out on the ward and away from isolation for fifteen minutes or so. Take them in and out of isolation, and they can talk over what the other patients have said. (The anthropologist asked how the other patients react to a patient who comes back from isolation.) With fear, mostly. If they are newly admitted, they are terribly afraid, but if the patient has been here quite a while, and we, the staff, talk about the patients, then they, the patients, ask us how he or she is doing today, and we should tell them. Keep up the contact. I've seen the women greet a patient back from isolation with open arms, almost have a party. As it was on the men's locked ward last year, we had a group of four or five who had been in isolation and we used to have little sessions on the ward where we'd sit and chat, and the topic would get around to isolation, and they would say, "I bet I was worse than you," and we got a group discussion of isolation. We talked quite openly about it. With Dick Earle, we set up housekeeping in isolation. He was in there for six weeks, and we let him visit on the ward, and this spring when he was leaving, he said: "Now you can rearrange the furniture again." . . . The attitude held of isolation by the patients depends entirely on the attitude of the staff. I think we should use isolation more, especially as a place where they can go and be alone with the door closed if they want it. Then, when the day came when they became acutely ill, they wouldn't be so frightened of it. We had a postpartum psychosis in. She saw Dr. Ryan and was frightened to death of him. She and I talked, and finally she said that the night she was admitted Dr. Ryan took her to a terrible dungeon. And I told her I thought she should come with me and see the place, and she said, "Oh, no," but I insisted, and after we had seen the place she burst out crying and was so relieved to find out that it was just around the corner. There are some sweet potatoes in the sound proofing on the ceiling in isolation. A patient threw the food up there, and we can't get it out of the little holes. She had thought that this was blood dripping, and was scared to death. And now she is relieved and can go up and see Dr. Ryan. I think we should use isolation more.

That's why I had Walt take his examinations out there this fall for his schoolwork. My ward now has three men who have been in isolation, and the other two are about ready to go. They talk about it, and we can have a real family group out there.

The attitude expressed by Miss Nicholas that seclusion can be used positively and is often more therapeutic than drugs, was an unusual one among the staff. On the whole, the nurses disliked using seclusion and felt that the patient resented it. Thus Miss Noyes said: "I think most nurses have considerable feeling about putting patients in isolation; we might have the same feelings a patient would about being put in a barren room, and a good many of the patients couldn't help but feel it's more like a jail than a room."

What is interesting here is that the seniors, residents, and nurses tended to show considerable guilt over their participation in the use of seclusion, as when Dr. Rolfe said: "That's isolation and it shouldn't happen. You know how I am fighting against isolation. . . . I feel guilty, assisting in something that's wrong." On the other hand, the patients had a much less guilty and more accepting view of seclusion. In addition, as did the other role groups, the patients stressed that seclusion was feared as an unknown, that it was punishment, and that it accentuated loss of control. These latter aspects can be seen in the following three excerpts from interviews with patients:

(Picture 5, Miss Prescott) Well, this girl is obviously disturbed . . . it's probably necessary for people who are very disturbed so they don't injure themselves. . . . Everybody's scared of going upstairs. People who have never been upstairs are afraid of the unknown, and people who have been upstairs know what hell it is. In a mental hospital you're dealing with too much of an unknown, and it's very disquieting to anyone with a disturbed mind. . . . You don't know exactly what's wrong with you, how long it will take to get well. You don't know if you'll get well, or if the psychiatrist can help you, that's the unknown. . . .

(Picture 5, Mr. Edwards) That's so obvious it needs no comment. Somebody's just been brought in and put in isolation. Suggest a new patient, suggest the unaccountable ravings that occur on the locked ward, that die down, that are usually quickly silenced. . . . Also I don't have any clear idea exactly where isolation is. One gentleman down on the open ward got drunk, and they took him up there, and in telling it to me, when he woke up he wondered where he was. Well, the doctor arrives and says: "Do you think you can behave now?" And the patient, having had enough of it, just says: "Yes." I think even a very sick person would consent to get out of that place—an awful place to be—that's what I would say is the ending.

(Picture 5, Miss Farrell) . . . She is feeling that I am in such a mess I have to get myself out of this immediate situation of being locked in a room, being forced into such a situation. I think I would feel hatred for humanity, and even if the doctors did expect me to be reasonable, finding myself in such a situation, I'd lose control of myself; or else secondly, I'd play the game and get myself out of this environment as quickly as possible, do what was expected of me. I would try to hide my neurotic symptoms because it would be up to the doctor to get me out and hence I would try to appear rational. Everybody talks about whether you've been on the locked ward, and if you've been there, as I have, you've really been through all. . . .

The pressures for conformity expressed in the last excerpt by Miss Farrell are related to similar attitudes that arose as one sort of topic on Picture 4, which is the final picture to be discussed in terms of the interaction of the patients with the hospital-in-general.

In general, on Picture 4—a patient either entering or leaving the hospital—the seniors were rather pessimistic, while all other role groups were optimistic. The distribution of topics was: seniors—2 optimistic and 3 pessimistic, residents—4 optimistic and 1 pessimistic, nurses—8 optimistic and 1 pessimistic, and patients—15 optimistic and 5 pessimistic.

On the optimistic side among the seniors, Dr. Shaw stressed the anxiety of the patient on leaving or entering the hospital, but saw the patient as able to overcome this and carry out the matter well:

(Picture 4, Dr. Shaw) . . . I think there's a lot of anxiety that the patients have as to how they appear going in and out of the hospital, as though this was the point at which they display themselves and their accomplishments to the outside world. Whether they do it smoothly or with uneasiness is of a good bit a concern to them. If the patient is returning to the hospital after the week end, I feel that the patient has been here long enough so that he feels a real sense of achievement and therefore is himself glad to be back. . . . This is always a struggle for the patient to return to the hospital. I think this is a real narcissistic blow, and perhaps it is one of the reasons that if they are going to do it, damn it, they are going to do it with poise, or with as much poise as they can, in order to maintain their own self assurance. . . .

Dr. Scott, on the other hand, viewed the patient as leaving, and felt that the hospital had not participated sufficiently in this: that is, there was no one who really saw the patient off and bade him good-bye. Both Dr. Shaw and Dr. Scott, as well as the other seniors, however, interpreted the picture in terms of the patient's struggle to maintain contact with, or return to, the outside world. The residents also interpreted the picture in this way and emphasized the outward direction of the patient despite his opposing feelings of dependency and depression at leaving. For example, Drs. Ryan and Reynolds said:

(Picture 4, Dr. Ryan) . . . It isn't quite as happy leaving as he hoped it would be—he really leaves the hospital with a sort of dejected feeling, but finally comes out of this depression and goes up to the cab driver and puts the bag in the car, and gets in and takes a last look at the hospital. . . . He knows he had good treatment, made friends in the hospital. He's had similar periods of depression before, and knows life is quite different in the hospital than it is on the outside, and that this is a pretty big step for him to take.

(Picture 4, Dr. Reynolds) Well, this patient seems to be returning late at night from a week end with his family. . . . He is an extremely dependent person who really in some ways feels more at home in a regimented situation than he does on the outside. The pressure of having to maintain the normal masculine role in the community was a tremendous strain on him. Yet, the longer he stays in the hospital, the more ambivalent he becomes. . . . It seems necessary for him to assert some feeling of independence and definition of himself as an individual; he is so much afraid of his tendency to sink into the situation and accept it that he has to fight all the time to show people that he is a person. . . . If he were my patient, I think I would feel that there were a number of aspects to the problem. One aspect would be to examine with the patient his feelings about the hospital, and about the world, and about himself. I think the hospital can be used in a situation like that to point out to the patient what his feelings are in relation to himself and the people around him. On the other hand, I think that he also has to be encouraged to remain aware of the fact that there is a world outside, and in so far as he is able, to keep himself in touch with it. . . .

The tendency among the seniors and residents to see the patient as moving toward contact with the outer world was quite the reverse of the general position taken by the nurses, who emphasized the need of the patient to remain within the security of the hospital. The nurses were perturbed by the leniency and frequency with which patients were allowed to leave the hospital for activities in the city or for visits home, and they felt the patients would do better if they remained inside the hospital.

The emphasis placed on the security of the hospital was evident when Miss Nagle said: "Maybe he's going home for the week end and is worried about it. Maybe he'll change his mind before somebody comes after him. He probably can't wait to get back to the ward again. . . . He'd probably feel uneasy and would feel more comfortable in the security of the hospital where he has the doctors and nurses to talk to." Equally, Miss Nye said: "He is really anxious to get back in"; while Miss Noyes said: "He was glad to get back to the security of the hospital where he feels protected again and doesn't have to try to control himself." Also Miss Nicholas, in this case, expressed the same viewpoint as the other nurses when she said: "No matter how unpleasant they say the hospital is, they are grateful. . . . He has a feeling of wanting to be back in the hospital." She then went on to discuss her opinion that the patient often left before he felt ready to do so, or, indeed, before he should leave.

In general, the nurses were strongly opposed to certain therapeutic and administrative policies which, in their minds, resulted in too much activity of the patient outside of the hospital. While this point of view is implied throughout the nurses' material on Picture 4, it is stated unequivocally in their responses to Picture 3—the picture of patients signing the book indicating their outside activities. Although in one sense, this anticipates the discussion of interaction in the administrative area of hospital life, it is useful here to indicate the opinions of the nurses concerning the effect on the patient of a policy permitting relatively free access to the outside world. Miss Nicholas, for example, was concerned about the added strain on the patient and believed that such outside activities serve to gratify the needs of the staff for indications of therapeutic progress (as in the case of Dr. Ryan in Chapter 3) more than to help the patient:

(Picture 3, Miss Nicholas) . . . I think this is a patient signing out to go home with her husband. Probably for the week end. . . . I have the feeling the nurse looks a little bothered by the whole thing. Maybe she doesn't approve of this patient's going out, not too pleased by this. A patient she didn't feel was ready to go out and who has been allowed to go. Somehow she is thinking, this isn't going to turn out, but if that's the way they want it, let them go ahead; see if I care. . . . The nurse feels there is too much going out, and I feel so too. The patient should stay in the hospital situation. Having them in a few weeks, and then letting them go out, means that we've not really improved things. We're not fair to the patient or to the family. . . . We have the feeling that if the patient goes home for the week end, he is better. I don't think that the patient is better. It means we have mobilized them enough so that they can set foot outside of the door. . . . I can't see where going home for the week end is such a big deal. It is almost cruel to them. . . . The family goes through the period of getting the person to the hospital, and then when they are there, the family heaves a sigh of relief, and then the telephone rings, and the patient says, "I'm coming home for the week end," and the family says, "Oh, God, not again." There is much, much too much going out on the week end. (The anthropologist said: "You mention that we mobilized patients enough to get them out of the door.") I think of David Isherwood. He has no real desire to be out. I think most of this going out stems from our own need. Going out means that the patient is better, and that we have done something for the patient. We say unconsciously, we will be pleased if they go out, and so the patient feels it would be wonderful if I should go out, and he pulls himself together in some sort of fashion and goes out. I met Doris Murdock in a department store, and she was just wandering around, just lost, and I had the feeling: "Ye gods, why do we think this is so good for the patients to be out unless it's under some sort of organized program." . . .

While they agreed with Miss Nicholas, the other nurses had quite different reasons for feeling that the patients should not go out of the hospital, such as the opinion expressed by Mrs. Nixon that the patients were likely to get in trouble with the police, or the opinion of Miss Newcomb that the patients' outside activities placed the nurse in a difficult position where she did not know what was going on, and hence she wished for greater restrictions so as to bring about more order and routine:

(Picture 3, Mrs. Nixon) This looks like the signing-out book. . . . It's for when the patients are given permission to go out. They either assume responsibility for themselves, or a staff member assumes responsibility for them. Of course, some patients resent this very much because it makes them feel incompetent, like jailbirds. You tell them it's just a matter of routine, they check in and out of a hotel, don't they? . . . Also, it becomes important if anything happens while they are out. I remember one instance while I was on duty. The patient's brother took him out. They went for a ride, and he shot himself, and the physician in charge asked me if I'd had him sign out, and to be sure not to let anything happen to that sign-out slip. . . . It's a matter of routine, and you do have to follow a certain amount of routine, and frequently it's not good for the patient to be out more, though they don't think so, and neither do their families. . . . The patients may not want to go, but can't say no. . . . The time out wasn't enjoyed too much, and they were both relieved to have it over with. He comes back in upset, wanting to see the doctor, wanting to talk with someone about the situation. . . . He doesn't sleep well and requires some sedation that evening.

(Picture 3, Miss Newcomb) . . . From the nurse's stance, it looks like she's worried about something. Probably the patient doesn't have permission to go out. After much telephoning and annoyed waiting, the doctor says: "Oh, well, let him go." I suppose so far as the patient is concerned, going out means a great deal, but I think it gets to be quite a problem. Once it was only allowed on certain days with the doctor's permission. But now since they are not used to that routine, and let the patient go out anyway, there is hell to pay. They let him go out and discover he needed special permission, and then it gets to be an issue, and you can't deal with it as openly as you'd like to, and you express resentment toward the patient even though you don't want to. You ask yourself: "What's going on here, or why is it going on?" And if you've been here for years, you ask for the good old days when things were easy. If you have elasticity, you think that perhaps the patient gets things out of this, but it leaves you in a spot. I don't know if I'm coming or going at times.

The individual differences of opinion just cited between nurses, but all falling within a shared general pattern of attitudes, bring into focus once again a basic position taken in this book: the need to know *both* individual variation and the shared general pattern within which this takes place. Thus, Miss Nicholas shared with the other nurses the opinion that patients went out too much, but she had quite different reasons for wanting the patients to stay in the hospital. In this sense, as was discussed at the end of Chapter 5, it is not sufficient to know either the individual variation or the shared general pattern, but rather it is necessary to have both kinds of information in order to predict the structure and nature of the "interpersonal field" at any given time, and to evaluate the effect of certain combinations of personnel who may be on duty.

Returning to the analysis of Picture 4, the patients were predominately optimistic. They stressed the security of the hospital and the importance of friendships formed during their stay, and showed considerable ambivalence about activities outside the hospital and the problem of leaving for good. In this latter attitude, the patients were much *closer* to the opinions of the nurses than to those of the seniors or residents. Indeed, it seemed that the nurse was often able to assess more accurately the feeling of the patient about entering or leaving the hospital than was the senior physician or resident. For example, Mr. Osgood was in accord with Miss Nicholas when on Picture 4 he said: "Leaving for good, all cured and that sort of thing. Kind of afraid to get out and sorry to leave in a way. Probably not quite sure the doctor is right in letting him out."

For some patients, entering the hospital was an immediate relief, as it was for Mr. Armstrong, who said: "They will tell him what they think best for him. . . . Once I had entered, a lot of pressure was relieved in my mind." Other patients, however, and this was more usual, had to struggle to come to terms with their illness. This took Mrs. Lasker about a month:

(Picture 4, Mrs. Lasker) . . . He's entering, beginning to doubt how he ever did it, but then he said: "Of course, I can always get out in ten days," and of course most doctors tell you when advising you to come to a place like this: "Well, if you don't like it, you can always leave." . . . He gets inside and the doctor says: "Well, what are you here for?" And he says: "Well, something's wrong. I'm not sure." He's not sure what's wrong, but he doesn't think it is so terrible as long as he can sign out. The first week he's in he keeps saying he'll only stay a week. The second week he keeps saying he'll only stay two weeks more, and then the third week it becomes a month, and about at the end of the third week he usually tries to sign out and then finds out he can't. He's in. He's just stuck. He's there. He goes through so many different reactions. One day a lot of nonsense, and the next day, "what am I doing with all these crackpots?" Eventually he gets convinced there is something wrong with him, and then he worries about it, and he begins to accept the situation. That's the hardest thing. If he has any sense, he usually starts to work with his doctor. That takes a month.

Most patients, throughout their stay, both valued the security of the hospital and disliked the dependence and loss of self-esteem they came to feel. Thus Miss Prescott said: "At the beginning you sort of hate the place for what it's done to you. The feeling of dependency it's instilled in you, and also the feeling of security maybe, the outside world can't touch you if your doctor doesn't want it to touch you." These sorts of contrary feelings were perhaps best expressed by Mr. Erskine:

(Picture 4, Mr. Erskine) The guy is packed up to go home for the week end. . . . He's in a situation where he's asked for a privilege, and it was granted, and he can be happy or nervous and tense to get out on his own. He doesn't have the security. Can either be elated, or full of fear of what will happen when he gets there. . . . Or, I could take it he's just come back and is scared about coming in. He doesn't look too happy, and he wasn't looking forward to coming back to this security. He's either happy to get back, or sad to get back to the security. Security means discipline, means doing what the hospital says at the time the hospital says it. You can't tell by the expression. I smile when I feel the lousiest. He probably has mixed emotions. . . .

A final aspect of Picture 4 emphasized by the patients was that, upon leaving, the patient feels the loss of the companionship he had developed with other patients during his stay in the hospital. Miss Farrell said this succinctly: "I have established a circle of friends that I am comfortable with. I guess that is security. The problem of insecurity for me will be making a new circle of friends and not having the bond of mental illness in common. Instead of being an integral part of a group I will be isolated while still knowing I'm not yet well."

Several other pictures contributed their share to the total of topics concerning the interaction of patients with the hospital-in-general. This additional material, however, would only serve to corroborate what has already been discussed. In summary, this type of interaction was seen relatively pessimistically by the seniors, residents, and patients, and somewhat optimistically by the nurses.

INTERACTION OF STAFF WITH THE HOSPITAL-IN-GENERAL

Turning now to the interaction of the staff with the hospital-in-general, Table 8–1 shows that this type of interaction was viewed with uniform pessimism by all role groups. It is interesting that the patients produced only 4 topics on this type of interaction, whereas they produced 80 topics concerning the interaction of the patients with the hospital-in-general. The following discussion, therefore, is predominantly in terms of the responses of the staff.

The pessimistic topics on the interaction of the staff with the hospital-in-general can be divided roughly into three categories indicating concern over: (1) the rigidity of the hierarchy in the hospital, (2) the lack of integration and the uncertainty of procedure, and (3) the difficulty experienced by various role groups in carrying out their work because their training had inadequately prepared them for the kinds of problems they would face—this latter was particularly true for those topics dealing with the nurse's role. All the topics in these three categories were spread throughout the various pictures without a concentration on any particular picture.

Dr. Scott's analysis of the difficulties encountered in the rigidity of the hierarchy of the hospital reflects fairly well the opinions expressed by the seniors. Dr. Scott said:

(Picture 11, Dr. Scott) . . . First of all, I think that the whole problem of accepting the implied atmosphere of the administrative rounds hits the resident particularly, in terms of his struggle for status and some reasonable autonomy, and I think that much of the expectation on the part of the resident is that he comes to the staff in order to petition for what he wants to do, and his expectation is that some authoritative person will categorically say, "You can't do that," or "That isn't acceptable." So he then already feels an anticipatory resentment and may react to this either with silence, camouflage, or maybe judicious spacing of his activities so that somehow he diminishes the possibility of getting an authoritative refusal for something that he has already partially, or even openly, committed himself to. So, too, I think from the standpoint of the nursing staff, communication in this kind of atmosphere is definitely conditioned and inhibited by the expectancy on the nurse's part that, if a doctor says something which is contradictory to what she believes in terms of her observations of the patient on the floor, she feels she cannot and will not say anything about this, but will nevertheless be angry toward the doctor about it. This, of course, can easily generalize to the doctor's patients, so that what may happen in such a circumstance is that either the nurse stays silent and swallows her own feelings about what she thinks is inadequate reporting on the doctor's part, or she suddenly explodes in anger and is then angry about the patient, because the feeling is that the doctor doesn't see the patient as she sees the patient, and therefore she dislikes the patient and the doctor together in this. And I think, too, on the other side, the leader of the administrative rounds can also have his own defenses in terms of making authoritative pronouncements on inadequate information, or covering up his own feelings of insecurity by being quite categorical about what he says. As a matter of fact, the utilization of the so-called "rules of the house" can certainly function in this way. A blanket kind of referral to these rules may mean that "I don't really want to make individualized decisions because of my anxiety," and so I simply say: "Well, that's how the rules are." So I think that the ending of most of the rounds is on the basis of the feeling that things have never really been talked out enough, that arbitrary kinds of decisions have been made, and also some anxiety that decisions that have already been communicated to the patient will have to be undone because the already legislated decision by the resident has been overruled in the administrative conference. The nurses go out many times feeling that the doctors just don't know what the hell is going on, and there is frequently a general air of this kind of dissatisfaction and resentment. This doesn't always have to be the case, because some administrative rounds end on a note of clarity and some collective affirmation about the goodness of a decision.

In addition to the over-all problem of the rigidity of the hierarchy, a number of special points were raised by the seniors. One of these was the difference in underlying values—stemming mainly from the different social class backgrounds—between nurses and residents, which heightened the difficulty of making administrative decisions. Dr. Shaw noted this when he said:

(Picture 11, Dr. Shaw) I think the general permissiveness that goes on around here bothers some of the nurses because the patients are allowed to behave in ways that are in general socially unacceptable, and in ways which the nurses have had to struggle with in their own development. The doctor is caught in the need to support the nurses, and yet he has a feeling that this is somehow trivial . . . and he also has a tendency to do as his supervisor did with him—that is, to interpret the response of the nurse as evidence of psychopathology and as an area that can't be frankly discussed because of the unconscious motivation and the intangible determinants.

Dr. Simmons also indicated the influence of social class differences between nurses and residents when he said:

(Picture 14, Dr. Simmons) . . . I think these two patients are probably just grateful for each other's company, and it is a kind of an oasis. I think the feelings of the staff vary a good deal. I think the therapists probably regard these patients' relationships rather benignly. . . . Among the nursing staff, I think there is always a tendency to look askance at any situation in which any male and female patient spend time alone together, and there's probably a certain amount of snickering comment which tends to be suppressed more or less in the presence of the doctors, who, the nurses feel, condone more of this thing than is really right. I think there are two primary reasons for this: one is the social class difference between the doctors and nurses. Each group has a somewhat different set of sexual attitudes and the nurses are, I think, more of the straight-laced lower middle class variety. The second reason is, I think, that the doctors tend to regard the situation more in terms of individual dynamics and in some ways to blot out current reality.

Much the same attitude was expressed by the residents as by the seniors on the matter of the rigidity of the hospital hierarchy. Dr. Rivers, for example, said:

(Picture 11, Dr. Rivers) . . . I think the routine is always too conservative and restrictive, and frequently too much along the lines of a military institution, so that things that never have been done just never get tried. The nurses have very little to say. I don't think they dare say very much and, unfortunately, when they do say something they are confronted with it and asked to speculate about it as if they were in the patient's chair, and this makes the nurse defensive, and that is the end of that. . . . It leads to resentment and general discomfort, to the feeling that you'd better keep your mouth shut.

Dr. Rolfe echoed Dr. Rivers' concern over the fact that the administrative hierarchy led to the concealment rather than the dissemination of information:

(Picture 11, Dr. Rolfe) . . . The general feeling is: "Let's get it over with without being picked on." We have a tendency to make the nurse or doctor responsible if the patient doesn't do what he is supposed to. Dr. Ramsay always gets hell, for example, when Miss Miller behaves badly, and this is a pretty frustrating feeling, because you know you have no chance really to influence the behavior. . . . A good deal of inter-staff fighting goes on. The nurses feel defensive and they pick back at you. When I notice a clear mistake in nursing and mention it to the nurse, then five minutes later I hear that my patient threw something at someone else. . . . You have to think over carefully what you bring up at administrative rounds, when you bring it up, and how you bring it up. I think first, you should not bring things up that you are sure will be answered negatively. Then the routine things—I speak about little decisions—you base on whether you think you have enough personal prestige to have them get through. . . . And then, of course, you can take a short-cut and avoid a long and fussy discussion when you just invent a good psychodynamic reason. I get regular hell about Mr. Erskine's behavior. I can take an honest and open approach or I can take the dishonest way and say I will explore what it means to him, and then everything is fine and he can do what he likes.

The second category of material on the interaction of staff with the hospital-in-general was concerned with the lack of integration and uncertainty of procedure. This material had two broad aspects: (1) a sheer lack of acquaintance by various role groups with certain of the physical features of the hospital as well as a lack of knowledge of hospital rules; (2) the fact that many of the hospital rules and procedures were inconsistent and caused confusion in the minds of the staff.

As to the first aspect, the seniors were simply unacquainted with the details of the physical makeup of the hospital. This was similar to the state of affairs noted earlier for nurses, where a nurse working on the open ward would not have any real knowledge of what life was like on the locked ward. The seniors frequently were stumped as to the location or meaning of a scene which the other three role groups recognized immediately. This can be demonstrated by the initial reactions of many of the seniors to Picture 3, which is an everyday scene in the nursing station on the open ward where the patients signed out and in. In response to this picture, Dr. Sloan said: "I don't know where this next scene takes place, I'll have to venture a guess; hence what I have to say now is a supposition. . . ." Equally, Dr. Sutton said: "That's new to me. I can only guess what that is. I wouldn't exactly know. I suppose the patients have to sign a book when they go out or when they come back. . . . I don't know." Lastly, Dr. Scott said: "Well, I'm not quite sure, I was a little puzzled initially by this one. . . . The actual locale, I'm not certain, all I would say is that it seems to be the angle of a ward and presumably somewhere near a door, although if this is supposed to be the nursing station. . . . I must confess that I don't really know about this procedure."

The lack of integration in the second sense of conflicting goals and rules was reflected in what Dr. Scott had to say about the supervisory relation between seniors and residents on Picture 10:

> (Picture 10, Dr. Scott) . . . I simply have the general feeling that they don't really get together about what is the crucial problem. . . . This must be so because the supervisor is usually not somebody who is engaged in the hospital context of treatment, but who is in part-time private practice, and who therefore tends to think almost entirely in terms of the therapeutic relationship itself as it exists between him and the patient. The resident has wanted to get fairly definite advice about "what shall I do about the patient," and he has gotten this, but in not too clear a way. He departs with a somewhat mixed feeling about what really is the most definite thing to do. This may be enhanced by the fact that he may also have talked this over with the director of the hospital, who has said something else, and the whole problem is to be able to harmonize the conflicting opinions that he is left with. . . . I think the senior man would feel again as if this had been a rather perfunctory experience for him. He feels he hasn't really known enough about the patient, that he may or may not have satisfied the resident's need for certainty, but that he has only a part-time obligation to the hospital and he has discharged it. . . .

The residents in particular brought up the problem of the lack of real involvement with the hospital on the part of the supervising physicians. Dr. Ryan, for example, on Picture 10 said: ". . . By and large the resident is going to feel the supervisor doesn't have much contact with the hospital, and this is going to be so much theory, and the actual management of the patient is going to be up to him or the chief resident or the head of the hospital. . . . I think this relation makes for rather difficult integration of policy, and the resident, who is just beginning to learn, is torn between many possibilities that he isn't really equipped to integrate."

The nurses also saw a problem of integration in terms of the remoteness of the senior physicians, with whom they felt they had little contact. This can be seen in what Miss Nicholas and Miss Noyes had to say:

(Picture 10, Miss Nicholas) Ah. The supervising hour, and this supervising hour to me is a complete farce. Mainly because the supervisors have never even seen the patients they are supervising, and they are merely going by a secondhand telling of what the patient is like. I feel many of the plans and decisions they make in the supervising conferences are completely unrealistic. I think definitely that junior residents need very close supervision. . . . I think they need someone to direct them, to explain to them, to help them grow in their handling of the therapeutic situation, but I think that the person who is doing it should have much more contact with the patient and the setup in the hospital. . . . In this situation the resident is probably wishing he had more help. I can't tell you much about the senior, because I don't know any of the senior men. I have never talked to any of them, and I've never seen any of them down on the ward except Dr. Sloan to pick up Joe, or Dr. Saunders to pick up Ellen. But, if we had the staff available to take these patients up to their offices, they wouldn't even come down for that. They call down to ask if we have someone, and if not, they come down to pick them up. . . .

(Picture 10, Miss Noyes) . . . My own feelings are that these senior doctors should have a little contact with the patients in order to help these resident doctors with the cases. And if they didn't have direct contact, they should at least get down and read the nurses' notes and talk with the nurses about these particular patients. Of course, this might be a resident who is just the administrative doctor. He is trying to find out from the senior man what is going on in therapy so he will know some of the meaning of the patient's behavior on the ward. Also, the administrative doctor wants to know how the senior man wants the patient handled, that's providing the senior man wishes to fit in with the hospital. I don't think they know the policies of the hospital, which they should if they are to be in the situation. If they are acting as the therapist, and the resident is acting as the administrator, they often tell the patients they can do something that is against the policy of the hospital, such as going out or having certain things in the hospital which are not permitted. These things should be up to the administrative man, but I don't think we have a definite line drawn there, not straightened out completely. . . .

There are several things that should be pointed out specifically in the material just cited. First, both nurses insisted that the supervising physician should have had more contact with the patients and the procedures of the hospital. They were unaware of the possible usefulness involved in the supervisor's not directly knowing the patients, in order that the resident might have an objective third person who was not part of the situation with whom to talk. Be that as it may, the nurses were probably correct in their observation that the seniors needed to know more than they did about the daily work of the hospital.

Secondly, the rather slighting reference in Miss Noyes' material to "a resident who is just the administrative doctor" represents an over-evaluation of the technique of psychotherapy and a depreciation of the administrative resident's ability (as well as probably her own) to understand the behavior of patients on the wards except in terms of what was going on in the psychotherapeutic sessions. As indicated in Chapter 2, the hospital under study, like many psychiatric hospitals today, was in a state of transition, with an increased emphasis on psychodynamic principles. The nurses were confused about their own worth and role in this setting, and had come to believe, somewhat vaguely, that they could understand what was "really important" if only the doctors would tell them what went on in psychotherapy. Some of the results of too exclusive an emphasis upon the meaning of individual psychodynamics were discussed in Chapter 5.

Both these matters—the lack of contact between role groups and the depreciation of administrative functions—are pertinent to thinking about the future structuring of a psychiatric hospital and about changes in the training of residents and nurses. Whatever the pros and cons of these matters may be, the fact remains that the residents and nurses felt the senior physicians were not in touch with the daily work of the hospital. The patients seemed to share this feeling (see Chapter 5), although they did not comment upon it very often in their interviews. Mr. Edwards, however, did say:

(Picture 10, Mr. Edwards) . . . Strikes me as somebody interviewing the boss. . . . The doctor who comes here is a resident and is interested in getting himself a good recommendation wherever he chooses to go. As for doctors who are seniors—well, I know of no single senior doctor with the exception of Dr. Scott, and who is that woman doctor, I don't remember her name, but maybe she has the same rank as Dr. Scott. I would surmise that she has the same rank as Dr. Scott. (The anthropologist asked why.) Well, for one thing, she's rarely seen; she's not seen much more than Dr. Scott, and that would suggest she's in the higher echelons. I suppose from that it's quite obvious she is in the higher echelons.

The lack of integration and the uncertainty about procedure in the hospital blends into the third category of topics—the discomfort experienced by the various groups in carrying out their particular roles. Especially this was true for the nurses who said they preferred working on the locked ward, where they could utilize more of their previous training, to working on the open ward, which was seen as an unknown, threatening, and hostile place. The discomfort of the nurse on the open ward seemed to cause her to defend herself by criticizing the types of patients who were admitted—mainly the "character disorders" were a target for hostility—and by retreating into the busyness of routine duties. Miss Nicholas was again very perceptive on these matters as well as on the effects of the change in the therapeutic program of the hospital:

(Picture 6, Miss Nicholas) . . . The nurses who work on the locked ward usually don't like the open ward. The feeling is that the locked ward patients are psychotic, their behavior is caused by their psychoses, and the reason for the behavior makes it easier to work with it. . . . I would absolutely refuse to work on the open ward under the setup as it now is. From my view, I have a feeling that the open ward is going in all directions. There is no order or plan from the top down about what should and should not be going on. . . . Another thing is the continuous, subtle hostility on the open ward. . . . The main bone of contention is what we label the character disorders. So far we have not helped one of them, and hospitalization is not the answer. If the open ward is supposed to be for psychotics who are better, then the open ward is a step to the outside, and that would be my view. I could see the neurotic patients there, but the character disorders, no, because of their need to act out toward authority. If you've spent eight months on the locked ward working with a psychotic patient, and then send him to the open ward, after working with him to get him to the point where he can believe in love, and then throw him into that mess where there is nothing but rejection and hostility, it is saying to him, in essence: "Look at the nice, pretty place you were, and people liked you, and now we are going to put you right back where life was before." There must be a place, but I don't know where it is, for the character disorders—they are nasty and intolerable, the hospital isn't the answer. Maybe we need another war and commando troops for the sake of the other patients and the staff. . . . The whole problem of the open ward is so complex. It involves the change in régime, and the emphasis in the hospital of a new type of therapy. Conflict between the older nurses and the newer residents. The nurses have been here for ten years or more and have seen a lot of changes. I think they are a flexible group, but by this time they just say: "Well, they'll come and they'll go, try a lot of new things, but they won't really work." (The anthropologist asked Miss Nicholas to tell him a bit about how things were on the locked ward.) From my point of view, it's an interesting place, a very warm place. The staff on the locked ward have a really genuine interest in the patient, and are interested in their work. . . . The locked ward is an easier place to be, the behavior is so different. You can put your finger on it and say: "Here is the symptom." It's not this everlasting delving into details. I think the open ward mirrors more than any place else the conflicts and lack of coordination in the whole hospital. . . . Also, the locked ward is easier, as it is much more what the psychiatric nurse knows as a mental hospital. You couldn't find a psychiatric nursing textbook anywhere that could tell you about the care of the neurotic patients unless you went to a child growth and development book. I don't think the nurse has any security. No definite body of knowledge to hang her hat on with neurotics. With psychotics, you can read and study what their behavior means. There are innumerable books about how to handle psychotics, but nothing for nurses on neurotics. (The anthropologist said to Miss Nicholas that she mentioned that the open ward mirrors the confusion in the hospital.) It mirrors the lack of direction. Probably because of the constant testing by the patients to see how far they can go. No definite limits. Their hostility toward the nursing staff. They've picked up a lot of feelings of the residents and probably of the higher-ups too, that there really isn't anything to psychiatric nursing. The residents have conveyed this to the patients. . . . It also reflects just how the very top fits into this, although I'm not sure. The nursing staff feel that there are those grandiose powers up there who make the decisions, and there is no way of fighting back at them or of working with them—it's all so intangible. I date a lot of this business about decisions from the time some months ago when somebody decided that we were going into the hole financially. Somebody decided that the first place to cut down was the nursing staff. I think that this brought to a head a lot of the frustrations the nurses were feeling. . . . I think it mirrors the panic we are now in as we are losing three full-time staff nurses—two pregnancies and one leaving who has gotten a job on straight days. . . .

Miss Noyes echoed the feelings of Miss Nicholas about the types of patients on the open ward when she said on Picture 9: "It's the types of patients who come in, the types of patients we get on the open ward. We've always had these situations, and I think we always will, but we've got to learn to get around them. I think if we were rigid in the beginning, we'd have no problem, but that isn't the way we are, so we have to work through each one of these situations."

The use of routine busyness as a defense against relating to patients will be discussed in more detail later. It was indicated when Miss Nash said on Picture 9: "You think about going into a patient's room, but the phone rings. If you do get in to talk with them, you have to run off, and anyway they don't seem to want to talk to you."

It was particularly interesting that some of the residents saw the nurse in difficulty with her fellow nurses because she was able to form a warm relation with the patients. This can be seen in the material given by Dr. Ryan in response to Picture 9:

(Picture 9, Dr. Ryan) . . . I think the feelings the doctor would have is that this is a helpful relation, and that this nurse will turn out to be one of the more significant relations for the patient. This may be frowned upon by the other nurses, who feel that they should not in any way lend strong personal feelings to relations with patients, and because of this the relation between this nurse and her superiors may be a strained one. (The anthropologist asked why such a situation might be.) In part because of their nurses' training that they should be professional at all times, and in part because of their own anxiety about what would happen if they were actually to discuss the patient's problems and find that their own problems were not too dissimilar—this would be very disturbing to them. Also, they may fear that the doctors would not approve of a close relation in spite of the fact that the doctors continually say that this is something they would like the nurses to do. The doctors and the other nurses also may give the nurse the feeling that she is trying to solve her own problems by discussing them with one of the patients. (The anthropologist asked Dr. Ryan what he felt might be some of the answers.) Some of the answers, or one, might be a more helpful orientation of the psychiatric nurse in the sense that she could be taught more about what psychiatric treatment is, and with a playing down by the doctors of so much emphasis on dynamics and the erotic elements in the relations of nurses with patients. And in another way, by loosening the formality of the nurses' organization. Nurses could be without caps, allowed to smoke on duty, and much less emphasis put on routine, such as note-keeping. All this would free the nurse from a rigid schedule and allow her to be warmer with the patients, more genuine. . . . This over-maintaining of external appearance is a manifestation of inner insecurity, and if you are not sure of your individuality, then you have to use all sorts of methods of presenting it to the outer world. . . . The threat of criticism is a very strong threat, and until the group is loose enough and friendly enough so that criticism can flow freely, we are going to lose a lot of valuable spontaneity, going to dampen down a lot of new ideas.

Under the circumstances described by Dr. Ryan, the role of the nurse was a difficult one because of the negative and somewhat punishing attitudes expressed toward nurses whose own feelings became involved in their relations with patients. A similar difficulty was mentioned by the residents, who felt that their contacts with the senior supervisors were made less rewarding by the tendency of the supervisor, since he was not in touch with the reality of the hospital, to interpret matters too much in terms of the resident's own personal problems. For example, Dr. Reynolds said:

(Picture 10, Dr. Reynolds) . . . This resident has seven or eight patients, and he has found himself in considerable difficulty with the management of two or three of them. He has a tendency to be overidentified with the patients, and has some hostility toward the policies of the hospital. . . . The resident is trying to get some feeling as to how much of the situation is really related to his personal problems, which he recognizes, and how much is due to a basic feeling of disagreement with some of the hospital policies on a reality basis. He feels there is too great a tendency on the part of the supervisor to make everything into a personal problem on the part of the resident. . . . The supervisor has very little contact with the ward and with the patients. His involvement in the ward policies is not great, and he can have very little understanding of the reality situation, although he appreciates the amount of emotion on the part of the resident that goes into it. . . .

Just as Dr. Ryan felt that the threat of negative criticism blocked communication with the nurses, so Dr. Shaw felt that the same thing was true in the supervision of the resident's therapeutic work. Dr. Shaw also noted that such a blocking of communication led to defensiveness and identification with the patient on the part of the resident, as was mentioned by Dr. Reynolds and discussed as one of the factors in the history of the collective disturbance in Chapter 5:

(Picture 10, Dr. Shaw) . . . I think in the setting that I describe, the supervisor feels the need to add the wisdom of his experience, and I say that a little critically, because I think there is a need to maintain status that creates an awkwardness and adds to the need of the resident to make himself appear to be as near equal in competence as possible, without feeling at ease to explore and discover what his errors and mistakes are. There is a kind of smug assumption that the problems that the resident is having in dealing with his cases have to do with the resident's psychopathology, . . . and this must be very difficult for the resident. It's a thing against which the resident reacts critically because he has a feeling that he's treated like a patient, whereas many of the things that he omits and doesn't handle skillfully, he could have a learning experience from, despite the fact that behind it there might be some neurotic problem on his part. . . . It means that there are some subjects that are scarcely broachable. I think this really intensifies the empathy of the doctor for his patient, and a kind of sense of defensiveness about his patient. . . .

The matter of supervision, with its difficulties and successes, was a very important one for the residents, as they felt this was potentially the most rewarding area of their training in the hospital. Therefore, they were much concerned over working out a good relation to the supervisor. Dr. Rolfe indicated this problem very well when he said:

(Picture 10, Dr. Rolfe) . . . The junior resident doesn't know that his presentation is too long, is not focused on important data, and he gets the feeling that the supervisor makes a decision, gives advice, or touches the case without even listening to the full story, and without seeing the patient. The short outcome will be that the supervisor will leave ten minutes before the time is supposed to be up. The junior man will feel kicked out, and that he didn't get something that he was supposed to get. Because supervision is like pay in the hospital. Practically speaking, you work here for the supervision that you are getting, and for some courses. In the long outcome, I think the junior resident will improve his presentation, and make an adaptation to the supervisor. The supervisor will get more acquainted with the resident, which will reduce his tendency to think that he is getting too much stuff, and they will come to a reasonable cooperation. Part of the resident's feelings comes from the fact that there is a tendency of all the supervisors to cut down on time. . . . All the residents have these experiences—each money of the supervisor—each minute, that's a good slip, has real value. The more the supervision develops, the more you appreciate the value of what you get and not the time; a quantitative approach is changed into a qualitative one. . . .

As for the patients, they were quite aware that the resident, as well as the nurse, had a difficult role to play in the hospital. The patients were sometimes critical, yet showed considerable understanding, of the difficulties in the way of the development of a fairly free relation between the resident doctors and the patients. This role relation between residents and patients seemed to founder on much the same shoals as did the relations between nurse and patient, or between supervisor and resident—the rigidity of the hospital hierarchy, the lack of integration of policy and procedure, and the questions in role identity of "who and what am I." Mr. Osgood indicated some of these problems when he said:

(Picture 11, Mr. Osgood) . . . I suppose in a way, it wouldn't do for the doctors to let the patients know that they are human too, I suppose the doctor has got to play the role of a demigod in order to keep his position of authority, and if that was knocked down, it would really play hell. . . . I suppose half of the time the doctors don't like what they're doing either. . . . Once in a great while you feel sorry for them—they walk in the room and everybody stops talking. Not too many say hello, makes them feel awful lonely. Just twice as bad, considering the fact they are trying to help the patients. . . . (The anthropologist asked why the patients stop talking.) It's just the idea, with no doctor around, of sitting down and enjoying themselves, and I suppose the patients transfer their feelings about authority to the doctor; they are afraid of the doctor and expect the same treatment that they were accustomed to before they came to the hospital. The poor doctor walks in not thinking about it, and gets it in the neck. The doctor walks in hoping he'd get a cheery hello for a change, and gets met with a lot of stony silence and stares. . . . The doctors are bound to react to the attitudes of the patients. It doesn't just bounce off, and they are in a pretty rough spot sometimes. It depends on how well adjusted the doctor is, the more well adjusted he is, the easier the relations would be between the patients and the doctors. . . .

In summary, then, the interaction of both patients and staff with the hospital-in-general was viewed rather pessimistically. Relatively speaking, however, there was a good deal more optimism about the interaction of the patients with the hospital-in-general. In no other area of life—therapy, administration, or human relations—was the world of the hospital seen so pessimistically. And it is to these other areas that the discussion now turns.

CHAPTER 9

Therapy, Administration, and Human Relations

Life in the hospital may be divided, somewhat arbitrarily it is true, into matters of therapy, administration, and ordinary human relations. The distinction between these becomes sharper if the main goal of an action is considered—whether the purpose is getting well, getting work done, or getting along with other people. On the one hand, a major aim of this book is to show the interrelatedness of actions in the hospital—how administrative actions have therapeutic consequences, or how ordinary human relations on the ward affect the progress of patients. On the other hand, it is also an aim of this book to show the difficulties that are encountered when the main purpose of one type of action is obscured by treating it as if it were part of another type of action, as in Chapter 4, when a meeting on the ward for the transmission of an administrative decision to the patients was handled as if it were a group therapy session. Both the interrelations between areas of life, and the usefulness of a clarity of purpose in actions, are evident in the picture interview material focused on interaction in the three areas of life to be discussed in this chapter.

THERAPY

As indicated in Chapter 6, topics were scored in the area of therapy if they were concerned with a conscious attempt on the part of one person to participate with, influence, or evaluate another person with reference to the problem of getting well. As such, therapeutic interaction could occur between residents and patients in psychotherapy, seniors and residents in supervision, nurses and patients on the ward, and patients in their life with each other.

TABLE 9–1. Number of persons and topics showing optimism or pessimism about therapy, by role group and type of interaction

Type of interaction	Seniors (N=6)		Residents (N=5)		Nurses (N=10)		Patients (N=18)	
	Persons	Topics	Persons	Topics	Persons	Topics	Persons	Topics
Seniors with residents								
Optimistic	3	3	2	2	7	8	14	14
Pessimistic	3	3	3	4	3	3	4	5
Residents with patients								
Optimistic	3	4	5	8	1	2	10	12
Pessimistic	3	3	0	2	9	12	8	10
Nurses with patients								
Optimistic	3	5	2	2	9	24	2	3
Pessimistic	0	4	0	0	1	3	7	12
Patients with patients								
Optimistic	2	3	2	2	1	1	7	8
Pessimistic	0	0	0	0	2	2	1	1

As can be seen from Table 9–1, the therapeutic interaction between residents and patients was viewed optimistically by the residents; the seniors and patients were about equally divided in their opinions; and the nurses were quite pessimistic. It is interesting that the residents, who did the therapy, were the most optimistic.

The majority of topics on the therapeutic interaction of residents and patients came from Picture 2. The manifest content of this picture of a psychotherapeutic hour was such as to cause interviewees to start their topics rather pessimistically. This became apparent during the pilot study referred to in Chapter 6, and if it had been possible another picture would have been substituted in the actual research interviewing. As it was, there proved to be a considerable difference of opinion between role groups regarding the outcome of the hour. In this sense, the seniors were equally divided as to the outcome of Picture 2, with 3 optimistic and 3 pessimistic. The residents had a different proportion, with 4 optimistic to 1 pessimistic. This proportion was reversed for the nurses who had no optimistic topics and 10 pessimistic. The patients, like the seniors, were about equally divided, with 10 optimistic and 8 pessimistic.

The quality of the seniors' topics can be seen in the following examples, where Dr. Scott was optimistic while Dr. Sloan was somewhat pessimistic:

(Picture 2, Dr. Scott) . . . The psychiatrist seems to be relatively relaxed, the patient less so. The patient gives the impression of some tension and uneasiness in his posture in the chair. . . . I feel that this might be somewhere near the beginning of a doctor-patient relationship. . . . I have the feeling, however, that there is some kind of an air of expectancy, as if the psychiatrist were waiting for the patient to speak. My impression is that there is some attempt being made to allow the patient to tell his story, but that the psychiatrist is rather expectantly structuring the situation so that some information gets out that would be useful in the creation of a case history record. . . . I would see this in terms of the beginning of a psychotherapeutic process. I would foresee a progressive relaxation on the part of the patient, and a progressive increase of interest by the patient in the interaction with the psychiatrist. I would anticipate this as happening over a period of several weeks with these kinds of interviews going on. . . . As to this particular session, I would have the temptation to say that it ends with increased interest, and maybe even hope on the part of the patient, and that, in other words, I would simply say that I could narrow down my optimistic prognosis of this even to the ending of this particular interview. . . .

(Picture 2, Dr. Sloan) This is a rather carelessly dressed patient in the psychiatrist's office. His posture is limp, and the patient seems to be a little perplexed and not altogether happy, which is an understatement. . . . I personally don't care especially for the arrangement of doctor and patient. There is a certain formality about the arrangement which I think would make this patient quite uncomfortable. I don't know how much the doctor will get out of this interview. I have the feeling that he's asking a lot of questions for information, and perhaps he is not getting replies to them, or answers that are not quite satisfactory. . . . I think that the patient will slump out of his office, annoyed, not very happy about the whole thing, and in all likelihood the doctor himself will feel somewhat uncomfortable about what happened in the interview.

The residents were the most optimistic of all groups; yet, at the same time, they often felt uncertain in their role, since they were having their first experience in psychotherapeutic work. For example, Dr. Reynolds said:

(Picture 2, Dr. Reynolds) This picture shows a patient and a doctor starting out in a treatment relationship. The patient seems to have a rather sullen, withdrawn expression. . . . The doctor looks comfortable and relaxed, and seems to be prepared to give the patient whatever time he needs to get oriented in the situation. The feeling on the part of this patient is one of weariness. He's very anxious to get established in a good relation with the doctor; he has a great many problems that he is willing and anxious to discuss; however, he feels that he can't really enter into the situation until he has achieved some kind of an estimate of what kind of doctor he has, and how the doctor is going to respond to him. The doctor is not highly experienced in the techniques of psychotherapy, and he probably doesn't feel quite as secure as his posture seems to suggest. On the other hand, his basic feeling toward the patient is one of a desire to help him, and also a desire to size up the patient and get some kind of a line on what direction his therapy should take. . . . This young doctor hasn't treated a great many patients and has some conflict between his need and desire to help the patient, and his relation to his immediate supervisor. . . . The doctor finally breaks through the reticence and the insecurity of the patient by some encouraging remark which leads the patient off into a discussion of his problem. The doctor feels somewhat uncertain as to how to proceed, and very wisely says very little or nothing, and the interview terminates with a pretty good feeling on the part of both the patient and the doctor. I think the patient feels that the doctor basically wants to help him, and even though he still feels somewhat uncertain and insecure in the situation, the balance of his feelings is positive, and he feels that eventually, when he and the doctor get to know each other, they will be able to get somewhere.

In the light of the pessimism expressed by the nurses about the outcome of the therapeutic interaction between resident and patient, it is interesting that 3 of the 10 nurses suggested that the patient in Picture 2 should receive electric shock treatment. This suggestion was not found in the responses of any of the other role groups to this picture. Indeed, there was nothing in the manifest content of any of the pictures to suggest shock treatment, and an analysis of the material given on all twelve pictures revealed that the question of electric shock was introduced by the seniors 3 times, by the residents 5 times, by the nurses 16 times. Expressing these numbers as a percentage of each role group's total topics (see Table 7–1): the seniors had 2.5 per cent, the residents 4.2 per cent, the nurses 8.5 per cent, and the patients 0.7 per cent. The greater emphasis on the efficacy of shock treatment among the nurses was indicated in their topics on Picture 2. For example:

(Picture 2, Miss Noyes) This undoubtedly is a doctor's office—the patient being interviewed. He is certainly very untidy, looks almost unresponsive. I don't think this doctor got much out of this interview. He looks more like a locked ward patient who is extremely hostile and doesn't communicate. . . . He seems angry and rather determined not to help out in the situation any. He acts as if he doesn't want to be there. After he has been here a while, his attitude might change in his interviews, but that would be a long time after this interview. Of course, he might have a few shock treatments, and he improves. Certainly looks like a long-term patient to me.

(Picture 2, Miss Nye) That's the doctor interviewing his patient, I would say. Looks like a catatonic schizophrenic, yet it could be a depression. Couldn't be a catatonic because he couldn't get in that office. It looks like a depression, could be a form of schizophrenia, maybe a form of both. Looks like a very sick man. Electric shock would help him if psychotherapy doesn't work. He's the kind of patient who looks as though he could be helped. Shock isn't always permanent. Right now the doctor is trying to interview him, but I don't think he's getting much response. . . .

It is reasonable to believe that part of the pessimism expressed by the nurses about the doctor-patient therapeutic relationship was owing to their lack of understanding of the process of psychotherapy. An interesting facet of this was the frequent reference made by the nurses to their suggesting to the patient that he "write down what to tell the doctor." Psychotherapy was thought of much as a "thing" which could be given to the patient, similar to a dose of medicine. The nurses tended somewhat to think of their own activities in these terms, as when they spoke of "giving reassurance to the patient," or that the patient "would not accept reassurance." This confusion about the nature of the psychotherapeutic relationship may be seen in the following topic:

(Picture 2, Miss Nagle) This is the doctor's office. The patient goes in for a conference. He doesn't look like he's going to say much. . . . Not accepting treatment too well. He might come back on the ward and tell all the things he should have said, and I'd suggest he write them down, which I think is a good idea. He might say more to the nurse after the conference, and in that way the doctor could get to these things through the nurse. He doesn't care much about his appearance. His shirt's not buttoned, the sleeves are half rolled up. His pants are half up, no socks, only slippers or loafers on. . . . After a few minutes the conference ends, and the patient goes on the ward and tells the nurse all the things, but he'll later realize that the doctor is the one he should be talking to. (The anthropologist asked what the nurse does in such a situation.) Offers reassurance. And as I tell them, to write it down, as the only way they can remember what they did want to talk about. Actually, they are afraid to mention things to the doctor, and through the nurse they can tell the doctor about it. (The anthropologist asked: "How does the situation turn out for the patient?") Well, I don't know. If he did stop to realize he should make use of his conferences, he might get well. It will take a long, long time.

As noted, the patients were about equally divided in their opinion of the doctor-patient therapeutic relationship, although the balance was on the optimistic side. A very interesting aspect of the patients' topics on Picture 2 was that 10 of the 18 patients concerned themselves at some length with the problem of "time," often beginning with a reference to the incongruity of the patient's wearing a watch. This concern with time on the part of the patients was exclusive with them, as none of the seniors or residents, and only one of the nurses mentioned this problem. In the following remarks about time by the patients, Mrs. Lange handled the matter rather philosophically, whereas Mrs. Lasker was aware of it but not in as symbolic a sense:

(Picture 2, Mrs. Lange) I'll have to rummage around here. The first thing that occurs to me, the doctor looks much more at ease as an interlocutor. Many times I didn't have time to think how my hair was looking, or my shoes, and the general baggy appearance of the poor patient strikes me strongly as I often found myself in this situation. The doctor looks conciliatory, amused, while the patient looks confused, hesitant, and blank. He wishes he weren't there. . . . His attitude as he sits in the chair has a temporary quality, as if he were about to be picked up bodily and taken somewhere else. One often has the sense here of being deposited in places bodily. The impression that pervades the whole thing is a loss of autonomy that the patient feels—no choice that will be recognized. . . . All sorts of aggressive movements are wrong, or are put in the wrong, in the hospital. One is forced into a receptive, subjective mood and can't express even the more wholesome forms of aggression. His clasped hands look as though he were handcuffed, while the doctor has perfect ease of gesture. I often remember having my hands in that position, as if trying desperately to communicate something, and wasn't able to get my hands apart. . . . The patient has a watch on his arm, and that must indicate something, as if he had some comprehension. He is at one level, and has difficulty getting into the next level. Time has a very important symbolism. There were times in the hospital when it indicated to me emotional and sexual development in a sort of time-space concept. Without time there is no emotional balance. The fact that I didn't have a watch at the time on the locked ward indicated this to me. Very few people wear watches there, and any indications by the doctor of time had a very important bearing on the thing. Also the doctor's wearing eyeglasses, and the patients on the locked ward do not have their eyeglasses. The doctor has on glasses here, and the patient has not, and they got mixed up with symbolism for me too. As if the possession of lenses gave the ability to look at past and future. . . .

(Picture 2, Mrs. Lasker) Naturally it's a conference, and he's very uncomfortable, isn't he? I can tell by the awkward way he's sitting. He's scared to death. There's some mistake in this picture—where's the watch on the doctor's arm? The doctor will say: "Oh, here's another one." He's beginning to wonder why he didn't take up dentistry or engineering or something. The patient looks awkward and quite worried at the whole business. . . . The doctor wants to win his confidence. Wondering how to go about it. After all, the doctors don't like failing. Also, please put in a wristwatch; I don't know why the patient has one on, he's not going anyplace.

While the matter of time was important for the patients, only one of the staff, Miss Nicholas, spoke of the matter in her interview material. What she had to say from her observations as a nurse was close to what the patient, Mrs. Lange, had to say about time on a locked ward. Miss Nicholas said:

(Picture 2, Miss Nicholas) . . . This is a doctor's appointment for, I would say, a locked ward patient. . . . His clothes look wrinkled and mussed up. He does, however, have a wristwatch on, which gives you the feeling that all is not abandoned so far as adulthood goes. I notice the watch because when patients get—well—I don't know how to put it—sick, they don't seem to want to wear watches. I have two or three of them out in the cabinet now. It's not that I take them away, but that they just don't want to wear them. I don't know what this means to them. Perhaps—well, a watch is usually a present that most of us get on graduation from high school or college. It means, you're grown up and responsible. Have to be concerned with time. A symbol of adulthood, and when patients give us their watches, it's not that they are concerned with smashing them, but that they are telling us: "Look, don't expect me to be an adult, right now I am a child, or at least I want to be a child." I'm thinking of a hostile paranoid patient we had here. He wore his watch all day long. He smashed it to bits. I tried to pick it up, but he didn't want me to touch it. He wanted it in his room, even though it was smashed to pieces. I took the glass away, but he took the pieces of the watch. When he left here for another hospital, he packed the pieces in a box and sent them along. I don't know just what this meant to him, except he was a very mathematically compulsive personality, and interested in figures, and I sort of think of this compulsive business as having to do with the watch. It symbolized to him when he could be on time, and when he smashed it, he felt that he could no longer do that, and yet didn't want to be parted from it completely. . . .

Another aspect of Picture 2 that was frequently pointed out by the patients was the continued "cheerfulness" of the doctor, oftentimes when the patient felt it was not appropriate. For example, Mr. Osgood said:

(Picture 2, Mr. Osgood) Reminds me of when I just got here, very hostile, and you can't help me here. Immediate outcome is that they did. The doctor seems to be smiling, and saying: "We know. We know." Like Jerry Colonna. Brings to mind you're feeling as low as can be, and the doctors are just so cheerful about it. Well, I suppose this has got nothing to do with the picture. Still, I have the feeling once in a while when I'm not making out too well, and I've got the feeling I'm never going to be cured, and the doctors don't act the way you feel—sometimes they can be the most optimistic bunch. . . .

The patients were, however, on the whole fairly optimistic about the therapeutic relationship between resident and patient and felt that whatever was happening, it would turn out satisfactorily in the end. For example, Mr. Erskine said:

(Picture 2, Mr. Erskine) The situation is that a patient is being interviewed by a psychiatrist in a psychiatrist's office, and the people are the physician and the patient, who are there for analytic treatment. The doctor is there to treat the patient. The doctor is well dressed, and the patient is sloppily dressed—to me that is a very important thing. I used to dress this way, and they say when you dress sloppily, you tend to think sloppily. It's very important. What's more, that looks like me, only somewhat thinner. Well, the patient is there with his problem, and the doctor is sympathetic but firm in his decisions. . . . The patient has a drab face, the things he is bringing up are bothering him. Usually you don't smile when you get as deep as that. . . . It's the doctor's job to see that the patient gets well, and the patient's job to work with the doctor. Both have the same goal—to get one person well. . . .

As can be seen in Table 9–1, the seniors were equally divided, while the residents were more pessimistic about the interaction between the senior physician and resident in the supervision of psychotherapy. The wider context of this relation has already been discussed in the previous chapter on the hospital-in-general. As noted there, the senior man often felt that the resident could not see the underlying dynamics of his patients very clearly; and the resident, on his part, felt that the senior man was not in sufficient contact with the day-to-day work of the hospital, and tended to overemphasize the personal psychopathology of the resident in accounting for difficulties he might be having with his patient. Despite these problems, the resident valued very highly his contact with the supervisor, as was evident when Dr. Rivers (on Picture 10) said: "I think such a discussion is very helpful to the resident, and he gets the right kind of mixture between criticism and encouragement—he is told in a nice way that he might be doing things wrong without crushing him."

Some of the seniors saw the supervisory relationship fairly optimistically, as did Dr. Simmons, whose response to Picture 10 also indicated some of the problems in this type of interaction:

(Picture 10, Dr. Simmons) . . . It's a consultation between the resident and the supervisor. . . . They are both making a considerable show at informality, both are smoking. The supervisor is covering up in this way the sting of rather harsh criticism that he feels he ought to make in terms of the patient's therapy, but realizes that there is not much point in making these points in terms of the resident's inexperience. So he decides on a kind of compromise, he tells the resident largely what he thinks he can take, in as friendly and benign a way as possible. I think that the patient will get well in spite of the problems that are obvious. . . . One of the most prominent problems is the unrealized countertransference of the doctor for his patient, and that is often, even in a *tête-à-tête* situation, a difficult thing to discuss. . . . Sometimes this is still further complicated by the fact that it's displaced from some administrative figure in the hospital hierarchy who has perhaps told the resident that the patient should have shock or should not be moved to the open ward, or something like that. In this instance, the supervisor is in an especially difficult situation because he cannot really side with one or the other, regardless of his own feelings. And in this instance I assume the supervisor is a psychoanalyst, or someone in analytic training, and I see this as a very clear representation of what I have encountered, and his feelings are usually in the direction of greater freedom for the patient, greater emphasis on psychotherapy, rather than shock. . . . I think that the confusion arises in the resident's mind as he tries to serve three masters: his supervisor—four masters, really: his supervisor, the administrative psychiatrist, the patient, and all the things that he himself has learned while growing up and in medical school. I think that this confusion is very frequently passed on to the patient, but it can be worked out to the patient's ultimate benefit if the resident and his supervisor actually talk about this divided responsibility situation. . . . I think that in this particular session whatever current crisis they are talking about will be resolved; that the resident will talk out his conflicting feelings during this hour, and probably at the end of it the supervisor will offer one small concrete suggestion which the resident will then try. He will probably come in next time saying that it did work. I think that the motivation of the supervisor there is at least twofold, and undoubtedly there are many more, but the two on the surface would be: (1) his knowledge that the resident often feels better if there is some direct concrete suggestion; and (2) his feeling that if the resident decides definitely on at least one concrete move during the next week, the sense of definiteness will be passed on to the patient, who is probably at this point feeling that his resident is very indefinite.

Both the nurses and patients were more optimistic about (and further removed from) the supervisory relationship than were the seniors and residents themselves. Most of the nurses reported on the relationship in a rather stereotyped way in terms of the resident's gratefulness at being told what to do. Some nurses went beyond this and felt the resident ought to be told what to do, especially that he ought to be told to deal more firmly with his patients. These aspects can be seen in the topics given by Miss Nagle and Mrs. Nixon:

(Picture 10, Miss Nagle) . . . Some problem has arisen, and he's come to seek further advice from one of his superiors. . . . And the doctor will find out how he should deal with the patient. . . . I should imagine the superior would certainly feel helpful and offer all that he can, and the other doctor feels more at ease, knowing how to handle this situation as it stands. The doctor would take the advice and carry it out as fully as possible.

(Picture 10, Mrs. Nixon) . . . Could be a resident and a man who's directing him in therapy. We only suppose what goes on. The resident is sure his patients are the only ones. He finds it hard to curtail their privileges or to admit they are sick, and it's up to the person who's guiding him to lead him to see just what is going on. Some of the senior men look on them as sons and feel very paternal towards them. . . . It usually puts the junior man in a position of a schoolboy, and he can profit a great deal by it if he can see his mistakes and profit by them. This particular person, he wants to be told. He turns out fairly well. . . .

The patients, in their topics on Picture 10, felt that by and large, the relation between the senior physicians and the residents was a good one. For example, Mr. Onofrio said: ". . . What I am thinking of is the idea that two doctors' talking over a situation makes for a better diagnosis—less chance of error; the head doctor can pick up things overlooked by the ward doctor and get it straightened out." As did the nurses, Miss Peters saw "a teacher-pupil relationship, and working together." She went on, however, to express an attitude more generally held among the patients that the resident staff were too restricted in their exercise of authority: "There is the feeling that the junior staff can't do too much on their own. They have to discuss it in staff meeting, which isn't always good for the patients. A delay in an answer makes the patient wonder if the doctor is evading, or can't decide anything on his own." Finally, a number of the patients felt that the resident doctor must alter reality in order to obtain the desired results from the senior staff. This was evident when Miss Prescott said: ". . . However, I don't think the junior staff is entirely helpless, in so far as they can heighten or lessen the color of a situation to get the result that they want. They can sort of change the story slightly if they think the answer should be yes. They will change what the patient says, which is all right as they know what is better for the patient. . . ."

Turning to the therapeutic interaction between nurse and patient (Table 9–1), the first thing of interest is that proportionately so much more of it was seen by the nurses than by the other role groups. Secondly, the nurses were highly optimistic about such interaction, whereas the patients who gave topics were unequivocally pessimistic.

A good part of this difference of opinion lay in the fact that the nurse was optimistic if she could somehow place the patient in a traditional patient role, and then react to him therapeutically in this context. She was more uncomfortable with the patient if he was in less of a "sick" role. Thus, on pictures of the locked ward or seclusion the nurse could see a therapeutic relationship more easily than she could on pictures of the open ward. Along these lines, it has already been discussed in the preceding chapter how Miss Nicholas, working on the men's locked ward, was able to develop a creative use of the seclusion rooms, and how she was able to calm the fears of a patient who, after an initial experience upon admission, thought of seclusion as a dungeon. In such situations, and with patients who are closer to the traditional state of illness, the nurse has both the protection of the routines of the hospital and a feeling that the patient will be grateful for a warm and often motherly approach. Such an approach to patients was most successful on the locked wards, where the patients were more disturbed, but was less satisfactory with the open ward patients. Nevertheless, the nurses who worked on the open wards, in terms of their training and in lieu of anything else, often used such an approach and were optimistic about it without apparently being aware of the negative feelings it aroused in the patients. For example, an open ward nurse, Mrs. Nolan, said:

(Picture 6, Mrs. Nolan) . . . In comparison, the patients on the open wards are demanding, self-centered individuals. It's not surprising when so many of them are such immature, unhappy little children. I seem to enjoy the open ward patients, and it almost seems as though I can understand something and feel quite comfortable with them most of the time. I've been on the open ward for years, and seem to feel quite capable in handling their little immature demands and in settling their little differences. With some people with whom I am not familiar, I can't call a spade a spade, but I can point out how some of their ideas are ridiculous, and we are able to discuss them as such. . . .

In regard to the uncomfortableness of the nurse in trying to establish a therapeutic relationship with patients on the open wards, Picture 9—showing a nurse talking with a patient in a private room—was particularly troublesome for nurses, and this was a quite unexpected result of the interviewing. On Picture 9 the nurses could not readily see the nurse as a regular staff nurse, but instead often interpreted her role as that of a private duty nurse. If there was some way of putting the patient in Picture 9 in a "traditional sick role," the nurse could talk about the relation more easily—for example, calling the patient an insulin patient who needed special care because of her treatment. Many of these aspects can be seen in the responses of Miss Newcomb and Miss Nagle:

(Picture 9, Miss Newcomb) The first thing is that the nurse must be a special nurse, as general duty nurses don't get settled quite so comfortably. If we have any dealings with the patients, they are usually on the run. I fail to see why that nurse is there anyway. The patient seems busy and not to have any restrictions on her. But again, you could do a lot with a patient like that. Maybe it's a patient on the open ward who doesn't join the group, and the nurse is trying to get her out to join the group. Maybe she's going to succeed in getting her out, but the patient looks awfully comfortable. A setup like that, you wonder why it was necessary for a nurse to come in and talk to a patient, except to try and get her out of the room. She strikes me as not being very comfortable, the nurse does. The patient is much more comfortable than the nurse. I don't know why unless she was told to get the patient out and feels defeated before she starts. . . .

(Picture 9, Miss Nagle) . . . It could be a private duty nurse with either a suicidal or an insulin patient. She looks pretty good, I'd say an insulin patient. This looks more like afternoon after the treatment, and the nurse spends time with her to make sure she doesn't have any delayed reactions, because they both look pretty relaxed. . . . You just have to make sure she's all right. Sit and talk to her and take her out for a walk. . . . Maybe the nurse is just sitting with her with a sort of protective feeling, to make sure she is all right through the afternoon. . . . Well, I've seen some pretty good insulin patients, so I guess she goes along having treatment and gets along pretty well, and goes home.

The patients on the open ward were not willing to accept a therapeutic relationship with the nurse in her traditional role, but did not know how to make any other sort of relation because of the defenses against communication erected by both nurses and patients. Mrs. Lasker, for example, felt that nurses did help patients, but at the same time got a wrong impression of them. Somewhat more pessimistically, patients frequently said they kept their mouths closed when the nurse was around. These, and other, problems in communication between nurses and patients are evident in following excerpts:

(Picture 9, Mrs. Lasker) She has "on constant?" Do they have that here? Or it could be one of the regular nurses visiting you in your room—they do that once in a while. I don't know which it could be—it could be both, as I see the nurses visiting on the open ward for ten minutes or so. Well, she'll come in and try to get all the gossip about all the other patients. That's what they usually do. It all depends on which nurse. Some of the nurses stop in just to ask how things are. I think it's a good idea. It's not done very often, but I've seen it done. They used to visit Mrs. Patterson a lot when she lived next door to me, and I remember someone visited me. It's especially a good idea when you are low, as you don't see a doctor unless it's a vital emergency or you throw a tantrum. If the nurse comes in and she's a decent egg, it makes you feel a lot better, but it depends on the nurse. . . . There's only one trouble. In the beginning you appreciate it, but you talk too much, and everything is charted in the way that the nurses feel, which may not be quite how you feel, and after a while you learn to say nothing. I used to talk a lot and have just about stopped now. Most of the patients try to be very careful when the nurses are around. . . .

(Picture 9, Miss Farrell) Well, if it were me in the same situation, I'd keep my mouth shut. I'd have more the feeling that the nurse is very curious, but that there is no possible way she could help me. I am taking this situation as of a time when I'd feel rather depressed, and the nurse is coming in to help, and I'd watch everything I'd say, knowing that everything I'd say would be put on a report and read, not only by the doctor, but by other people. If the nurse would give more of herself and be more of an individual, it would make the situation even more difficult. I wouldn't know how to act toward her the next day, if she ceased to be a nurse and became a person who was affecting my life. And then again though, it all depends on the nurse. I would appreciate some of them wanting to help me at the time I was having a great deal of difficulty.

(Picture 9, Mr. Erskine) . . . The patient is pouting and griping, and the nurse comes in and tries to comfort her. The nurse doesn't like it too much. Had to rush in and wants to get back to the office. The patient is less pouty, though, since the nurse came in and she had her wish granted. The nurse will go back to her office where she wants to be to get her report written up. I have seen the nurses sitting on the edge of their chairs, wanting to get back to the office many times. The nurses don't very often go in the men's rooms, mostly with the women, although on the locked ward they did come in and visit with the men. The nurse goes away with the thought: "Thank God that's over with." They probably do it other ways, and she might be sympathetic, although I haven't seen it. . . .

The patients, as well as the nurses, were quite conscious of the difference in the relations between nurses and patients on the locked and open wards. The patients felt that the nurse was able to establish a therapeutic relationship on the locked ward, and they wished that she could do so on the open ward. Since she was unable to, the patients indicated that they turned more to each other for such help. For example, Miss Prescott said:

(Picture 9, Miss Prescott) On the locked ward in a woman's bedroom. She isn't feeling too well so the nurse comes in with a cheery word. They don't do that on the open ward. Their talk is probably along the lines of how do you feel, and the patient starts talking about herself at great length, and the nurse listens. If the patient is in a talkative mood, she's probably quite happy that someone came in, or if she wants to be left alone, she is probably annoyed at the nurse's intrusion. . . . On the open ward you can rot before a nurse will come near you. I guess they are not supposed to show any sympathy. Either you get it from your fellow patients, or you don't get it. . . . Well, in this situation the nurse leaves and goes to her office, and the patient was quite glad to have the nurse come in.

As to the therapeutic relationship between patients, the staff saw very little of such interaction, while the patients spoke of it more frequently and were optimistic about it (Table 9–1). This situation was similar to that of the therapeutic interaction between nurses and patients, where the nurses proportionately gave more material than any of the other role groups.

What few topics on therapeutic interaction between patients were given by the seniors and residents were presented optimistically. For example, on Picture 14 Dr. Scott said: "It strikes me as a fairly happy kind of circumstance which might exist between two patients. They are not erotically involved, but are using each other in some sort of sharing way by talking, and are making this more comfortable by drinking and eating. They are discussing mostly the boy's problem; he is talking about his unhappiness and his difficulties, and the woman is listening and trying to share, somewhat passively it's true, but still she's trying to allow him to use her for talking out some of his moodiness." Along the same lines, a resident, Dr. Ryan, said: ". . . The general mood is one of relaxation. The boy and girl seem to be comfortable, relaxed, enjoying each other's company. . . . They have similar interests, and this relationship is a meaningful one to them; it has been healthy for them in their treatment and in helping them to adjust to the hospital. They are able to discuss their problems with each other, and share their views on their problems."

The nurses were much less willing to see the patients in a useful relationship to each other. Miss Nicholas, despite her rather creative thinking in other areas, said on Picture 14: ". . . Once something like this gets started, you find patients in the rooms pouring out their difficulties to each other, and trying to work them out with the other patients instead of with the doctor, who can really help them. . . . I feel that if they are sick enough to be in a hospital, they are certainly not adult enough to carry on any sort of emotional relations. Eventually it comes to a point when they are trying to prove to themselves their own sexuality. . . . You can't tell the patients, 'You can't sit in the room because we think you'll have intercourse,' so it's good to be able to say that the hospital doesn't permit it." The same feelings were expressed by Miss Nagle, who said: "I don't like this situation. . . . Maybe here they are trying to help each other and not seeking help where they should. . . . Someone always does this visiting, but we have the authority to tell them it's not permissible. They have to talk in the living room."

The results of these attitudes held by the staff were that the seniors and residents paid little attention to the therapeutic efforts beween patients except to feel rather benignly about such actions, whereas the nurses were strongly disapproving, especially when men and women were together. Since the patients approved of such interaction up to a point, this was a source of friction with the nurses. These things can be seen in what Mr. Onofrio and Mr. Ashton said:

(Picture 14, Mr. Onofrio) They are visiting and talking, and the nurse comes in and tells them they can't visit. It happened to me once. I thought it was a silly rule. We were talking about the way sickness had affected us, comparing notes on the visits with the doctors. Whichever patient had made the most progress would be the patient who was helping the other one more. It is sort of pulling along the other person, and I am thinking here about my moving from the locked to the open ward. Other patients followed me, and gradually the group situation built itself up again, and I believe that a good group situation helps to make a speedier recovery. . . .

(Picture 14, Mr. Ashton) . . . They are talking about something to do with the hospital. It's pretty serious. How long one of them has been in. They are discussing the guy and his future in there. . . . They are very sympathetic to one another. They have the same tastes, the same sense of humor. While she is sympathetic with him, she is also telling him that the doctor knows best, knows what he is doing. Well, I think he feels better afterwards, it does anybody good to get it off your chest.

In general, while all role groups tended to see the area of therapy fairly optimistically, the various groups differed in their opinions about the adequacy of certain kinds of therapeutic interaction. As to the psychotherapeutic relationship between resident and patient, all groups except the nurses were optimistic in the balance of their material. On the other hand, the residents were rather pessimistic about their relation with the seniors, while the other groups were optimistic—the more so the further they were removed from the actual interaction. There was a considerable difference of opinion between nurses and patients about the therapeutic effect of their relations—the nurses being optimistic particularly when their interaction could be within a traditional nursing framework. As for the therapeutic effect of patients on each other, the patients saw more of such interaction and were optimistic about it. In what attention they gave this matter, the seniors and residents were optimistic, the nurses pessimistic.

ADMINISTRATION

As can be seen in Table 9–2, the pictures elicited material mostly with reference to administrative interaction between staff and staff, and between nurses and patients. The administrative interaction of staff with staff was interpreted optimistically by seniors and patients, opinion was more divided among the nurses but the balance was pessimistic, while the residents were uniformly pessimistic. Most of the material on this type of interaction came from Picture 11, which represented the daily administrative conference.

Those senior physicians who did not attend the daily conferences saw them as running rather routinely and smoothly. For example, Dr. Simmons said:

(Picture 11, Dr. Simmons) . . . Of course I have never attended the morning conference under these circumstances. . . . I suppose the various doctors will report on the problems of their patients, and the nurses will tell about the problems that they have encountered. One or two specific difficulties involving such things as moves from one floor to another, telephone privileges, and so forth, will probably be resolved, but the chief function here is

TABLE 9–2. Number of persons and topics showing optimism or pessimism about administration, by role group and type of interaction

Type of interaction	Seniors (N=6)		Residents (N=5)		Nurses (N=10)		Patients (N=18)	
	Persons	Topics	Persons	Topics	Persons	Topics	Persons	Topics
Staff with staff								
Optimistic	4	5	0	0	4	6	12	12
Pessimistic	2	2	5	8	6	11	4	5
Nurses with patients								
Optimistic	5	11	2	8	4	20	13	30
Pessimistic	1	7	3	11	6	23	5	25
Residents with patients								
Optimistic	0	0	1	1	1	1	2	2
Pessimistic	0	0	2	3	0	0	0	0

the passing on of superficial information. The mood is, I think, one of a routine meeting without special enthusiasm. . . . Well, the session will probably end as all other sessions do, with people being a little more up to date than they were on the preceding morning, but with nothing dramatic being achieved. . . .

Among those senior physicians who were involved in the day-to-day administrative work of the hospital, the tensions and problems of making decisions were much more evident. Many of these have been discussed in the preceding chapter in connection with the interaction of the staff with the hospital-in-general (see Dr. Scott's response to Picture 11 in Chapter 8). The residents expressed the same dissatisfactions as did the seniors: they felt that communication was difficult, status relations were left unresolved, and decisions were not clear-cut.

Similar to the seniors, those nurses who regularly attended the administrative conferences were the ones who were pessimistic, whereas those nurses whose work usually prevented them from being present were optimistic. The interviews of the former group contained such opinions as:

(Picture 11, Mrs. Nixon) Each one sits around waiting for the next one to speak. They talk about these things, but nothing is ever settled. . . .

(Picture 11, Miss Newcomb) Well, I suppose Dr. Shaw is going to start by saying, "Is there anything to bring up?" and we'll all sit in stony silence thinking a lot, probably. You probably think of a lot of stuff to bring up, but wonder if it's worth while. Often it is brought up and is discussed, and nothing is done about it, so you say, why bother. Maybe nothing can be done. I don't know. I think altogether they are a good idea; when something unusual or particularly troublesome comes up, it is brought out. You get to know how other people feel about it, and that changes your own attitude toward it. . . .

(Picture 11, Miss Noyes) This looks like one of our morning meetings, and nobody looks too interested in what's going on. . . . Where things should be communicated about what went on on the ward, but often are not communicated. . . . Sometimes the situation clears itself up before we really get around to it. I think we really take too long in making our decisions. . . .

(Picture 11, Miss Nicholas) . . . I think that it's often true on Monday rounds that the doctor's impression of what went on over the week end is opposed to the nurse's impression. Some Monday mornings it's an awful shock to find out how quiet the week end has been, when you have just torn your hair out over it. . . . I think there is an awful lot more information that could come out at these conferences. I think they are a good step, and having them each morning is good as far as planning goes, but I don't think we use them enough.

The nurses whose work permitted their attendance at the conferences only about once a week were more optimistic and found the conferences useful as a place to obtain specific directives from the doctors. Among these nurses, Mrs. Nolan, for example, said:

(Picture 11, Mrs. Nolan) . . . Well, I think sometimes these conferences are quite helpful and sometimes they aren't. When we heard that Mrs. Fox's husband decided to take her back, we found out why she began to giggle and carry on. Dr. Rivers made the announcement that day, and it was very helpful. We understood why Mrs. Fox has a different slant on the world today. When announcements like that are made, it's passed on to all the other nurses, of course. . . . When we hear what has gone on in therapy, we can realize why the patient presents such a picture, and if we understand it, we feel more adequate in handling the patient. When the patient stays in *status quo* for such a long period of time, we know then it's because nothing, or so little, goes on in therapy. . . . Also it's helpful to have Dr. Scott tell us how to handle situations, to give me a specific statement to fall back on. . . .

By and large, the patients, who said they knew little about it, saw the administrative conferences in an optimistic light. Mrs. Lange's response was fairly typical, when she said: "I can only guess, but the nurses may give their points of view as to the reactions of the patients during the day, and the psychiatrists listen and offer suggestions on how to handle different individuals. . . . They review each case thoroughly and arrange for a meeting to discuss the reactions of patients again." The few patients who were pessimistic brought up such matters as the difference in importance attached to the conferences by doctors and nurses. For example, Miss Prescott said: ". . . As for these conferences, the doctors don't think they are important enough to mention anything very much, and the nurses think they are too important and secret ever to talk about."

As is evident from the above, opinions varied regarding the usefulness of the daily administrative conferences. In fact, the conferences, as well as the wards, provided a sensitive place for gaining understanding of what was happening in the flow of day-to-day life in the hospital. A detailed analysis of the interaction and content of sixty-three consecutive administrative conferences is made in Chapters 10 through 12.

The material on the administrative interaction of nurses with patients did not come from any particular picture, but was spread throughout the interviews. It is useful, however, to discuss this type of interaction in terms of Pictures 17, 12, 3, and 14. In this order these pictures form a series from traditional to quite untraditional situations with which the nurse must cope administratively. Thus, Picture 17—the nurse bringing sedation to a patient at night—is in accord with the nurse's usual conception of her role. Picture 12—evening activity on the open ward, and Picture 3—patients signing a record of their excursions outside the hospital, represent situations which, while not part of the traditional nursing role, are at least more or less in line with other kinds of administrative duties the nurse might perform. Picture 14, however, presents the nurse with the question of how she is to respond administratively to the relations of male and female patients with each other, and this is a situation for which her training has done little to prepare her.

In terms of this series of situations, Picture 17 was seen optimistically by all role groups, with emphasis being placed on the routine nature of the interaction and the comfortableness of the nurse in her role. These aspects may be seen in the following excerpts, one from each of the four role groups:

(Picture 17, Dr. Shaw) This is night rounds. The patient has a repeat order of sedation, and the nurse brings it with her rather than having to go back and leaving the patient awake and waiting in case he should need it. . . . In this situation, the patient is asleep, and she comes in and looks, and then retreats.

(Picture 17, Dr. Reynolds) . . . I think of it as a situation in which she is making one of her routine checks of the patients on the locked ward who have their doors open throughout the night, and are periodically peeked in upon by the nurse. . . . Ordinarily the patient comes to accept the routine and to deal with it in terms of whatever it means to him as an individual. . . .

(Picture 17, Mrs. Nixon) . . . She has an order to give him sedation and she is bringing it with her to see if he is awake. The patient is apparently asleep, so what will happen, when she gets back and finishes her rounds, the patient will wake up and say he hasn't slept at all tonight, and she'll come back with the sedation a second time. . . . He says he's just been lying with his eyes closed. So, he'll take it, and let's hope that he'll be asleep within the next half hour.

(Picture 17, Mrs. Lasker) . . . Whoever it is, is upset or sick, and the nurse is bringing the sedation. The person probably had a rough day, is feeling dopey, miserable, unhappy, and depressed, I guess. I don't really know what the nurse thinks. I don't think this nurse here is feeling anything. She has orders to give sedation, so she is giving sedation. The patient goes to sleep, and is groggy the next day.

The administrative problems presented by the situations in Pictures 12 and 3 were less easily handled by the nurses in the opinion of all the role groups. All role groups were about equally divided between optimism or pessimism on these two pictures.

On Picture 12 the nurses expressed difficulty in knowing how to relate to patients during an evening of recreation on the ward. In such a situation the nurses frequently fell back upon their traditional role, and this created resentment on the part of the patients. These difficulties for the nurses were seen fairly well by the residents, nurses, and patients, but were not well known to the senior staff, who took a rather unrealistically optimistic view of the situation. Contrast, for example, the views of the seniors and the residents in the following excerpts:

(Picture 12, Dr. Scott) . . . The nurse stands with one arm draped over a chair, and I would say she is with this group because it is a happier group; it's less threatening in terms of interaction problems. . . . I would say that the three people who are playing cards after a time decide that they now want to have something to eat, and they suggest that to the nurse, and go together with the nurse to set up the refreshments, and the other patients then join in. . . . I would say that—well—I know this probably doesn't happen, but—my conception of it is that they go to the kitchen and actively help the nurse with the preparation of the food, and I would personally like to see a ward kitchen in all psychiatric hospitals available to the patients themselves, where there can be individual variation and execution of the kind of food that they want, and some preparation of it—in other words, approximating the possibilities of the home situation. . . . (The anthropologist asked what happens at bedtime.) I would have the feeling that almost everyone in this group would go to his room spontaneously—that is, sort of sensing the hour of retiring. . . . The nurse could either be anxious or not anxious about being able to put all the lights out at a specified time. I have the feeling here on the open ward that this nurse would not be unduly anxious if some of the patients had their lights on in their rooms beyond the accepted time for retiring, that she might tolerate this kind of individual variability. . . .

(Picture 12, Dr. Ryan) . . . There is a nurse there kibitzing, and she seems to be pretty well ignored by the three patients playing cards. . . . She's an administrator, but not a person the patients appreciate having around, though she's never been a real threat. . . . This whole scene isn't an infrequent one, except for the nurse sitting in the corner, that's unusual. I've never seen two nurses on the open ward living room at any one time. They rarely go into the open ward living room, as it's a pretty unwelcome spot in general for nurses. And the nurse standing up with her hand on the back of the chair would be an unusual thing, as by and large the nurse would be too much held in by her professional feeling to go so far as to make this much of a physical contact with one of the men patients. . . . It would be healthy if the nurses could act like this. (The anthropologist asked about bedtime.) There might be trouble in that the nurse turns out all the lights, and the patients glare at her, and she'll say, "It's bedtime," and the patients will say, "So what," and there will be a mutual exchange of glances. She comes back and nobody has moved, and finally she says: "You have got to go." They might say, "All right, no use causing trouble," or they'd say, "Go ahead and call the doctor," and the nurse runs to the phone and says, "Doctor, the patients on the open ward won't go to bed. What will I do?" And, as the doctor walks in, they go to bed, and the doctor is disgusted and asks the nurse what's going on, and she says, "The patients won't go to bed," and he says, "Well, they are going now," and the nurse is angry with the patients, and feels frustrated in calling the doctor, yet he's the only one who can handle it. This wasn't really planned by the patients, one of them decides to put up an argument, and they'll all go along with it—not to undermine the hospital, but just one way of showing how they feel about the lights' being out at 10 o'clock, which is a ridiculously early hour, as most of them are used to staying up pretty late.

The nurses were even stronger in their feelings about the discomfort of the nurse on the open ward during the evening. Only one of the nurses, Miss Nash, felt the situation was a comfortable one, while the other nine nurses stressed the administrative difficulties of getting the patients to bed and the tension between nurse and patient. For example:

(Picture 12, Miss Noyes) . . . Probably it's near time for nourishment, or time to go to bed, or this nurse might be trying to finish up the game so she can get the patients into their rooms. She might be asking them what they want for nourishment, but they probably wouldn't want anything the hospital has. At least it's a good time to break up the grouping and get all the patients to have nourishment, but I don't know if they'd stop playing bridge or if they would continue. . . . You might have a few who stall around and refuse to go to bed. One or two will go to bed and be annoyed that the TV is still on, and they complain because it is allowed to go on, and they want to go to sleep. Perhaps some of these people can't go to sleep, and they get a little more out of being able to see something on TV. And after that they are a little more relaxed and can go to bed later. . . .

(Picture 12, Mrs. Nye) . . . The nurse makes the half-hour check, makes refreshments, writes the chart, gives the sedation, and tries to keep them happy, but there isn't much we can do. They prefer to be by themselves and entertain themselves. They play bridge and sit around and talk and smoke. They complain about the refreshments as being monotonous. . . . At bedtime we put the lights off at 10 o'clock, and generally speaking they are good and go to their rooms. If they start breaking ash trays, and start acting up, Mrs. Nixon said she wouldn't go in the living room at all. She goes and calls the doctor, and then they tell him they haven't anything to do, and that's why they do it. . . .

(Picture 12, Miss Nash) . . . Well, perhaps they invite the nurse to join them, and she has to decline because of so many interruptions from the doors that have to be answered, and the telephone, and she can't stay with them long enough to play. She'd like to play, and she hates to refuse them. The patients play cards until 10 o'clock, and these patients who are conversing have gone to their rooms, and at 10 o'clock the nurse will turn the lights out in the corridor, and the patients will ask if they can finish the game, and she'll say all right. When she returns, the patients go to their rooms, and she turns out the lights and goes back to the office and starts sedations. . . . I've never had any trouble getting patients to go to their rooms. Occasionally they'll say, "Oh, we're going to stay up all night," but I say, "Oh, swell, we'll have a pajama party." And we kid, and I say: "Go to your room, and I'll come in and kiss you good night." And Mrs. Paul this morning said she had a bad night because I didn't come in and say good night to her last night. I think this approach is better than a blunt one of being told. After all, they are adults, and human beings.

The patients were a good deal less pessimistic than the nurses about administrative interaction between the two groups. The patients frequently said they realized the nurse was busy and had a rather difficult job to perform. At the same time, they also complained about the formality of the nurse and her lack of flexibility about rules. These two sides to the patients' opinions were evident in the interviews of Mr. Ashton and Mrs. Lasker:

(Picture 12, Mr. Ashton) This is nighttime on the open ward. Actually, it's a pretty typical scene—bridge or canasta going on. Two girls are talking, and one girl is looking out of the window. . . . Everybody seems to be having a pretty good time, enjoying themselves. . . . The two girls talking, one is on the locked ward and the other one is on the open ward. They became very close friends when they were both on the locked ward, and now one is on the open ward. They understand each other. . . . The nurse is just sort of looking in on her way back and forth from the desk, her post. She thinks everything seems to be pretty much under control. I don't think the patients are noticing her. It depends on who the nurse is. If the people like her, they will talk and kid around. If they don't, they will just say hi. At 9 o'clock the people from the locked ward go back there, and the rest go over and watch television.

(Picture 12, Mrs. Lasker) Everyone seems to be extremely social in this picture except that one—she seems restless. Why are all the nurses there? We never have them around. If they were, everybody would feel quite uncomfortable. Just a couple are welcome because they can bridge the barrier—I don't mean barrier—the bridge between nurse and patient. With the others, there is definitely a nurse-patient feeling, sort of a condescending air about them. . . . You know, we do a lot of things that so-called normal people do, but when we do them, they assume such great proportions. Lots of people blow up for a moment, it's just a temporary thing, a perfectly normal reaction. I think that the nurse's reaction is that the person is "excited" or "disturbed." If you could stand this place without losing your temper, there's something wrong with you. . . .

Much the same proportion between optimism and pessimism among the various role groups was evident on Picture 3 as on Picture 12. The residents, in response to Picture 3, emphasized that the nurse was often frustrated by being caught between the patient and the resident physician. Thus, Dr. Ramsay said:

(Picture 3, Dr. Ramsay) . . . The nurse's stance suggests the whole problem of the patients' going out. . . . I see the nurse as passive, and having to put up with it without being able to control it—caught between the patient and the order book. I think the patients would recognize the nurse's feeling of being caught between them and the order book quite clearly, and perhaps the woman signing out is almost feeling as if she were doing something the nurse disapproved of. Probably she is acting just a little bit upstage—the feeling: "Well, you know the doctor said I could go out." The nurse looks as though she has no leverage, even to the extent of protecting her own security. She has to take this kind of response, and can't handle it directly; she has to consider that much of what she does will be reported back by the patient to the doctor, and she will catch it on a personal level without a chance to work this through with either the patient or the doctor. . . .

The nurses expressed feelings similar to those of Dr. Ramsay, and often added that the nurse should insist that the resident write explicit orders for the activities of his patients. This was part of a more general feeling among the nurses that their duties kept them so busy that they were unable to relate to patients. They particularly resented what they felt was the inclusion of a domestic role as part of their duties. Such a domestic role was often linked with the additional work attending the departure or return of patients who were permitted activities outside the hospital. For example, Miss Neal said:

(Picture 3, Miss Neal) Two patients on the open ward returning from going out to buy food for the group. The fellow is probably waiting for the nurse to finish on the telephone, so she can put some of the food in the refrigerator, or have her give them the necessary things to serve it. The nurse is telephoning because the information desk just called to ask about one of the patients, and at this point she's wishing that she had a little assistance, as it's the night the patients are allowed out of the hospital, and she's running back and forth to the door. . . . The nurse doesn't mind if the food is brought in if it is food like pizza, but where it's such things as clams, it takes an hour and a half while the nurse has to stay out in the kitchen, and that's quite a problem because she's the only one on the floor. After they finish their food, they go watch a TV program, and leave the dirty knives and plates on the table. If some of the patients would begin to clean up, the nurse would help, but I don't think it's up to the nurse to clean up. It doesn't happen constantly, but sometimes you have a group of patients who think that after each meal the nurse should wipe off the table, sweep the floor, put the magazines back, and generally be a maid. . . .

On the other hand, despite being busy, some of the nurses indicated that they found time to express pleasure over the patient's evening out, as when Miss Nash said that she would comment on how nice the patient looked and hope that she would have a good time:

(Picture 3, Miss Nash) . . . Well, I think if it were a particularly nice evening and I were working, I'd make a comment on how nice she looked and hope that she would have a good time. Somewhere in the back of my mind I might feel: "I wish I were going out, too." She's telephoning, so probably a superior called for information about one of the patients, and I might be a little anxious to get this person out of the office so I could deliver the message. The patient looked quite pleased when I told her that she was dressed attractively. She'd probably say: "Oh, really, thank you, it's just an old suit, I've had it for five years." For some reason it always seems to be an old suit. (The anthropologist asked why.) Perhaps it is because they are paying so much here, I doubt if they can buy many new clothes. Well, they went out and had supper and went to the theater, and then they came back and she says: "I hated to come back, I was having such a wonderful time." And you'd say: "It's too bad you had to come back." No, I guess you wouldn't say that, but you might be thinking it, and they will tell you something about the meal, and the play they'd seen, and suggest that you see it if you hadn't. . . . The patient goes into her room and gets into bed, and asks for sedation, and you bring it in and exchange a few more words. The patient asks you if you are going to be on duty tomorrow, and if not tomorrow, they ask you when you are going to be on next, and you tell them. You've said good night, so that's all there is to it.

As on Picture 12, the patients also saw Picture 3 somewhat more favorably than did the nurses. In general, the main problem for the patients was that they felt the nurse was unpredictable. They did not know when she would be rigid or flexible, formal or relaxed. The problem was well brought out by Mrs. Matthews:

(Picture 3, Mrs. Matthews) . . . The patient has probably brought back a few personal things that are allowed on the open ward, but that she wasn't allowed to have on the locked ward—some food, and some personal things such as a mirror, lipstick, and cigarettes. . . . The nurse probably doesn't object as long as the things can be kept in her room. But, if they are things she wants to keep in the icebox, the nurse is probably very annoyed. I think this is a ridiculous rule, not allowing people to keep things in the refrigerator. . . . Still, the patient doesn't realize that the nurse doesn't make the rules. She probably gets a couple of things into the refrigerator if she promises to eat them the next day. It's funny, when I have things to share with the group, the nurses are so unpredictable—chase you out one minute, and the next come in themselves and join the group. One would say, "Everybody likes to go into Mrs. Matthews' room," and then come in and have candy; and then the same nurse two or three days later would say, "Girls, you are not allowed in each other's rooms." . . .

The most difficult situations for the nurse were those that bore little relation to her traditional training as a nurse. Such a situation was depicted on Picture 14, showing a male and a female patient talking together in one of the private rooms. All the role groups, in their topics on this picture, were pessimistic about the administrative interaction between nurse and patient.

The reactions of seniors and residents to administrative interaction on Picture 14 can be seen in the following excerpts:

(Picture 14, Dr. Scott) . . . I suppose that if this were two patients together, then a possible ending is that a nurse gets disturbed about this kind of intimacy and tells them that there is a rule that patients should not visit in each other's rooms. So this might, therefore, end on a rather unfortunate note, in the sense that my feeling here is that this is a good kind of exchange between two patients and the introduction of a kind of finger-pointing that this is somehow bad behavior would destroy the good effect that both of these people could have on each other. . . .

(Picture 14, Dr. Ryan) . . . The general mood is one of relaxation. . . . A nurse would open the door, express astonishment, some amusement, a semblance of a professional approach, and she would say that men are not allowed, they know the rules. The nurse feels caught up in the rules too. She can't do much about it. The nurse may feel that the hospital is intolerant, or too rigid, yet she feels compelled to break it up. She reports this to the head nurse, it is brought up in rounds, and each doctor is expected to take it up with his patient. The patients accept this rather grudgingly, and they go out together instead of visiting in each other's rooms. . . .

As was the case on Picture 12 in the discussion of administrative matters that arose during the evening on the ward, Miss Nash was the only nurse who reacted favorably to Picture 14 and felt able to cope with the situation. The other nurses were critical in that they felt the patients either did not know the rules, or were acting out their illnesses, or were violating canons of good taste. The context of these criticisms, as well as Miss Nash's acceptance, are indicated in the following topics:

(Picture 14, Miss Noyes) Well, this looks like there shouldn't be two patients there, it's against the rules of the hospital, and from the looks of it, the people know about it. They both look rather angry and disgusted, perhaps disgusted with the rest of the patients or with the staff, and maybe they just wanted to get away from the group for a while. . . . Some of the staff members might go in and break it up, it depends upon the personality of the person on duty. Sometimes it goes on regardless of policy. . . . They might want to talk, and there is no place to talk, and they don't want to sit in the living room with the rest of the patients, and the only other place they would have would be the room. Of course, these might be patients who don't know the rules. I don't think they are always made too clear to the people when they first come in; and many people wouldn't see any harm in talking to a patient in her room, even if it's considered her bedroom. Of course, one reason for the rule is to protect people who can't protect themselves, and consequently we have to have it.

(Picture 14, Mrs. Nixon) . . . Patients are not supposed to visit in each other's rooms, but it looks like a couple of patients having a midnight snack. . . . The first nurse who went by should break it up. It was very seldom they were allowed to visit in the bedroom. Should have their snacks in a different setting. It must be on an open ward to have bottles and knives and glasses. So, they are either alcoholics or psychopaths. Those are the ones who cause each other the most difficulty. . . .

(Picture 14, Miss Nash) This is a man's room, and this female patient went to visit, and they are discussing their problems and that's why they have retreated to their rooms. They don't want to discuss it in the living room, and one patient is telling the other what type of parents he has and how he was brought up. She is probably listening to his problems, and agreeing with him, and being sympathetic with the other patient. . . . So far as the visiting goes, I don't care. I don't know about the other nurses, but it's like when you are in college or in training, and we used to bring back food to our rooms and share it. . . . I don't make an issue of it. You know they aren't supposed to visit, and yet you know they are going to, and all you can do is remind them not to each time they do it. I think that it's just natural that they should visit if you are living in a place like this. In my own life, in training, we visited each other to borrow a cap, or a dress, or to talk together about a letter from a boyfriend. It's natural visiting. The situation is very similar here, the patients visit very innocently, not to break a rule, but just to tell each other that they got a letter or that they want to borrow something. They don't do it too frequently.

From the patients' point of view, the "no visiting" rule was something of a nuisance. They felt that some such rule was useful for maintaining privacy in one's room, but that the existing rules were too rigid and should be more flexible. Mostly, the patients indicated the lack of a place where they could be alone in two-person groups. They disliked the lack of an alternative to being either all together in the living room, or isolated in their individual rooms. Some of these feelings are indicated in the following excerpts:

(Picture 14, Miss Prescott) . . . Well, not only are the opposite sexes not allowed to visit, but even the same sexes are not allowed to, and people don't always like to talk when other people are around. Other people resent it when two are whispering, and it's much nicer to be able to say: "Come on in to my room for a while, and we'll have a talk." In a way, I think it prevents two girls from being as close to each other as they might be, because they are always subject to the public. Every time Betty comes down, she likes to come into my room, it's much cosier and we are able to talk much more freely. The minute the nurse finds out, she is kicked out. You can't really get acquainted in the living room. You don't want to open up your life to twenty people. . . .

(Picture 14, Mr. Isherwood) . . . I think a man and a woman patient in the woman's room, and I'd say the man patient has brought in some food. . . . The man patient is doing the beefing, and trying to get the sympathy or affection of the girl, and he's made an effort to get away from the group in the hospital and found somebody to talk to. . . . They'll get to talking more; she'll get more interested and so will he. Probably the nurse will come in and bust up the twosome, and both are resentful of the nurse yet realize she's got to do her job, and so the fellow will go back to his room, and they'll agree to do this again some time.

(Picture 14, Mr. Osgood) . . . Actually all very innocent, say a relief from the goldfish bowl, feel more free to express your emotions. If it was me, I'd be making a hard time out of it. Let's say a nurse walks in, and you feel guilty at being caught, and resentful of having it broken up, and at the same time you are relieved of the guilty conscience—more or less the idea that authority is easier to take than freedom. . . .

Mr. Osgood's feelings were those of many of the patients: a desire to be relieved of freedom of choice, yet a resentment of this. Such feelings were heightened by a sense of exposure, the "goldfish bowl" atmosphere. Most of the patients agreed with Mr. Osgood, when, on another picture, he went on to say: "From my point of view I am in a glass bowl and everything I do is noticed, and to hell with it, it's me, take it or leave it."

The manifest content of the pictures was such that it elicited only a few topics concerned with the administrative interaction between resident and patient. There were even fewer topics specifically about interaction between resident and nurse, and these few have been included in the interaction of staff with each other.

In summary, the administrative interaction of staff with staff was seen most optimistically by those role groups and individuals—such as some of the seniors and nurses, and all of the patients—who did not participate directly in this type of daily work. The residents and nurses who were engaged in this work saw it more pessimistically. In the interaction between nurse and patient, all groups saw the nurse as having the most success in traditional situations, with progressively less success in coping with situations for which her training had not prepared her.

HUMAN RELATIONS

In the area of human relations, Table 9–3 shows that the interaction between nurses and patients was viewed optimistically by the seniors and patients, while the residents and nurses were about equally divided in their evaluation. Much of the material in this area came from Pictures 6, 9, and 12.

As in other types of interaction, the seniors' opinions about human relations between nurses and patients seemed to be somewhat overly optimistic when compared with the responses of the nurses and patients themselves. For example, Dr. Sloan said:

> (Picture 9, Dr. Sloan) Well now, here's a female patient in her room. . . . She is conversing with a nurse seated near by. . . . I think the conversation is a friendly chat and probably unrelated to the patient's illness. They may be talking about some of the day's events, or something they read in the newspapers, perhaps about sewing or knitting or some such thing. I would say that it is a kind of formal friendliness, that they liked each other, and perhaps in other circumstances could even be friends. Both seem to be in a fairly good humor. I think that at the end of their little chat the nurse will just say good-night and leave.

The residents felt that good human relations between nurse and patient did occur, but that often the hospital system and the previous training of the nurse prevented such relations from developing very far. These aspects of the residents' feelings were illustrated in the material given by Dr. Reynolds on Picture 9, and cited as part of the scoring examples in Chapter 6.

Among the younger nurses who had been working for a shorter time in the hospital, the human relations between nurses and patients were seen as mutually satisfying. This was apparent in the enjoyment Miss Neal felt in sharing family anecdotes with the patient, as mentioned in her material on Picture 9, cited in Chapter 6. The older nurses had more difficulty with human relations, and stressed such problems as the loneliness of the nurse in her work, the situation in which only patients who

TABLE 9–3. Number of persons and topics showing optimism or pessimism about human relations, by role group and type of interaction

Type of interaction	Seniors (N=6)		Residents (N=5)		Nurses (N=10)		Patients (N=18)	
	Persons	Topics	Persons	Topics	Persons	Topics	Persons	Topics
Nurses with patients								
Optimistic	5	10	3	4	3	10	12	18
Pessimistic	1	3	2	3	5	13	4	13
Patients with patients								
Optimistic	6	11	3	7	2	2	15	29
Pessimistic	0	2	2	4	5	11	3	11
Residents with patients								
Optimistic	0	0	0	0	0	0	1	1
Pessimistic	0	0	1	1	0	0	0	0

were ostracized by other patients would talk to the nurse, and that the behavior of patients must be related to the fact that they were ill. These three problems for the nurse can be seen in the following topics:

(Picture 12, Miss Nagle) This looks like the open ward. I don't think I'd be standing there watching them play cards, but this is probably a friendlier group. . . . Doesn't seem to be any air of tension like there usually is. The nurse is accepted by the patients, and the patients seem glad to have her around. On certain days, complaining days, the patients just sit and wait till the nurse comes around so they can blow off at her; or if they are planning things they shouldn't do, then they hush up when you come around. It's not very comfortable to be here eight hours and have no one to talk to. If you sit down with the group in the living room, they won't talk to you, so the best thing is just to leave them. They are more relaxed, and you are more relaxed, too, if you don't go around them. The nurse might spend some time with the patients, and if they accept her, they'll tell her their problems, and she'll offer reassurance and help. Just like Kay Prescott—someday, she's going to come looking for me, and I'll not be there. One day I went into Kay's room, and Mrs. Nolan thought I was hallucinating. I said: "My God, there's a big black cat in Kay's room." I called the desk and said they had to get it out, and Kay called me all sorts of s.o.b.'s, and took the cat and went home with it, and since then she won't even give me a letter to mail. . . . We had a cat around here once before, and when you work nights and the cat jumps up on the desk, it's scary. You'd see those glassy eyes looking at you. . . .

(Picture 9, Miss Noyes) Well, this is a room on the open ward. Looks like a situation of a patient—I don't know if she's angry or not. She might be discussing one of her own problems with the nurse. She might be angry over the food, or annoyed with some of the other patients, or she might be angry because the doctor hasn't come to see her, or angry at what one of the nurses said to her. . . . She might be discussing a problem of the other patients, not being accepted by the other patients, feeling alone. If she's talking to the nurse, she must be out of the group. The nurse might be telling her she doesn't feel she has to stay out of the living room, she has the same privileges as anyone else, she can go on the ward where she wants to. The nurse looks like she's trying to give her reassurance about the situation and the other patients. She might be trying to explain to her why these patients are doing this. She might tell her about the other patients' needs, or why they are expressing their feelings the way they do. . . .

(Picture 12, Mrs. Nolan) . . . I'd say these three card players must like the nurse, as they are continuing to play, so in this case the nurse is considered as a friend and interested. Otherwise you get that blank expression they look up with, as if to say, "What do you want?" and it makes you wonder what you do want, what you are here for. . . . Everyone likes to be liked, but I don't think the patients really dislike the nurses, but they are ill, and most of us feel that way, that they react the way they do because they are ill. . . .

As may be seen in Table 9–3, the patients were more optimistic about human relations between themselves and nurses than were the nurses. This optimism, however, was frequently qualified by such a statement as: "But it doesn't happen very often." Such a wistful, or irritated, seeking for a relation which was only occasionally found, may be seen in the patients' responses to Picture 9:

(Picture 9, Mr. Osgood) First thing I thought of, a woman patient having a special nurse, and second thing, a woman patient on the open ward and the nurse just came in, and they got to chatting. The nurse forgetting her position, let's say—just happened to click and they forgot about their relative positions. It happens once in a while, but usually the nurse doesn't—most of them—for myself, every once in a while find it easy to have a little talk, I rather enjoy it when I talk with nurses, but for more than a few words, it doesn't happen too often, at least for me. . . . The nurse is probably doing what she would like to do more often. We're not all a bunch of stinkers. It could be one of two things, her duties prevent it from happening more often, or her personality could prevent it from happening more often.

(Picture 9, Mr. Edwards) . . . Suggests harmony, rapport, home-like scene. The way it's drawn it sort of suggests, "I found a home." I think I would say there are moments when one feels quite cozy and home-like. It might even be a scene of somebody who moved off the four-bed ward to a private room, and the nurse is saying: "How do you like it here?" It's nicer to live in a private room than it is in a ward. I'm not sure what else the nurse is saying. Nurses don't spend—well, I don't know—well, I suppose on the women's side you do see a good deal of visiting, but on the men's side they don't visit in the rooms. Sometimes they ask you what you are doing. But this seems to be more intimate, a chat. The patient looks happy. I don't have any fixed ideas about the hospital. I felt differently at different times. . . .

(Picture 9, Miss Lindsey) This is a nurse apparently sitting and chatting with the patient. The patient looks relaxed and as though she is enjoying the company of the nurse, and they seem to be having a pleasant conversation. I'd say it isn't the most common sight on the open ward, I think it would be more usual on the locked ward. As far as I can see, there is no reason why it shouldn't be a fairly familiar situation on the open ward, too, if the nurses were able to make the patients feel comfortable. . . . The nurse may feel she shouldn't be just talking and enjoying herself with the patient, but should be doing something else. She may think because she is rather enjoying sitting and talking to a patient that it isn't quite the thing to do. Well, she may think she's supposed to be straightening out the ward, keeping an eye on other patients, but just sitting and talking is not the thing to do. Or, it's not a good policy to get on too friendly terms, have to preserve a certain barrier. Probably she talks for a while and then gets up and leaves with some sort of excuse. . . .

(Picture 9, Mrs. Matthews) . . . Well, not too often one has a visit from one of the nurses. Looks as though a very pleasant little chat. Of course, she might just have come from the locked ward, and the nurse is there explaining the rules and regulations of the open ward to her. The nurses as a rule don't come in and visit, it would be nice if they did. Oh, they do come in if you are disturbed about something. Of course, I keep my room so cold they don't want to stay in long, but none of them make a practice of coming in. If they do, they don't sit down, but just stand by the doorway. I think feelings vary, according to the circumstances. I think nurses are all very nice and good to the patients in spite of their enforcing all the regulations. These two seem to be very comfortable in each other's presence, no tension there.

An important insight into the difficulties in human relations between nurses and patients came from a separate analysis of Picture 17—the night nurse making rounds on the ward. The following analysis does not appear directly in the scoring on any of the tables, but was developed to explore a particular point. The approach of all role groups to Picture 17 was divided into the following two categories: (1) the nurse was seen as engaged *solely* in routine administrative activity; (2) in addition to her routine activities, the nurse was also seen as responding emotionally and warmly to the patient in either a therapeutic or human relations sense.

When Picture 17 was scored in this manner, *only* the nurses gave material involving a warm emotional relation with the patient; none of the other role groups did so. The actual scoring by role group was: seniors—5 routine contact only, 1 emotional relation; residents—5 routine contact only, no emotional relation; nurses—4 routine contact only, 6 emotional relations; and patients—18 routine contact only, no emotional relation.

The point indicated by these figures is a very important one because, as has been seen in analysis of preceding material, the nurses stressed the traditional and technical aspects of their role and felt the need for firmer and more explicit rules and regulations. The figures just presented suggest the hypothesis that such a conception of their role was partly a defense on the part of the nurses and did not really represent what they wanted. Looking beneath the surface of the manifest content of much of the interview material, it seems that what the nurses actually wanted was to feel they were helping patients, enjoying experiences with them, and doing a productive and creative job on the ward.

It is interesting, in terms of Picture 17, that none of the 10 nurses who were interviewed were regularly on duty after 11 p.m., as the late night shift was rotated among a number of the staff nurses. Thus, the nurses, who worked mainly during the hours when patients were awake, seemed to be projecting into Picture 17 the kind of relation they would have liked to experience with the patients, and felt more at ease in talking about such a relation on a picture which showed the patient in a passive, receptive situation—in bed. This can be illustrated by the material given by Miss Newcomb on Pictures 12 and 17. On Picture 12 she spoke of the problems of the nurse in her contacts with the patients during the evening, while on Picture 17 she spoke of the warmer relation it might be possible to have with a patient at night:

(Picture 12, Miss Newcomb) . . . The nurse feels very comfortable with those patients. You wouldn't go and stand in back of a card player, unless you were sure of your reception. . . . I get the feeling they are getting along quite well. They accept her even if she is a nurse, and she must feel on a good footing with them, or otherwise she wouldn't be right there. Of course, maybe she's urging them to do something else. Maybe she's trying to break up the game. Maybe it's bedtime. She's standing there, hanging on to her chair to steady herself and get ready for the barrage; they don't like to go to bed. . . . I'd still like to see an institution where everything was carried out to the letter. . . . Well, if I were the nurse standing there, I would ask them to go to bed. I'd be a little rougher on these people playing cards than on this one who is alone by the door. I'd let her stay in the living room until the others were out. . . .

(Picture 17, Miss Newcomb) . . . I think it must be the middle of the night, because she's got her flashlight. The patient can't sleep, so she's asking for more medication, or the nurse has observed she's awake and is going to offer her more medication. If the medication is the right kind for that patient, she'll go back to sleep. . . . On the other hand, if it's a patient who asks for a great deal of sedation, I would try to reassure her without giving it. Try to find out why the patient is awake. At that time of night you have a closer bond to people than in the daytime. Every minute is an hour. The patients are insecure at night, and you can find out much more from them than in the daytime. Sometimes it even helps to hold a patient's hand. It sounds melodramatic, but it works, and they go to sleep. That's one time when firmness does not bring you anything. . . .

The material given by Miss Newcomb was typical for those 6 nurses who saw the nurse as relating emotionally to the patients on Picture 17. As previously indicated, however, the patients did not see the nurse in such a manner, so that the nurse's feelings were not reciprocated. For example, what Mrs. Lange said on Picture 17 was similar to the responses of the other patients: ". . . The patient is asleep and the nurse is coming in with a sedative that may have been prescribed for that particular time. Not much to tell except that the nurse comes in with the sedative, and the patient goes to sleep afterwards. The nurse is just going through her routine duties."

Turning to the interaction of patients with each other in the area of human relations, it can be seen in Table 9–3 that the seniors, residents, and patients were optimistic, while the nurses were pessimistic. In their optimism, neither the residents nor the patients were unrealistic in their evaluations; both groups saw the relations between patients as predominately good but capable of causing difficulty. On the other hand, the seniors were overly optimistic, and the nurses seemed to see little but difficulties.

On the positive side, the residents felt that the patients were able to do small things for each other which made life more pleasant in the hospital. On the negative side, they were aware of the administrative problems that could be caused by small groups of patients banding together on the ward. These points of view are evident in what Dr. Ryan and Dr. Reynolds said:

(Picture 3, Dr. Ryan) It is a picture of a young woman patient in her late twenties or early thirties signing in after being out with this fellow, who's about her same age. Probably signing for him, too, because he's carrying a bundle of food which he and she bought when they went outside. . . . This particular outing was for the sole purpose of getting food for the people on the ward. These patients knew where to buy the food. The girl knew what the girls would like, and the fellow went because he knows what the fellows would like. They didn't think of this as an occasion to do dramatic things—just bought food and came back. This whole thing began the night before when the group was sitting in the living room. They decided they might like to have a different type of food from the regular nourishment, and elected this fellow and girl to do the errand because they were sort of neutral people. . . .

(Picture 12, Dr. Reynolds) . . . This group has set itself up as the dominant group on the ward, and has caused some anxiety on the part of the staff because of its tendency to want to dominate the activities of the whole ward. Both doctors and nurses tend to resent this, and to have considerable hostility to the individual patients in this group. On the other hand, when a patient who has been on the periphery is allowed to enter into this group, it is often looked upon as a sign of social improvement and is therefore encouraged by the staff. . . . This particular little card-playing group is apt to be the one who ignores crackers and milk, or who wants to have its own little party by sending for food from the outside, and taking it elsewhere to eat it apart from the other patients. This, of course, creates considerable resentment among the other patients who are not included, but they knot together around the crackers and milk and verbalize their complaints about the other patients.

The nurses, in discussing human relations, were mostly concerned with the dissension on the ward brought about by arguments among the patients, which led to administrative problems for the nurse. For example, Mrs. Nolan said:

(Picture 3, Mrs. Nolan) . . . Well, for example, in planning one party recently they took a collection of money for lobster, and Elizabeth Farrell took over. Elizabeth Farrell doesn't know a thing about cooking. The patients were excited and looked forward to it. Elizabeth Farrell had ad lib permission to go out, and had taken all the money and found a sale of cheap crab meat. It smelled. Mrs. Matthews was disappointed and told Elizabeth so, because they had decided on lobster. Mrs. Matthews tried to make the best of a bad bargain, and she tried to fix it; she knows how, and Elizabeth made a nuisance of herself. Too many unauthorized people tried to help in the kitchen and got in the way. The party started out wrong, started with the crab meat. Even when they ate the snacks, they grumbled about this isn't lobster, and Elizabeth didn't show up—she was uncomfortable. It was much better when they were bringing in prepared spreads. Then you didn't have to suit different individuals.

Perhaps not unexpectedly, the patients, more than any of the other role groups, seemed aware of both the positive and negative aspects of their relations. They felt such relations were useful, yet they knew that emotions were close to the surface and likely to flare up, and that patients could be petty, jealous, and rejecting of each other. Frequently, both the positive and negative aspects of relations were commented on within the material given to a single picture. For example, on Picture 6, Miss Farrell and Mrs. Matthews gave sensitive portrayals of both sides of the question.

(Picture 6, Miss Farrell) . . . Well, during the time before I was sent to the locked ward, I had made a tremendous commotion. I was miserable and wanted everybody to know it. After two weeks on the locked ward, I felt terribly ashamed. I didn't know how everybody was going to accept me. I felt they would isolate me from the group, and it was impressed upon me that I had stirred up other people's illnesses—that is what Kay and Walt told me. It wasn't so much a question of creating a commotion and then having the doctors, who were on the other side of the fence, put me in an isolated place, it was that the feeling was given me by the patients that I was hurting others. On the locked ward, if someone starts to cut his wrists, everybody rushes to help; on the open ward, when your own neurosis is inflicted on others, the attitude toward me was that no matter how sick I was, I had no business creating such a disturbance. It wasn't anything specific that anyone said to me, but something that I felt, and I felt it even more strongly when Kay told me I shouldn't be embarrassed, that everyone would still like me regardless. When I came back to the open ward from the locked ward, I felt rather good because nobody paid much attention to me. My anticipation of coming back was a lot worse than actually coming back. During the first time I was sent to the locked ward, I was able to establish a relation with people on the open ward by dropping notes to them; but the second time, I had gone outside the rules of the group when I created such a commotion, and this gave others a chance to feel noble toward me. It would have been all right if I had just made myself miserable. The so-called leaders of the group took this chance to assert their authority toward me, and by leaders I'd say those better emotionally adjusted than others. I wouldn't go as far as to say when a patient is isolated it takes him that much longer to get well, but one of the needs is to feel the unity of the group. I felt this, and have seen it in others—the shining example is Joe. At first, Joe was not accepted by Walt and Kay, and they were against him. I know myself I was afraid to express my own opinion, and since Walt was prejudiced against Joe, rather than going against them, I went along with them. And Joe just met a stone wall. Then when he went to the locked ward and established a close relation with the men patients, as the other men were transferred to the open ward, he was able to come with the group, and it was easier for him to get into the group. I guess it is easier to talk about somebody else than yourself. . . .

(Picture 6, Mrs. Matthews) . . . Mealtimes on the locked ward were a horrible ordeal, as no one said "Boo," unless someone was trying to start an argument. For me it was worse, because I couldn't eat. I felt I'd be resented because the others were eating, and I wasn't. Also, I was more unstable emotionally than now. I attempted conversation and was put in my place by a couple of patients who since have been very nice. . . . I think on the locked ward you can't—well, it isn't isolate—you can't isolate yourself from the others. . . . You cannot live with them and not be influenced in some way. I was influenced to feel a great deal of pity and sympathy. In spite of the ruling that patients are not allowed in each other's rooms, it seemed as if my room was a meeting place and everyone, no, quite a few, ended up in my room. I found one patient sitting in there by herself one day because she said it was the only place she could relax. Everybody on the surface was gay and happy in my room, yet when they got out into the living room, they seemed to take on a different attitude. In my room we'd sit and talk and eat candy and I think—well, I'm not sure—I think my room was cozy. . . . On the locked ward everyone needs urging to join in the group activities, and on the open ward it's every man for himself. We don't mean to be cliquey, but there are certain ones who find they have more in common with another one, and yet they don't make one feel left out—at least I don't feel that way. . . . One time the canasta group asked me to play. I think if I'd said I'd like to play that they would have been perfectly agreeable, but I just didn't want to break up their foursome, and I don't think they would go out of their way often to ask someone. . . . When you first come to the open ward, you figure the sicker people are on the locked ward, and that the open ward is one or two steps nearer to going back into society, and yet, my goodness, when I got to the open ward, I never heard such foul language or behavior. You'd think that by the time they got to the open ward they'd have learned to control themselves.

As can be seen from the foregoing material, there was a good deal of pressure placed on patients by other patients to conform to certain kinds of behavior, and this was also noted earlier, in Chapters 3 through 5. It seems obvious from the material that has been presented that patients are not simply an aggregate of individuals, but form themselves into a small society, the structure of which definitely influences their behavior on the ward.

The detailed presentation in this and the preceding chapter of various kinds of interaction within the several areas of life has been as extended as it has because, while certain trends can be indicated by the numerical analysis in the tables, a real feeling for the material can only come from the direct interview data. It is, however, predominately the over-all *patterning* of attitudes that is the central concern of these chapters, and it is to this that the discussion now turns as a concluding summary for the picture interview material.

GENERAL PATTERNS OF PERCEPTION

In summarizing the patterning of the attitudes of role groups toward interaction in the areas of hospital life, the same procedure as was used in Chapter 7 will be followed. That is, the data in Tables 9–1 through 9–3 in this chapter are used to determine whether a role group's evaluation of a particular type of interaction in one of the areas of life was optimistic or pessimistic. As before, a role group was considered to be optimistic if 50 per cent or more of both persons and topics were optimistic within a category, and to be pessimistic if more than 50 per cent of both persons and topics were pessimistic.

Since a judgment of a role group's emotional evaluation of a type of interaction was made if there were at least three topics (see Tables 9–1 through 9–3) in a category, the following tables should be thought of

TABLE 9–4. General pattern of seniors' perception of hospital, by area of life and type of interaction

Type of interaction	Therapy	Administration	Human relations
Staff with staff	—	Optimism	—
Seniors with residents	Optimism	—	—
Residents with patients	Optimism	—	—
Nurses with patients	Optimism	Optimism	Optimism
Patients with patients	Optimism	—	Optimism

as more suggestive than definitive with reference to the over-all pattern of a role group. Also, because of the limitation on the number of pictures used in the interviews, as well as other factors, the material represents only a partial rather than a complete attitude pattern for a role group. The gaps in the material are indicated by the dashes in Tables 9–4 through 9–7. These tables are concerned with types of interaction in therapy, administration, and human relations; the area of the hospital-in-general has not been included, as it was treated in the preceding chapter and there was no variation in the emotional evaluations—all role groups were pessimistic.

As can be seen by comparing Table 9–4 with Tables 9–5 through 9–7, the seniors were the most optimistic of the four role groups. They were optimistic as to all types of interaction in the three areas of life. In this they were closest to the patients (Table 9–7), who also were optimistic in all their evaluations except with reference to the interaction of nurses with patients in the area of therapy. As mentioned earlier, this was probably related to the fact that neither the seniors nor the patients had very much to do with the day-to-day decisions that had to be made in the work of the hospital.

The residents and nurses were considerably more pessimistic than the other two role groups (see Tables 9–5 and 9–6). There were, however, differences of opinion between residents and nurses about the areas of optimism and pessimism. The residents, for example, were pessimistic

TABLE 9–5. General pattern of residents' perception of hospital, by area of life and type of interaction

Type of interaction	Therapy	Administration	Human relations
Staff with staff	—	Pessimism	—
Seniors with residents	Pessimism	—	—
Residents with patients	Optimism	Pessimism	—
Nurses with patients	—	Pessimism	Optimism
Patients with patients	—	—	Optimism

TABLE 9–6. General pattern of nurses' perception of hospital, by area of life and type of interaction

Type of interaction	Therapy	Administration	Human relations
Staff with staff	—	Pessimism	—
Seniors with residents	Optimism	—	—
Residents with patients	Pessimism	—	—
Nurses with patients	Optimism	Pessimism	Pessimism
Patients with patients	Pessimism	—	Pessimism

about therapeutic interaction between seniors and residents, whereas the nurses were optimistic. Similarly, the nurses were pessimistic about therapeutic interaction between residents and patients, whereas the residents were optimistic. Somewhat more vividly, the residents saw both of the types of interaction on which they concentrated in the area of human relations as optimistic, whereas the nurses saw the same two types of interaction as pessimistic.

A HYPOTHESIS CONCERNING RELATIONS BETWEEN ROLE GROUPS

One of the most interesting things about the pattern of attitudes held by the patients is that it was almost a complete reversal of the pattern of attitudes held by the nurses. Of the eight cells in Tables 9–6 and 9–7 in which the nurses and patients can be compared, they disagreed about their evaluation in seven of the eight cells. Thus, in the area of therapy, both groups were in accord regarding their optimism about the interaction of seniors with residents, but disagreed about the interaction of residents with patients—the patients being optimistic while the nurses were pessimistic. More importantly, where both nurses and patients were themselves parties to the interaction they were evaluating, there was a complete reversal of opinion. The nurses were optimistic about their therapeutic interaction with patients, but they were pessimistic about administrative and human relations interaction with patients. Patients, on the other hand, were pessimistic about their therapeutic relations

TABLE 9–7. General pattern of patients' perception of hospital, by area of life and type of interaction

Type of interaction	Therapy	Administration	Human relations
Staff with staff	—	Optimism	—
Seniors with residents	Optimism	—	—
Residents with patients	Optimism	—	—
Nurses with patients	Pessimism	Optimism	Optimism
Patients with patients	Optimism	—	Optimism

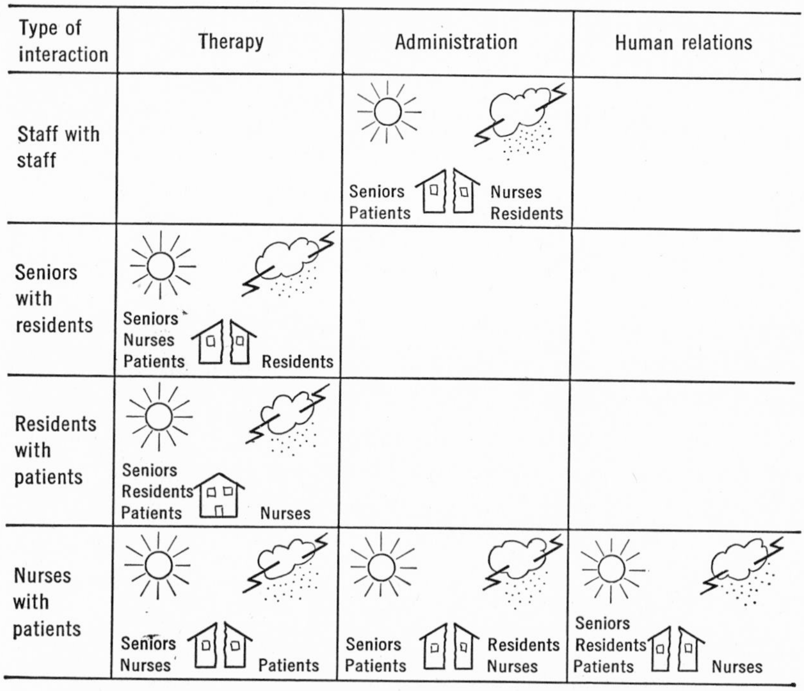

Type of interaction	Therapy	Administration	Human relations
Staff with staff		Seniors Patients / Nurses Residents	
Seniors with residents	Seniors Nurses Patients / Residents		
Residents with patients	Seniors Residents Patients / Nurses		
Nurses with patients	Seniors Nurses / Patients	Seniors Patients / Residents Nurses	Seniors Residents Patients / Nurses

FIGURE 9–1. Schematic summary of tendency toward optimism and pessimism in role groups, by area of life and type of interaction

with nurses, but were optimistic about their relations with nurses in the areas of administration and human relations. This mirror image reversal provides a good illustration of the somewhat separate attitude and value systems that existed on the various levels of the hospital. Such underlying differences would seem to contribute to the occurrence of problems in the daily life of the hospital which do not stem so much from the unique attributes of individuals as from the structural nature of the hospital as a social system.

In an attempt to follow this sort of phenomenon a bit further, Figure 9–1 summarizes (from Tables 9–4 through 9–7) the agreements and disagreements about emotional evaluation of interaction between role groups in three areas of life. The interaction of patients with each other has been omitted, since it concerns intra- rather than inter-role group relations.

If the reader will count the number of entries for optimistic evaluations which are indicated by the names of the various role groups appearing under the "shining sun," he will find that when all role groups are lumped together, the types of interaction in the three areas of life were seen optimistically 15 times, whereas a pessimistic evaluation was made only 8 times, as indicated by the entries under the "rain cloud." This positive balance would seem to suggest that by and large the hospital was seen in a favorable light. And, in this general sense, this appears to have been true. If this was so, why then, at the same time, did indications of tension and strife continually come up in the interview material given by all the role groups?

Part of the answer to this question would seem to be related to the underlying differences in emotional evaluation that existed between two role groups in the perception of their own interaction with each other. For example, the optimism of the nurses about their therapeutic interaction with patients contrasted with the pessimism of the patients about the same relation. These agreements or disagreements between the two parties to the interaction are indicated schematically by the nature of the "house" in Figure 9–1. If the house is shown as divided, the two parties to the interaction were in disagreement about their emotional evaluation; if the house is shown as whole, the two parties were in agreement. Looking at the types of interaction upon which data are available in this way, there was only *one* type of interaction where there was agreement between the two parties. This was the agreement between the residents and patients regarding optimism about their therapeutic interaction. In all other types of interaction, the two parties were in disagreement. This pattern should be clear from Figure 9–1, although perhaps the cell concerning the interaction of staff with staff in the area of administration needs a word of explanation. There the house is shown as divided because while the seniors were optimistic, the residents and nurses were pessimistic, and these three groups had to interact in carrying out the work of the hospital.

The over-all pattern in Figure 9–1 brings into focus once again the main point of this book. Taken singly, role group by role group, there was more optimism than pessimism about the hospital. Distressingly enough, however, where there was optimism in one role group which was a party to an interaction, there was pessimism in the other. Given this state of affairs, since actions at various levels of the hospital were interrelated (see Chapters 3 through 5), the operation of the hospital as a system was continually shaken by the effects of differences of opinion which were often hidden and difficult to trace to their sources. A lack of complement between roles in a social system (whether this be a hospital, a factory, or a family) leads to disequilibrium and faulty functioning. The rhythm of day-to-day work is disturbed; the necessary variations in everyday events are likely to turn into crises; and since good communication is disturbed, there is less chance that the system will regulate itself smoothly around a moving equilibrium. For such reasons, it would seem that a great deal further thought must be given to the way in which psychiatric hospitals are organized and to the effect of the operation of hospitals on the mental health of *both* staff and patients.

In closing, it is perhaps appropriate to suggest the utility of the interviewing technique developed in this research as a screening device for personnel selection in the psychiatric hospital. This sort of "projective interviewing" might enable the interviewer in a rather short time to tap underlying and often unconscious attitudes on the part of personnel. It also would seem that some such technique might be useful as one way of periodically evaluating the general balance or equilibrium of the hospital. A second possible way of gathering data on this latter problem will be suggested as a result of the analysis of the daily administrative conference material in Chapter 12.

At the end of an analysis of interview material, the question always arises that an interview produces data only on what people "say" they do. How is one to know whether such verbal expression is indicative of the way in which things actually happen in the hospital? In order to explore this question systematically, the next three chapters contain an analysis of what actually occurred during the course of sixty-three consecutive administrative conferences.

Section IV

ADMINISTRATION IN THE HOSPITAL

A Small Group Analysis

CHAPTER 10

Status and Role in Group Interaction

The focus of attention in this and the next two chapters will be on the actual day-to-day administrative operation of the hospital. The data to be analyzed consist of sixty-three consecutive administrative conferences which were held early each morning Monday through Saturday and lasted from fifteen to twenty minutes. The discussion in these conferences concerned such matters as: (1) the reports of the resident and the charge nurses who had been on duty during the previous evening; (2) questions of privileges, such as whether Mrs. Matthews might visit the beauty parlor or Mr. Esposito should be allowed to go to church; (3) the movement of patients in the hospital from the locked to the open wards; (4) the discussion of current admissions and discharges; (5) immediate therapeutic problems, such as a particularly disturbed patient who would perhaps need to be placed in seclusion; and so forth. One day a week, on Monday, the conference was of a somewhat different nature and consisted of a report on the recent progress and present status of each patient in the hospital. This discussion of the roster of patients was usually initiated by the chief resident, who asked for information from the resident physicians and the nurses. Thus, the Monday conference was longer than those on the other five days of the week and lasted from forty minutes to an hour.

These daily conferences were usually attended by the head of the hospital, the chief resident (classified here as a senior staff member because of his responsibilities), all the resident physicians, the supervisor of nurses, the charge nurses from both locked and open wards, and a number of other specialized personnel—the social worker, the group worker in charge of activities, and the occupational therapist. The writer was present at these conferences as an observer and had nothing to say except in the few instances where he had acted as a member of the hospital staff in escorting patients to and from various activities outside the hospital. In these instances he discharged his responsibility by giving a brief factual account of the events that occurred during the activity. During the course of the study, the size of the conference group on any one day ranged from seven to eighteen individuals, but the group most frequently included thirteen persons. More specifically, in the distribution by size of group in the sixty-three conferences, both the median and the mode fell at thirteen persons. The most usual composition of this group of thirteen persons, not including the writer, was: two senior staff members—the head of the hospital and the chief resident; five resident physicians; three nurses—the supervisor of nurses and two charge nurses; and three other personnel—the social worker, the group worker, and the occupational therapist.

The physical setting for the conference was much as it has been depicted in Picture 11 in Chapter 6. The individual members arranged themselves around a long table: the senior staff sat at the head of the table, flanked on either side by the residents, with the nurses and other personnel at the opposite end of the table. The writer, as observer, sat in a chair somewhat removed from the table.

Before beginning his observations of the conferences, the writer held a series of meetings (see Chapter 2) with all the various role groups in which he explained the work he would be doing and included the statement that he would be making verbatim notes on the daily administrative conferences. As always in such cases, it is difficult to assess the effect of the writer's presence on the interaction in the conferences, but his relations with all members were good and remained so throughout the study. There were never any requests that he not include certain kinds of material, and so far as he could tell the members of the conference simply accepted his presence, and the work of the hospital went on as usual. Two months prior to the beginning of the observations which make up the data reported in this chapter, the writer began regularly to attend the daily administrative conferences. During this initial two-month period he perfected his method of recording the data.

At the beginning of each conference the writer took his seat somewhat to the side of the table around which the members were grouped and wrote down verbatim the verbal interaction that occurred throughout the conference. In addition, he recorded outbursts of laughter, long periods of silence, and other types of essentially non-verbal communication on the part of both individuals and the total group. He had had extensive training in recording material in this manner in previous studies and had evolved an accurate and rapid personal shorthand. He found it was quite easy to record the exact words of the members of the conference because individuals spoke in turn, and there were very few times when more than one person would be speaking at once. Every day, within a few hours after the close of the administrative conference, the writer dictated his written account into sound-recording equipment, and this was subsequently transcribed by his research secretary.

Gathered in this manner, the material was as nearly verbatim as was possible without the use of elaborate technical equipment. The matter of sound recording the conferences on tape had been considered, but this was abandoned for financial and technical reasons. The technical reasons were the more important, particularly the difficulty experienced by secretarial help in identifying and keeping separate the various voices on the tape.

There were four reasons for gathering the conference material in as nearly verbatim form as possible: (1) The daily administrative conference was an important link in the chain of communication about events in the hospital. As such, it provided a sensitive place for ascertaining the information and attitudes held by various role groups: seniors, residents, nurses, and other specialized personnel. (2) The structure and content of the interaction at the administrative conferences provided actual behavioral material, which could be compared with the attitudes and role perceptions of hospital personnel obtained in the interviews to pictures (see Chapters 6 through 9). (3) Because of its nature, the daily administrative conference provided an excellent opportunity to study many aspects of "small group dynamics," which has increasingly become an area of interest in social science (Bales, 1950; Roseborough, 1953; Hare, Borgatta, and Bales, 1955). The conferences were in many ways ideal for this purpose in that they were composed of a relatively small number of persons who belonged to highly identifiable role groups and were participating in very meaningful decision-making processes. As such, the conferences provided a daily recurring "real life" small group situation which had advantages for study over experimentally created small groups. This broader theoretical interest in the conferences was closely related to Bales' (1950) work on the small group as an interacting system. (4) Equally, interest was centered on how the conference as a small social system reflected, and was geared to, the larger moving equilibrium of the total hospital system over time. At such a theoretical level the material takes on wider significance than simply an analysis of the administrative operation of the psychiatric hospital, and is related to recent thinking on the meaning of interaction in social systems (Parsons, Bales, and Shils, 1953). It is not possible in this book to explore fully both the theoretical and the practical implications of all these four reasons why the material was gathered in the way that it was. The first two areas of interest will be treated more fully here than will the latter two. Nevertheless, the more general problems of small group dynamics and the relation of the small group to the larger social system will be given some attention, and it is useful to pause a moment to consider these questions.

Following the line of thought developed by Bales (in Parsons, Bales, and Shils, 1953), it was possible to utilize the conference material in the study of the patterned sequence of phases followed in the discussion of a *single particular problem* during one of the conferences. As will be seen later, any one conference had approximately a dozen problems or "topics" which were discussed during the course of a meeting. Part of the analysis of the material was concerned with identifying what sort of sequence of phases resulted in coming to a concrete decision about a problem; and equally, what sort of sequence of phases resulted in *not* coming to a concrete decision about a problem, as when the matter was left "up in the air."

Secondly, the *entire conference* itself tended to follow a certain phase pattern from beginning to end, and this was of considerable interest. Thirdly, a *series of conferences* over time tended to develop a pattern of phases. This long-term phase patterning in the conferences seemed to depend, in part, on factors inherent in the daily administrative conference as a small social system, and also to depend, in part, on the state of equilibrium in the total hospital system over time.

In thinking about the analysis of the conference material, there was, therefore, a nesting of three problems, all of which involved a patterned sequence of phases: the manner of reaching a decision on a single problem in a particular conference; the course from beginning to end of any particular conference; and the phase movement in a series of conferences over time. These interests were a development, in one direction, of the theoretical ideas referred to in Chapter 1, where the hospital was thought of as a network of interrelated open systems in transaction with each other.

The use of such a transactional system approach to an analysis of the administrative conferences does not permit a logically valid conceptual distinction to be made between matters of structure and process. Structure and process are both aspects of a tendency toward regularity and equilibrium. A useful operational distinction can, however, be made in that structure denotes long-run and fairly stable regularities that are slow to change, whereas process denotes regularities that are more subject to change in the short run as part of the tendency of the system to maintain a moving equilibrium. Such a set of propositions needs to be stated in abstract terms, but in the specific material which is of concern here, the meaning of these propositions can be put very simply. The structure of the conferences consisted of relatively enduring patterns of interrelations between somewhat over a dozen individuals who represented four role groups in the hospital. During the period of roughly three months covered by the sixty-three conferences analyzed in this chapter, the structure of the conferences actually changed very little—though several attempts were made to introduce minor changes. The on-going processes in the conferences consisted of the attempts made by the dozen individuals to reach solutions to immediate problems and to get along harmoniously with one another. The nature of these processes shifted rapidly if the focus was on single problems within a conference, or on the pattern of one conference compared with the next. The nature of the processes shifted somewhat less rapidly, but at a much greater rate than changes in the structure, if the focus was on a sequence of phases over a period of several months.

The following analysis of the conference material will make use of the operational distinction introduced above. The remainder of this chapter will be devoted to the *form* of the structural regularities of the conferences. The form taken by the interaction in the conferences will be analyzed by making use of the interaction categories developed by Bales (1950). In Chapter 11 the structural *content* of the conferences will be analyzed by means of a set of content categories which were devised expressly for this purpose. Some discussion of short-run processes will also be included as part of the structural analysis made in this chapter and in Chapter 11. Lastly, Chapter 12 will turn to a consideration of long-run processes occurring over a period of several months.

METHOD OF SCORING FORM OF INTERACTION

It was necessary to find a convenient method of analyzing the formal characteristics of the daily administrative conferences. The method used, which was developed by Bales (1950), consisted essentially in the scoring of interaction by placing each "act" of interaction into one of twelve mutually exclusive "interaction categories." Such a method, described in more detail below, permitted the material to be analyzed in several ways. First of all, it was possible to analyze the sheer volume of participation by the various role groups in terms of the number of acts contributed by any role group or by any individual within a role group. For various reasons, including the possibility of later separating the acts into twelve categories, this was a technically more advantageous way of expressing the amount of participation than either a direct word count or a count by lines of type. Secondly, it was possible to indicate something of the nature and quality of the interaction by taking account of the categories into which acts fell, in addition to the sheer number of acts. After a description of the Bales system, and of the check on reliability, the over-all characteristics of the sixty-three administrative conferences will be examined—first in terms of the amount of participation by the various role groups, and secondly in terms of the nature of the participation as measured by the interaction categories.

The heart of Bales' method is a way of classifying behavior act by act as it occurs in small face-to-face groups. All the behavior that goes on in such a small group as the daily administrative conference can be viewed as a sequence of questions and answers, coupled with positive and negative emotional reactions to these questions and answers. This is the meaning of the four areas labeled A, B, C, and D in Figure 10–1. In terms of the sequence of events, a discussion will usually start out in the task area of questions (C), then move to the task area of attempted answers (B), and the cycle will be completed with some expression in the social-emotional areas—either positive (A) or negative (D). The twelve interaction categories are set up as follows. There are three types of questions: asks for orientation (7), asks for opinion (8), and asks for suggestion (9). Corresponding to these three types of questions are three types of answers: gives orientation (6), gives opinion (5), and gives suggestion (4). These answers are problem-solving attempts, and they usually call forth an emotional reaction. Negative emotional reactions include: disagrees (10), shows tension (11), and shows antagonism (12). On the positive side the corresponding emotional reactions include: agrees (3), shows tension release (2), and shows solidarity (1). The terms and phrases within the numbered categories in Figure 10–1 are *only* catch phrases designed to be concretely descriptive of the theoretical content of the categories. Actually there are extended definitions of each of the categories (see Bales, 1950).

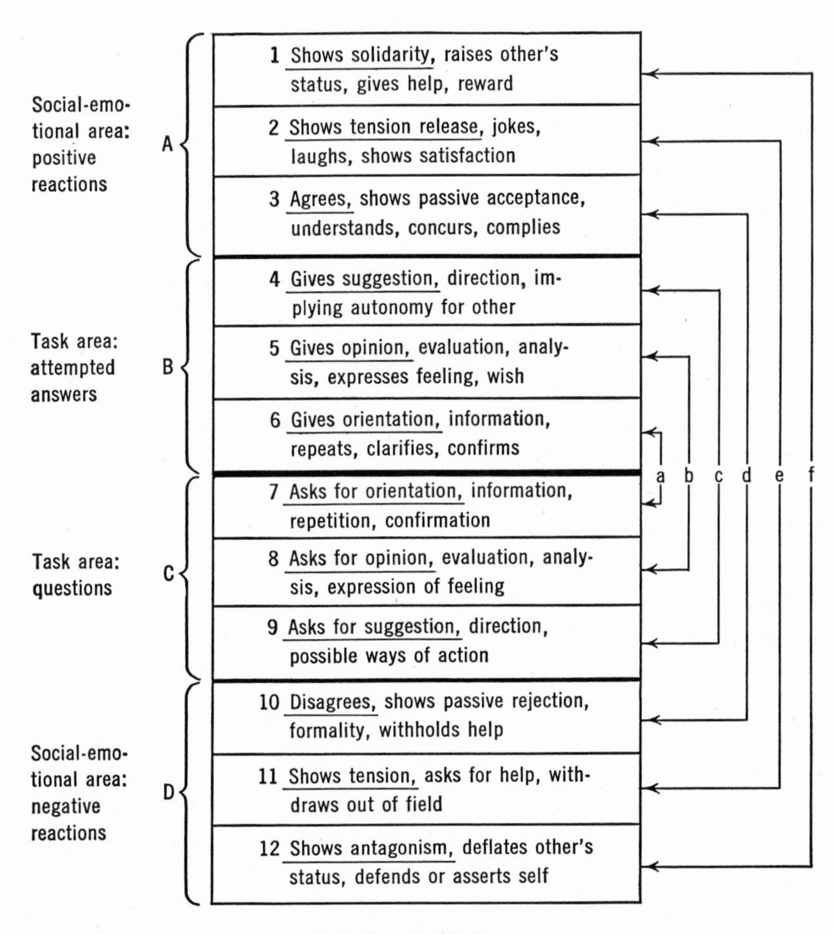

FIGURE 10–1. System of interaction categories used and their major relations (from Bales, 1950, p. 59)

As indicated in Figure 10–1 the set of categories includes six interlocking functional problems which are logically applicable to any concrete type of interaction system. These are, in one-word terms: problems of orientation, evaluation, control, decision, tension-management, and integration. There is a tendency, though it is something of an oversimplification, for these six problems to occur as "stages" or "steps" in a problem-solving sequence, as their order suggests.

In scoring all acts within the twelve categories, it is necessary to ignore certain qualitative distinctions which are of importance in the interaction. As Bales (1950, pp. 83–84) says:

> Thus in scoring we systematically ignore qualitative distinctions we know to be important. This we do in order to pierce through to more elementary similarities regarding the functions of acts in the problem-solving sequence. We hope that by obtaining reliable observations of these elementary characteristics and by noting the way in which these few major types of activity are *distributed between persons* we can reconstruct the main dimensions of the relationships between the participants: their relative access to resources, their relative control over each other, their relative status with regard to each other, and their relative solidarity.

As will be seen later in this chapter this proved to be a well-founded hope in terms of describing the role groups within the interaction of the conferences.

The basic unit to be scored in interaction is called the "act." More properly, it is a single interaction, since all acts in the scheme are regarded as interactions. This unit is the smallest discriminable segment of verbal or non-verbal behavior to which the observer, using the present set of categories after appropriate training, can assign a classification. Often the unit will be a single simple sentence expressing or conveying a complete simple thought. Usually there will be a subject and predicate, but sometimes these elements will only be implied. As an example, if the actor in a conversation says, "What?", the observer translates, "What was that?" or, "I do not understand you," or "Would you repeat that?" thus filling out both subject and predicate. Complex sentences always involve more than one score. Dependent clauses are separately scored. Compound sentences joined by "and" and "but" are broken down into their component simple parts, each of which is given a score. Several rules are used in determining into which category an act will fall if there is doubt in a scorer's mind. The first rule is to view each act as a response to the last act or as an anticipation of the next act regardless of whether the series of acts is produced by a single, or several, actors. If this rule were not followed, a client who came into a relief office to ask for funds might be scored in category 11 every time he spoke. Using the rule, he would be marked in category 11 only when he actually made an appeal. The second rule is to favor the category more distant from the middle in scoring, that is, to classify the act in the category nearer the top or the bottom of the list. Thus, if one person says, "It's hot today," and the other smiles and responds, "Over ninety," the possible dilemma is between classifying in terms of the function of giving information (category 6), or in terms of showing agreement (category 3), or in terms of showing still more active solidarity (category 1). These competing demands are resolved by favoring the category most distant from the middle and classifying the act in category 1. This rule has another implication relevant to possible hesitation about making classifications in area D (categories 10, 11, and 12). The rule helps the observer to avoid being inhibited about putting down a socially negative score.

Before turning to problems of reliability between observers, it is useful here to give an actual excerpt from a daily administrative conference scored according to the preceding explanation. In the following excerpt, the category into which an act falls is indicated by a number in parentheses following each act. The separation of the material, indicated by dots, refers to a classification of the content of the conference into topics which will be discussed in the next chapter.

Dr. Shaw: Who was on last night (7)?
Dr. Ryan: I was (6). Nothing happened (5).

. . . .

Dr. Shaw: The women's locked ward is full (6) so there will be no new patients taken in over the week end (4). (Dr. Shaw turned to Dr. Ramsay who would be on duty over the week end.) This means not to admit any new patients (4) because the "inn" is full (2). (There was no general laughter by the group at this so the only score is a "2" for Dr. Shaw.)

Dr. Sears: What is the census now (7)?

Dr. Shaw: It is quite low (5), about twenty-five or twenty-six (6), but it happens that our disturbed women's ward is the one which is jammed up (6).

. . . .

Miss Nicholas: Miss Lewis has been voted by the men on the open ward to come over and occupy the four-bed ward on their side (2). (There was general laughter from the group at this so each of the eight participants is given a score in category "2.")

Dr. Ramsay (who is Miss Lewis' therapist): I wonder what sort of recreation tax or fee we should look into if Miss Lewis moves over (2)? (General laughter from the group, so a "2" is scored for each of the eight participants.)

. . . .

Dr. Reynolds: Mr. Innes has written a letter to his family (6), and the contents are essentially that he's asking the family to get him out of here (6), saying that he has feelings like he was beginning to feel like a homosexual (6), and I am in doubt about whether I should send this letter (5), or just what

I should do about it (11). I can't seem to contact Mr. Innes in any sort of relationship (5), so I couldn't use the material if I were to send on the letter (5), and I'm not sure just what I should do (11).

Dr. Sears: It might be better to send the note (4), and then speak to the family about it (4).

Dr. Reynolds: Yes, I agree (3), withholding the letter is bad (5), but I am still undecided (11).

Dr. Rivers: Why don't you send a note along with the letter to the family (4)?

Dr. Sears: How far away do the family live (7)?

Dr. Reynolds: Smithville (6).

Dr. Sears: Well, they could come in and visit you then (4).

Dr. Reynolds: I have told the father not to visit for the time being (6), but it is true that he could come in and talk with me (3).

Dr. Ryan: It seems to me the note could be used in two ways (5), if we sent it on that might be one way to do it (4), on the other hand if we did send it it might disturb the family (5) so perhaps it would be better if we didn't send it (4).

Dr. Reynolds: I am ready to discuss with Mr. Innes the fact that I have to read his letters (5), and letters of this particular type (6), but I can't get in a relationship with him to do this (11).

Dr. Sears: We always have to work with and get the cooperation of the family before we can do anything with the patient (5), and I feel it would therefore be better to send the note on (4).

Dr. Reynolds: I just can't approach the patient (11).

Dr. Ryan: The patient seems to have had a history of several episodes such as the one he's in now (5), so that the letter might not be too different from others that he has sent to his family (5), and they might not be too disturbed by it (5).

Dr. Reynolds: The family does see the situation (5), but on the other hand has a great deal of guilt about putting the patient in the hospital (5).

Dr. Shaw: At this point I think it is necessary to say to the patient by our action that, look, we are not preventing you from communicating with your family (4), and if we were to prevent him from doing so we might never make any contact with him (5).

Dr. Rolfe: I don't see what we would gain by stopping the letter (5), the father knows that the son is sick (5), and he has already had to make a painful decision by putting the son into the hospital (5) and is therefore probably prepared for this type of thing which might come up (5). I feel we must send the letter (4), and if it is a fairly rational letter without too much delusional material in it, this is one thing (5). On the other hand, if Innes started to write to the President of the United States saying that he's being beaten up here (6), why that would be different (5), and we would have to stop that kind of letter (4).

Dr. Sears: In that case it probably wouldn't matter anyway (5), because the President probably has a secretary who stops just such letters (2). (There was no general laughter, so the only score is a "2" for Dr. Sears.)

Dr. Reynolds: Then you suggest that I send a note along at the same time with the letter (9)?

Dr. Shaw: Either that (4) or call up the family and talk to them and tell them that this letter is coming and explain the situation (4).

. . . .

Dr. Rolfe: I have a problem with Mr. Onofrio (6). He has permission to go to the football game with his brother this afternoon (6), and also in the normal course of events he has permission to go out on Sunday with his brother and sister-in-law (6). He has now asked me if he can't stay out with his family overnight and come back Sunday afternoon (6), rather than coming back to the hospital tonight and going out again tomorrow (6). I would like a decision on this (9). It seems a fairly reasonable sort of request to me (5).

Dr. Shaw: No (4). I don't think Mr. Onofrio should do this (10).

Dr. Rolfe (a little nettled): Why not (10)?

Dr. Shaw (looking perturbed and hesitating a moment (11)): Is the game here in the city (7)?

Dr. Rolfe: Yes (6), and the brother will take him home after the game (6). They would eat at home tomorrow (6), and then bring Mr. Onofrio back tomorrow night (6).

Dr. Shaw: I find it hard to say why I don't feel Mr. Onofrio should do this (11), but at this stage with Mr. Onofrio in insulin treatment (5), it seems best to me that he should not go home now (4).

Dr. Rolfe: Well, I am the one who has been giving the insulin treatment (12), and I don't feel that this is a break in treatment (5), or the fact that the patient is in insulin treatment will have any affect on his being out overnight (10). The brother and sister are both at home (6), and I don't like to bring up a privilege or a change which is against the policy of the house (10), but I think in this case it is all right (12).

Dr. Shaw: Well, it isn't exactly against the policy of the hospital (11), because we do want this patient to go home over week ends at a later stage (4). It's just that not right now (11).

Dr. Rolfe: All right (3). Well, not now then (11).

As can be seen from the above material, it was possible to collect the verbal material quite adequately, but probably certain non-verbal interactions were missed. For example, because the material was taken down largely in terms of the verbal interaction, certain non-verbal acts of agreement (category 3) and disagreement (category 10) were probably missed, as these may have been indicated by nods of the head and so forth. Also, certain acts of tension release (category 2) and tension (category 11) as manifested by smiles, frowns, and fidgeting were probably missed. However, the more pronounced laughter or long hostile silences were not missed, and, as can be seen in the sample material, these were scored. It is also likely, although more for reasons inherent in the Bales system, that certain "implied" or "hidden" emotional feelings were not included since they were veiled by statements of orientation, opinion, and suggestion. Admitting the lack of inclusion of such non-verbal interactions, it is felt that the effect of this factor was random, in the sense that these kinds of omissions were spread fairly evenly throughout the material.

A separate scoring in the twelve interaction categories was tabulated for each individual participant in each of the sixty-three administrative conferences. From this basic tabulation it was possible to show the interaction of a single individual during any particular conference, as well as this individual's pattern of interaction in terms of all sixty-three conferences, or to make any other division by time periods that one would wish. Equally, it was possible to summate the interaction of individuals within a role group and to compare the various role groups on a day-to-day or week-to-week basis.

The material for the sixty-three conferences was scored independently by two coders (the writer and his research assistant). Before this was done, the writer, who had had previous experience in the use of the interaction categories, trained his research assistant through the use of the manual written by Bales (1950), and practice scoring was carried out on administrative conference material other than the sixty-three conferences to be used as the data for this chapter. As recommended by Bales (1950), inter-rater reliability was checked during this training period by plotting the scores of the two coders against each other on binomial probability paper (see Bales, 1950; Mosteller and Tukey, 1949). This paper enables one to determine graphically the number of standard errors in the difference between the two coders in any interaction category. The coding is considered reliable when no point falls outside the plus or minus two-sigma range.

Having reached a satisfactory degree of reliability in training, the two coders then independently scored the sixty-three conferences utilized here. A reliability check on every twelfth conference of the sixty-three, indicated that the inter-rater reliability was within the plus or minus two-sigma range on all twelve categories. Indeed, it was within a range of plus or minus one-sigma for ten of the twelve categories.

A check on the internal consistency of the data provided a different sort of reliability test. As the sixty-three conferences followed one another in chronological order, the data were split into three periods of twenty-one conferences each. The figures obtained on all sixty-three conferences proved to be very consistent with those obtained on any one

TABLE 10–1. Number of individual participations and number of acts of participation in daily administrative conferences, by role group

Role group	First 21 conferences: Number of individual participations	First 21 conferences: Number of acts	Second 21 conferences: Number of individual participations	Second 21 conferences: Number of acts	Third 21 conferences: Number of individual participations	Third 21 conferences: Number of acts	All 63 conferences: Number of individual participations	All 63 conferences: Number of acts
Seniors	53	952	50	823	36	532	139	2,307
Residents	103	1,612	102	1,682	97	1,054	302	4,348
Nurses	68	325	74	348	68	258	210	931
Other personnel	43	191	48	259	44	178	135	628
All groups	267	3,080	274	3,112	245	2,022	786	8,214

of the three separate periods of twenty-one conferences each. The reader can check this internal consistency by inspection of the tables in the following material. Frequently, in addition to the general similarity in the three periods when compared with the over-all total, the reader will note tendencies toward change from one of the three periods to another. The change that is discernible over time, even in such a gross breakdown as a sequence of three periods of twenty-one conferences each, represents processes inherent in the material, which will be considered at greater length in Chapter 12.

EFFECT OF STATUS AND ROLE ON FORM OF INTERACTION

Certain aspects of the sheer amount of participation will be considered first; that is, the total number of acts given by an individual or a role group without regard for the particular interaction categories into which the acts were classified—in short, a measure of the amount of talking done. Table 10–1 shows the number of acts of participation by role groups for the three consecutive periods and for the total sixty-three conferences. The heading "number of individual participations" in Table 10–1 means that, for example, in the first period of twenty-one conferences there were 103 resident representatives present. Since there were 5 residents in the hospital, this means that roughly all 5 residents were present at all of the twenty-one conferences. If this were actually the case, there would be a total of 105 resident representatives during the first period. In reality, there were two conferences when only 4 residents were present. Thus, the "number of individual participations" does not refer to 103 different resident doctors, but rather to the number of times the 5 residents were present during twenty-one conferences—the number of

TABLE 10–2. Index of average individual participation per conference, by role group

Role group	First 21 conferences	Second 21 conferences	Third 21 conferences	All 63 conferences
Seniors	18.0	16.5	14.8	16.6
Residents	15.7	16.5	10.9	14.4
Nurses	4.8	4.7	3.8	4.4
Other personnel	4.4	5.4	4.0	4.7

role representatives. The same logic applies, of course, for the other role groups.

Since the number of role representatives during a period varied from one group to another, it is necessary to correct for this in order to make the number of acts comparable from one role group to another. The most expedient way of making this correction is to compute a simple average for any one role group during a period. For example, in Table 10–1 the seniors in the first period had 53 participations and produced 952 acts. This gives the seniors an average of 17.96 acts or, rounding off, of 18.0. By following this procedure for each of the role groups, the resulting average may be thought of as an "index of average individual participation" per conference within a role group. That is, what a representative senior physician, resident, and so forth, would produce on the average per conference during one of the three periods, or during the entire sixty-three conferences. The result of this adjusting process can be seen in Table 10–2.

Table 10–2 shows the four role groups from greatest to least average participation (see also Table 10–3). A second point to be noted in Table 10–2 is that all four role groups showed a *decrease* in average participation during the third period. For example, the seniors dropped from 16.5 in the second period to 14.8 in the third period, and the residents dropped from 16.5 to 10.9. These phenomena will be discussed later in this chapter. At this point it is only desired to remind the reader that the three periods of twenty-one conferences followed each other in chronological order, and hence the third period fell approximately at the time the events described in Chapter 5 occurred. As will be remembered, this was the period of mutual withdrawal on the part of the four role groups. These phenomena are empirically reflected in the data in Table 10–2. In the present discussion, however, the focus of attention is on the over-all form characteristics of the conferences, and the data are divided here into three periods merely to provide an indication of internal consistency.

TABLE 10–3. Ranking of role groups according to amount of participation in daily administrative conferences

Conferences	Seniors	Residents	Nurses	Other personnel
First 21 conferences	1	2	3	4
Second 21 conferences	1.5	1.5	4	3
Third 21 conferences	1	2	4	3
Total of ranks	3.5	5.5	11.0	10.0

Coefficient of concordance = 0.80 ($p < .05$).

If the data in Table 10–2 are converted to rank orders, from most to least talking role groups, the result may be seen on Table 10–3. For example, the rank order in the first period was: 1—seniors, 2—residents, 3—nurses, and 4—other personnel.

The consistency in rank order by role group shown on Table 10–3 has a coefficient of concordance of 0.80, with a probability of less than .05. That is, this distribution would be likely to occur less than 5 times out of 100 by chance.[1] The coefficient of concordance, usually termed W, is tested for significance by using Snedecor's distribution for F. The coefficient of concordance is designed so that it can vary from 0, signifying complete randomness in the allocation of rankings, to 1, signifying complete agreement among the judges. It is therefore possible to say with some confidence that the seniors talked most, the residents second, the other personnel third, and the nurses least (see "total of ranks" in Table 10–3). These results are in line with the work of others showing that higher status persons tend to participate more heavily in group discussion. For example, much the same method was used with similar results in a large state hospital by Apple and Arnason (unpublished paper) and in a study of jury deliberations by Strodtbeck and Mann (1956). The work presented here is also in accord with that of Mishler and Tropp (1956) in their study of status and interaction in a psychiatric hospital.

The same procedure which has been used in comparing role groups may also be used to compare intra-role status differences. For example, among the seniors, the head of the hospital may be compared with the chief resident. Table 10–4 gives the actual figures for subcategories of seniors, while Table 10–5 adjusts these data for average individual participation. As can be seen from Table 10–5, the head of the hospital talked more on the average than the chief resident during the first and second periods. This was true even though it was the chief resident's job actually to run the daily administrative conference. Secondly, in Table

[1] For a discussion of these matters, see Moroney, M. J. *Facts from Figures,* pp. 336–340. London: Penguin Books, 1953.

TABLE 10–4. Number of individual participations and number of acts of participation in daily administrative conferences, by subcategory of seniors

	First 21 conferences		Second 21 conferences		Third 21 conferences		All 63 conferences	
Subcategory	Number of individual participations	Number of acts	Number of individual participations	Number of acts	Number of individual participations	Number of acts	Number of individual participations	Number of acts
Head of hospital (N=1)	13	350	11	317	8	121	32	788
Chief resident (N=1)	21	520	21	463	20	396	62	1,379

10–4 it is interesting to note the drop in the number of individual participations by the head of the hospital from the first to the third period. It was also during the third period that the chief resident exceeded the head of the hospital in average number of acts per conference (see Table 10–5). Attention is called to these facts only in passing in order to indicate how the dynamics of process in the material show up even in such a gross breakdown as the three periods.

The main point of Table 10–5 is that the head of the hospital talked more than the chief resident, thus suggesting that subcategories of status within a role group also have an effect on the amount of participation. This can equally be seen among the nurses, where there were three subcategories of status: supervisor of nurses, charge nurse, and staff nurse. The number of acts of participation by these subcategories of nurses can be seen in Table 10–6, while the index of average individual participation within these subcategories is given in Table 10–7.

The staff nurses are included in these two tables—even though they were present infrequently, and the data are of no statistical importance—mainly to emphasize the point that the staff nurses did not attend the daily administrative conferences and hence had to rely on what the charge nurse told them about the conference when she returned to the ward. As was evident from the picture interview material given by nurses, the staff nurses felt the charge nurse did not communicate fully with them about

TABLE 10–5. Index of average individual participation per conference, by subcategory of seniors

Subcategory	First 21 conferences	Second 21 conferences	Third 21 conferences	All 63 conferences
Head of hospital	26.9	28.8	15.1	24.6
Chief resident	24.8	22.0	19.8	22.2

TABLE 10–6. Number of individual participations and number of acts of participation in daily administrative conferences, by subcategory of nurses

Subcategory	First 21 conferences		Second 21 conferences		Third 21 conferences		All 63 conferences	
	Number of individual participations	Number of acts	Number of individual participations	Number of acts	Number of individual participations	Number of acts	Number of individual participations	Number of acts
Supervisor of nurses (N=1)	16	113	13	88	14	107	43	308
Charge nurses (N=5)	51	212	60	258	51	151	162	621
Staff nurses (N=3)	1	0	1	2	3	0	5	2

the conference, so that in effect the staff nurses were blocked from one source of information concerning decisions and attitudes at higher administrative levels in the hospital.

Just as it was noted that the head of the hospital talked more than the chief resident, so it can also be seen from Table 10–7 that the supervisor of nurses consistently talked more than the average charge nurse. The main point in showing the breakdown by subcategories of seniors and nurses is to underscore the fact that the status hierarchy was not only related to which group talked most *among* the several role groups, but was also related to the subcategories of status *within* a role group. Such an analysis can be carried a step further in order to show that the same phenomena held true for *persons* within a role group. For this purpose, the 5 persons within the role group of residents will be used. For identification, the 5 residents are listed simply as Drs. A through E. Table 10–8 gives the number of acts of participation by each resident in the conferences over the three periods. Table 10–9 adjusts the data given in Table 10–8 for differences in the number of participations, although this factor was relatively negligible for the resident physicians.

TABLE 10–7. Index of average individual participation per conference, by subcategory of nurses

Subcategory	First 21 conferences	Second 21 conferences	Third 21 conferences	All 63 conferences
Supervisor of nurses	7.1	6.8	7.6	7.2
Charge nurses	4.2	4.3	3.0	3.8
Staff nurses[1]	0	2.0	0	0.4

[1] With so few cases, figures are not reliable and are only very roughly indicative for staff nurses.

TABLE 10–8. Number of individual participations and number of acts of participation in daily administrative conferences, by each resident

Resident	First 21 conferences		Second 21 conferences		Third 21 conferences		All 63 conferences	
	Number of individual participations	Number of acts	Number of individual participations	Number of acts	Number of individual participations	Number of acts	Number of individual participations	Number of acts
Dr. A	21	438	20	623	15	389	56	1,450
Dr. B	21	397	20	387	21	226	62	1,010
Dr. C	21	371	20	305	19	217	60	893
Dr. D	20	206	21	208	21	111	62	525
Dr. E	20	200	21	159	21	111	62	470

Table 10–9 contains some extraordinarily interesting findings. Perhaps the most striking is the consistency in the rank order of Drs. A through E in terms of most to least talking over the three periods (see also Table 10–10). A second point is that the 5 residents tended to form three groups. That is, first of all, Dr. A talked far more than any of the other residents. Below him, Drs. B and C formed a second group, while Drs. D and E formed a third and least talking group. Neither the rank order of talking nor the three subgroupings bears any relation to differences in length of previous training among the residents. Dr. E had had a preceding year on the inpatient service, and this was her second year of residency. Drs. A, B, C, and D were all experiencing their first year on this particular inpatient service. However, Drs. B and C had had previous clinical experience with patients elsewhere, whereas neither Drs. A nor D had had any previous clinical experience treating patients. Drs. C and E were women; Drs. A, B, and D were men.

The material in Table 10–9 is also interesting when compared with the material in other tables. First of all, when compared with seniors (in Table 10–5) it can be seen that Dr. A talked on the average about the same as the senior physicians, but that all the other residents talked less than either of the two seniors. On the other hand, the least talking resi-

TABLE 10–9. Index of average individual participation per conference, by each resident

Resident	First 21 conferences	Second 21 conferences	Third 21 conferences	All 63 conferences
Dr. A	20.9	31.2	25.9	25.9
Dr. B	18.9	19.4	10.8	16.3
Dr. C	17.7	15.3	11.4	14.9
Dr. D	10.3	9.9	5.3	8.5
Dr. E	10.0	7.6	5.3	7.6

TABLE 10–10. Ranking of residents from most to least talking in daily administrative conferences

Conferences	Dr. A	Dr. B	Dr. C	Dr. D	Dr. E
First 21 conferences	1	2	3	4	5
Second 21 conferences	1	2	3	4	5
Third 21 conferences	1	3	2	4.5	4.5
Total of ranks	3	7	8	12.5	14.5

Coefficient of concordance = 0.90 ($p < .005$).

dent, Dr. E, talked more than the most talking nurse—the supervisor of nurses (see Table 10–7). This is intriguing, as the least talking resident was a rather passive, withdrawn person, whereas the supervisor of nurses was an assertive person, who was willing to express her opinion in unequivocal terms.

In these data, then, it is possible to see the interplay between role group membership and individual personality characteristics—a topic of considerable theoretical importance. Even though Dr. E was a rather passive person, she was forced to speak because of the pressure on her, in her role as resident. Equally, the supervisor of nurses' tendency to dominate interaction was held in check by the position of her role within the status hierarchy of the hospital.

In general, these data show the existence of a continuum of interaction from most to least talking in terms of the relations among the various role groups, among subcategories within a role group, and among individuals within a role group.

It is difficult to leave Table 10–9 without again pointing out the tendency for process dynamics to show up over the three conference periods. Just as in Table 10–2 there was a drop in participation for all role groups in the third period, so also in Table 10–5 there was a drop in participation for both the head of the hospital and the chief resident, and equally there was a drop in participation for the charge nurses in Table 10–7. Finally, in Table 10–9 there was a drop in participation for *each* of the 5 residents during the third period. This is again strong empirical evidence for the mutual withdrawal of the four groups, as described in Chapter 5.

The results of converting the data in Table 10–9 into rank orders of most to least talking resident can be seen in Table 10–10. The coefficient of concordance for this table is high, 0.90, with a probability of less than .005. It is thus possible to accept the rank order from Dr. A as the most talking resident through Dr. E as the least talking resident as consistent over time.

TABLE 10–11. Ranking of residents according to seniors' evaluation of over-all ability

Senior doctor	Dr. A	Dr. B	Dr. C	Dr. D	Dr. E
Dr. Sutton	2	1	3	5	4
Dr. Scott	1	2	3	5	4
Dr. Shaw	1	2	3	5	4
Dr. Sloan	1	2	3	5	4
Dr. Sears	1	3	2	5	4
Dr. Simmons	1	2	3	5	4
Total of ranks	7	12	17	30	24

Coefficient of concordance = 0.93 ($p < .005$).

The remarkable consistency over time in the rank ordering of most to least talking resident was not anticipated, and became apparent only after the data were analyzed. After analysis of the data, the writer was struck by the correspondence between the rank order of most to least talking resident and what he felt would probably be the senior staff's estimate of the general clinical competence of a particular resident doctor during the year. He therefore predicted that the rank order of most to least talking resident would correspond with the rank order that would be assigned to the resident by senior physicians when they were asked to give a relative evaluation of the residents in terms of most to least competency after a year's work in the hospital. To test this prediction, he wrote to each of the six senior physicians who had taken part in the training of the five residents, giving the names of the residents in alphabetical order, and asking the senior man to rank the residents according to their general competence. The seniors were requested not to have any ties and to make the ranking independent of consultation with other physicians. These rankings were made by the six senior physicians two months after the residents had completed their year on the inpatient service, and seven months after the observations for this study had been concluded. The seniors' ranking of the residents according to over-all ability after completing a year's work can be seen in Table 10–11. There was a remarkable degree of consistency among senior physicians in the way in which they ranked the competency of the residents. The coefficient of concordance is high (0.93), and the probability is less than .005. It can be concluded that the six senior physicians agreed in ranking the residents from most to least competence as follows: 1—Dr. A, 2—Dr. B, 3—Dr. C, 4—Dr. E, and 5—Dr. D. The correspondence between the rank order of most to least talking resident (from Table 10–10), and the ranking by senior physicians according to all-around competence (from Table 10–11), can be seen in Table 10–12.

TABLE 10–12. Comparison of ranking of residents according to amount of participation in daily administrative conferences and evaluation by seniors

Ranked by	Dr. A	Dr. B	Dr. C	Dr. D	Dr. E
Amount of participation in daily conferences	1	2	3	4	5
Evaluation by seniors	1	2	3	5	4

It is obvious from Table 10–12 that there was a considerable correspondence between the amount of a resident physician's participation in the daily conferences and his evaluation by the senior staff. There was only one exception to the agreement between these two rank orders: the residents who were ranked fourth and fifth as most to least talking (Drs. D and E) were reversed regarding evaluation of competence.

It is difficult to know exactly what these results may mean. It is not felt that in any simple sense the most talking person was necessarily favorably evaluated because he spoke more during the conferences. In any case, this criterion could not enter directly into the judgment of three of the six senior staff physicians because they never attended the daily administrative conferences and only saw the resident physicians in supervisory sessions concerning psychotherapeutic work. Perhaps one answer, which would be operative in both the daily conferences and the supervisory hours, is that the most talking resident tended to be qualitatively different in his interaction when compared with the least talking resident. That is, Dr. A, in the administrative conference, would not only consistently transmit the requests of his patients for approval, but would also state his opinion about the advisability of these requests. For example, Dr. A would say: "Mr. Edwards wishes to go to the library this afternoon to return some books, and I feel that this is a reasonable request." Dr. D, on the other hand, would simply say: "Mr. Oliver asked me to bring up the request that he wants to go shopping today." Thus, Dr. A was willing to take a personal position in support of his patient and to defend his opinion at greater length than was Dr. D. Equally, Dr. A probably showed his greater interest in his patients in his supervisory hours as well as in the administrative conferences, so that he was likely to talk at greater length in both places. Dr. A was also likely to be more personally involved in the problems of his patients.

This brings up a further point which can be shown empirically from an analysis of each resident's participation in the administrative conferences: the residents who talked at greater length (Drs. A, B, and C) were engaged in more heated discussion with the senior staff than were the least talking residents (Drs. D and E). That is, the sparks flew more frequently between Drs. A, B, and C, and members of the senior staff. Clinically speaking, this meant that at any one time in the work of the hospital, there would be a stronger opinion—either positive or negative—held by the senior staff members about Drs. A, B, or C. At the close of the year, when asked to evaluate the residents, the seniors most favorably evaluated those residents with whom they had had the most interchange, whether their relations with the residents had been positive or negative. In this connection, and in terms of Table 10–12, it is interesting that the most heated disagreements occurred between the seniors and Dr. A, and yet Dr. A was the most favorably evaluated at the end of the year, and he became the chief resident during the following year.

Beyond the speculative ideas given above, it is hard to know exactly what to make of the correspondence shown between the amount of participation by residents and their evaluation by seniors except to note that it occurred and that it is consistent with the results found in very different small group interaction settings by other workers. Much the same sort of phenomena are reported by Bass (1949) in his analysis of leaderless group discussion, in French's (1950) work on verbal ouput and leadership status, and by Blau (1954) in his study of patterns of interaction among a group of officials in a government agency. For example, Bass (1949) reports a correlation of 0.93 between the time a participant in an eight-man group spent talking and the votes he received from observers for having demonstrated leadership. As this question could easily lead to an extended discussion of the general meaning of these phenomena in terms of small group dynamics, their correspondence must simply be noted in passing.

It is now time to turn to the analysis of the data within the twelve interaction categories, rather than discussing only the sheer number of acts as has been done so far. Table 10–13 shows the total number of acts of participation in the sixty-three conferences, by interaction category and role group.

As with the number of acts without regard to categories, the data in Table 10–13 must be adjusted for differing numbers of role participations by role groups. The simplest way to handle this adjustment is to express the number of acts generated by a role group in a category as a percentage of total acts for that role group. For example, among the seniors there were 434 acts of "gives suggestion," and an over-all total number of 2,307 acts. Thus acts of "giving suggestion" constituted 18.8 per cent of the total. The percentage distribution of acts within categories, ex-

TABLE 10–13. Number of acts of participation in 63 conferences, by interaction category and role group

Interaction category	Seniors (RP=139)[1]	Residents (RP=302)	Nurses (RP=210)	Other personnel (RP=135)	All role groups (RP=786)
1. Shows solidarity	36	48	13	8	105
2. Shows tension release	84	151	84	50	369
3. Agrees	62	72	25	9	168
4. Gives suggestion	434	168	28	16	646
5. Gives opinion	638	1,345	207	149	2,339
6. Gives orientation	509	2,051	358	313	3,231
7. Asks for orientation	163	67	54	23	307
8. Asks for opinion	89	43	19	3	154
9. Asks for suggestion	15	150	27	18	210
10. Disagrees	75	70	35	11	191
11. Shows tension	103	95	23	17	238
12. Shows antagonism	99	88	58	11	256
All categories	2,307	4,348	931	628	8,214

[1] Indicates number of individual role participations (RP) by role group in 63 conferences.

pressed as a percentage of a role group's total number of acts, may be seen in Table 10–14.

Some of the outstanding aspects of Table 10–14 occur in categories 2, 4, 10, and 12. In category 2 (shows tension release) the nurses and other specialized personnel were much higher than the seniors or residents. Since the acts in a particular category are expressed as a percentage of total acts for a role group, the higher figures for nurses and other personnel in the category of tension release reflect, in part, their lack of participation in other interaction categories—that is, they tended to remain silent.

Category 4 (gives suggestion) is quite interesting, as it shows that the seniors were a great deal higher, 18.8 per cent of their total, in this category, than the other three role groups, among which the highest percentage was 3.9 for the residents. Such a disproportionately greater percentage of suggestions on the part of one role group indicates a rather authoritatively run conference.

Category 10 (disagrees) and category 12 (shows antagonism) are interesting in that the seniors and nurses were considerably higher in both these categories compared with the other two role groups. This would seem to reflect the discontent felt by both seniors and nurses with the way the residents were handling their patients, particularly in administrative matters. It also reflects the feeling on the part of seniors and nurses, which was particularly acute for these two groups, of not being

TABLE 10–14. Distribution of acts of participation in 63 conferences, by interaction category, expressed as a percentage of total acts for each role group

Interaction category	Seniors	Residents	Nurses	Other personnel
1. Shows solidarity	1.6	1.1	1.4	1.3
2. Shows tension release	3.6	3.5	9.0	8.0
3. Agrees	2.7	1.7	2.7	1.4
4. Gives suggestion	18.8	3.9	3.0	2.5
5. Gives opinion	27.7	30.9	22.2	23.7
6. Gives orientation	22.0	47.2	38.5	49.8
7. Asks for orientation	7.1	1.5	5.8	3.7
8. Asks for opinion	3.9	1.0	2.0	0.5
9. Asks for suggestion	0.7	3.4	2.9	2.9
10. Disagrees	3.3	1.6	3.8	1.8
11. Shows tension	4.5	2.2	2.5	2.7
12. Shows antagonism	4.3	2.0	6.2	1.8
All categories	100.2	100.0	100.0	100.1

quite sure in their own minds that they knew what was going on. This is likely to be a problem in a psychiatric hospital where the major therapeutic technique is psychotherapy, as was true in the hospital under study. In terms of the observations in this study, the therapist—in this case a resident—could not report fully on what was going on with his patients because often he was not sure himself, and equally, much of the material was of a necessarily confidential nature. Nevertheless, considerable pressure was placed on the resident by both seniors and nurses to divulge information that might be used for administrative decisions (see Chapter 5). This often placed the resident in a dilemma.

With reference to the other categories: category 1 (shows solidarity) indicates that all the groups were about evenly divided in this respect, and this was also true for category 3 (agrees). In category 5 (gives opinion) the residents and senior doctors were higher, reflecting their higher status, than the nurses and other personnel. However, the percentages for category 5 were quite high for all groups, and this is indicative of the nature of the conferences. That is, these were communication and decision-making conferences, and hence the percentages in the category of giving opinion were high, as they also were for giving orientation (category 6). It is interesting that the people who had the most orientation to give about patients (the residents, nurses, and other personnel) were highest, while the seniors were lowest.

The reader should note the qualities of categories 4, 5, and 6 (gives suggestion, gives opinion, and gives orientation). By and large it takes more "push" to give an act of opinion, and somewhat more still to give

TABLE 10–15. Distribution of acts of participation in 63 conferences, by major area of interaction, expressed as a percentage of total acts for each role group

Area of interaction	Seniors	Residents	Nurses	Other personnel
Social-emotional area: positive	7.9	6.3	13.1	10.7
Task area: attempted answers	68.5	82.0	63.7	76.0
Task area: questions	11.7	5.9	10.7	7.1
Social-emotional area: negative	12.1	5.8	12.5	6.3
All areas	100.2	100.0	100.0	100.1

an act of suggestion, than it takes to give an act of orientation. This is reflected in Table 10–14 in the greater percentage of acts in categories 6 and 5 than in category 4.

In category 7 (asks for orientation) the seniors and nurses were high, and this is indicative of the tendency of these two groups to ask the residents for information about patients in the areas of administration and psychotherapy. Much the same is true for category 8 (asks for opinion).

In category 9 (asks for suggestion) the residents were highest, followed by the nurses and other personnel. The seniors were lowest in asking for suggestion, in contrast to being by far the highest in giving suggestion. Again this suggests the somewhat authoritative nature of the conference procedure. That the seniors experienced difficulty in playing their role in the conferences would seem to be indicated in category 11, where they showed a greater proportion of tension than any of the other groups.

Much of the material in Table 10–14 can be summarized by combining the categories in each of the four major areas of interaction. That is, the percentages in categories 1, 2, and 3 may be added to obtain an over-all percentage for the positive social-emotional area. Similarly a summation of categories 4, 5, and 6 results in an over-all percentage for the task area of attempted answers; and so on. The results of such a summary of the four major areas of interaction can be seen in Table 10–15. The residents were lowest and the nurses highest in both of the social-emotional areas. The balance between positive and negative emotion was on the positive side for all role groups except the seniors, where it was negative (12.1 per cent negative and 7.9 per cent positive). The residents confined themselves the most of any of the groups to the task of giving information, with 82.0 per cent of their total being attempted answers.

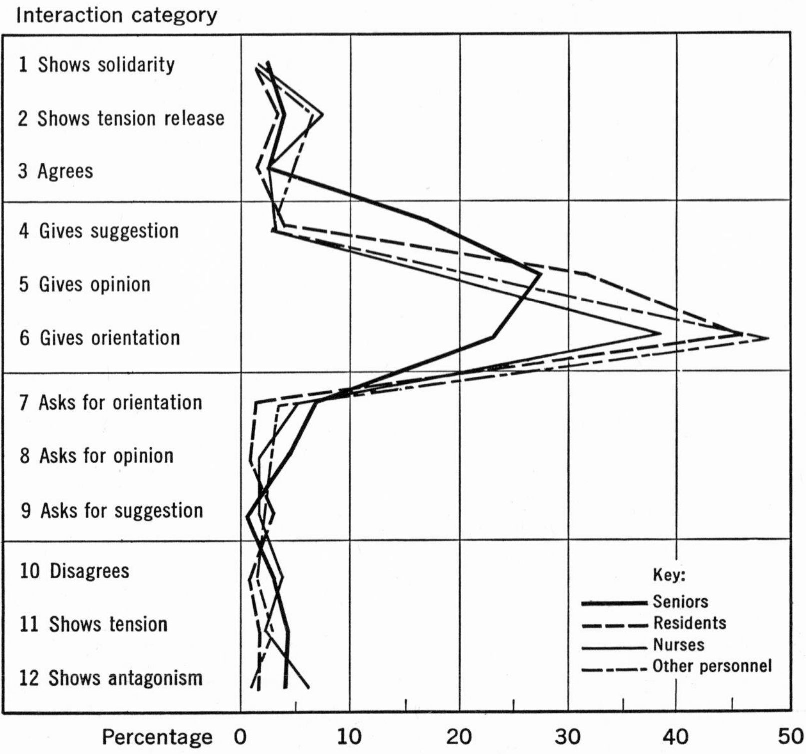

FIGURE 10–2. Profile of each role group's participation in 63 conferences, by interaction category. (Acts of participation in a category are expressed as a percentage of each role group's total acts.) Source: Table 10–14

The seniors and nurses were highest in the task area of asking questions with 11.7 and 10.7 per cent, respectively.

The material presented in Table 10–14 is summarized in Figure 10–2, which shows a profile of each role group's acts of participation. Although there are important differences between the profiles of the several role groups in Figure 10–2, the general configuration for each role group is roughly the same. This is in considerable part owing to the fact that the twelve interaction categories were devised to score *interaction*. In any kind of on-going interaction, an act in any one category by a person is most likely to call forth an act in the same category, or in its reciprocal, from the answering person (see Bales, 1950). For example, an act of giving orientation on the part of a nurse is likely to be answered by a further act of giving orientation on the part of a resident or another nurse. Alternatively, the giving of orientation often calls forth the asking for further orientation. Similarly, antagonism begets antagonism, agreement begets agreement, and asking for suggestion begets the giving of suggestion. This principle does not always hold true, but there is a strong tendency for it to do so, and as such it is manifested in the data when acts in a category are expressed as a percentage of the total acts for a group, and then one group is compared with another.

To carry the discussion further, it is necessary to return to the basic data in Table 10–13 and consider another method of analysis. The twelve categories may be considered as posing a set of "problems" in interaction. That is, when the conference discussion has progressed to a point where a need for suggestion comes up, which role group acts to meet this problem most frequently? Or, when a need for orientation arises, which role group provides it most frequently? Or, when antagonism is expressed, which role group is highest in its expression? Considered in this way each of the categories poses a particular problem, and it is possible to compare the various role groups regarding their relative participation in the "solution" of the problem.

In order to present the conference material in terms of the above discussion the data in Table 10–13 must first be reduced to average individual participation within the various categories, following the same procedure used for total acts (see Tables 10–1 and 10–2). As an example the giving of suggestion (category 4) may again be used. In Table 10–13 it can be seen that the seniors gave 434 acts of suggestion during 139 role participations, or an average of 3.12 acts per individual role participation for a representative senior physician. Similarly, the residents gave 168 acts of suggestion during 302 role participations, or an average of 0.56 acts per individual role participation for a representative resident. Treating the data in this way results in an index of average individual participation per conference within interaction categories by role groups, as can be seen in Table 10–16. The reader will note that the totals of these indexes correspond to the "all 63 conferences" column in Table 10–2. It would be simple to remove the decimal point from the figures in Table 10–16 by multiplying all figures by 100 and thus making the table less formidable, but this was not done because it might have been more confusing than helpful. Two decimal places have been retained for the purpose of later computing percentages and rank order within a category. The statistical reliability of the data in Table 10–16 is high as will be seen later (Table 10–19).

It is now possible to use Table 10–16 to discuss what happens when a "problem" represented by an interaction category arises, because the

TABLE 10–16. Index of average individual participation per conference, by interaction category and role group

Interaction category	Seniors	Residents	Nurses	Other personnel
1. Shows solidarity	0.26	0.16	0.06	0.06
2. Shows tension release	0.60	0.50	0.40	0.37
3. Agrees	0.45	0.24	0.12	0.07
4. Gives suggestion	3.12	0.56	0.13	0.12
5. Gives opinion	4.59	4.45	0.99	1.10
6. Gives orientation	3.66	6.79	1.70	2.32
7. Asks for orientation	1.17	0.22	0.26	0.17
8. Asks for opinion	0.64	0.14	0.09	0.02
9. Asks for suggestion	0.11	0.50	0.13	0.13
10. Disagrees	0.54	0.23	0.17	0.08
11. Shows tension	0.74	0.31	0.11	0.13
12. Shows antagonism	0.71	0.29	0.28	0.08
All categories	16.59	14.39	4.44	4.65

data for the various role groups are now comparable within a category (and the table can be read across the rows as well as down the columns). For example, it was noted earlier (in Table 10–14) that the seniors gave suggestions much more frequently than the other role groups, even when this was expressed as a percentage of the role group's total output. In terms now of a comparison between role groups when the problem of suggestion arises, it can be seen from Table 10–16 how thoroughly a representative senior physician dominated this problem, compared with a representative resident or nurse. The index in Table 10–16 for seniors in category 4 (gives suggestion) is 3.12 as compared with 0.56 for the residents, 0.13 for the nurses, and 0.12 for other personnel.

Carrying this method of analysis a step further, it is possible to convert the index of average individual participation across the rows in Table 10–16 to the percentage contributed by each role group to the solution of a problem represented by an interaction category. In these terms, when the problem of giving suggestion (category 4) arose in the conferences, the seniors gave 79.4 per cent of the suggestions, while the residents gave only 14.2 per cent, the nurses 3.3 per cent, and the other personnel 3.1 per cent. The results of such an analysis for each of the twelve categories can be seen in Table 10–17.

Table 10–17 shows that whenever any of the problems represented by the categories (1, 2, and 3) in the positive social-emotional area arose, the seniors were highest, the residents next, the nurses third, and the other personnel least expressive in this area. The problem of agreement (category 3) is particularly interesting because the seniors were so much higher than the other groups. This, in part, probably shows where the "power" was in the administrative conferences, and equally it indicates who felt "free" to participate and who remained more "constrained." Again, this is a reflection of the status hierarchy in the conferences.

In category 4 (gives suggestion) the seniors were overwhelmingly dominant. In category 5 (gives opinion), however, the seniors and residents were equal in contributing the bulk of responses to this problem, whereas the nurses and other personnel contributed very little. As in the problem of agreement, these differences in the giving of opinion show which role groups felt free to participate, and which did not.

The proportions among role groups shifted for the problem of giving orientation (category 6) with the residents highest, the seniors next, then the other personnel, and the nurses least. In a way, this problem of giving orientation reflects the general consensus in the conference about which role group "knows most about the patient." As indicated, the residents gave the most orientation, a fact that was probably related to the very high evaluation placed on psychotherapy, while the nurses apparently felt they had "little to contribute" or that "it wouldn't be recognized anyway" if they reported on the behavior of patients on the ward. This kind of attitude, lying behind the differences in proportion of giving orientation, tallies with the attitudes of the nurses toward the daily administrative conference which were presented in the picture interview material in

TABLE 10–17. Percentage distribution of the contribution by each role group to the solution of the problem represented by each interaction category[1]

Interaction category	Seniors	Residents	Nurses	Other personnel	All role groups
1. Shows solidarity	48.1	29.6	11.1	11.1	99.9
2. Shows tension release	32.1	26.7	21.4	19.8	100.0
3. Agrees	51.1	27.3	13.6	8.0	100.0
4. Gives suggestion	79.4	14.2	3.3	3.1	100.0
5. Gives opinion	41.2	40.0	8.9	9.9	100.0
6. Gives orientation	25.3	46.9	11.7	16.0	99.9
7. Asks for orientation	64.3	12.1	14.3	9.3	100.0
8. Asks for opinion	71.9	15.7	10.1	2.2	99.9
9. Asks for suggestion	12.6	57.5	14.9	14.9	99.9
10. Disagrees	52.9	22.5	16.7	7.8	99.9
11. Shows tension	57.4	24.0	8.5	10.1	100.0
12. Shows antagonism	52.2	21.3	20.6	5.9	100.0

[1] As indicated in the text, these percentages have been arrived at by considering each interaction category as a problem in itself, and then reading across the rows in Table 10–16 in order to ascertain the percentage an average individual member of each role group contributed to the interaction that went into the solution of a problem.

Chapters 8 and 9. Thus, the greatest amount of orientation was given by the residents—46.9 per cent. The seniors followed with 25.3 per cent, reflecting their contributions regarding contacts with the patients' families and broad policy matters. The other personnel were next with 16.0 per cent, and apparently felt freer to talk about the patients in occupational therapy or activities than the nurses felt free, with only 11.7 per cent, to talk about the general behavior of the patients on the ward.

The next two categories were dominated by the seniors. The seniors gave 64.3 per cent of the total in asking for orientation (category 7), and 71.9 per cent of the total in asking for opinion (category 8). Thus, whenever these problems arose it was the seniors who pressed the issue. The low percentages in both these categories for the other role groups essentially reflect the "passivity" of the residents, nurses, and other personnel, and the desire of these three role groups to "get the conference over with," as against the desire of the seniors to find out "what's going on." In contrast to categories 7 and 8, category 9 (asks for suggestion) was primarily taken over by the residents, who contributed 57.5 per cent of the total to this problem.

In the negative social-emotional area the seniors had over 50 per cent of the total in all three categories (10, 11, and 12). It is interesting that in categories 10 (disagrees) and 12 (shows antagonism) the seniors, residents, and nurses were all relatively high, while the other personnel were low. This would seem to indicate that the sparks were flying between these three role groups over matters under discussion, whereas the other personnel remained more passive.

The material in Table 10–17 can be shown graphically in terms of a profile of each role group's average individual participation within interaction categories. This is done in Figure 10–3, and (in contrast to Figure 10–2) a fairly distinctive profile emerges for each role group. A number of patterns are evident from the profiles in Figure 10–3. The first is the similarity in profile between the nurses and other personnel. The low percentage of participation in all categories is the outstanding attribute of both profiles. Within this pattern of low participation, both nurses and other personnel had their highest percentage in the category of tension release—that is, they tended to respond with laughter more than any other single type of response. Perhaps the best way of labeling the pattern shown by both nurses and other personnel would be to call it one of "passive minimal participation."

A second pattern is formed by the reciprocal nature of the profiles between the seniors and residents. When the seniors were high in giving

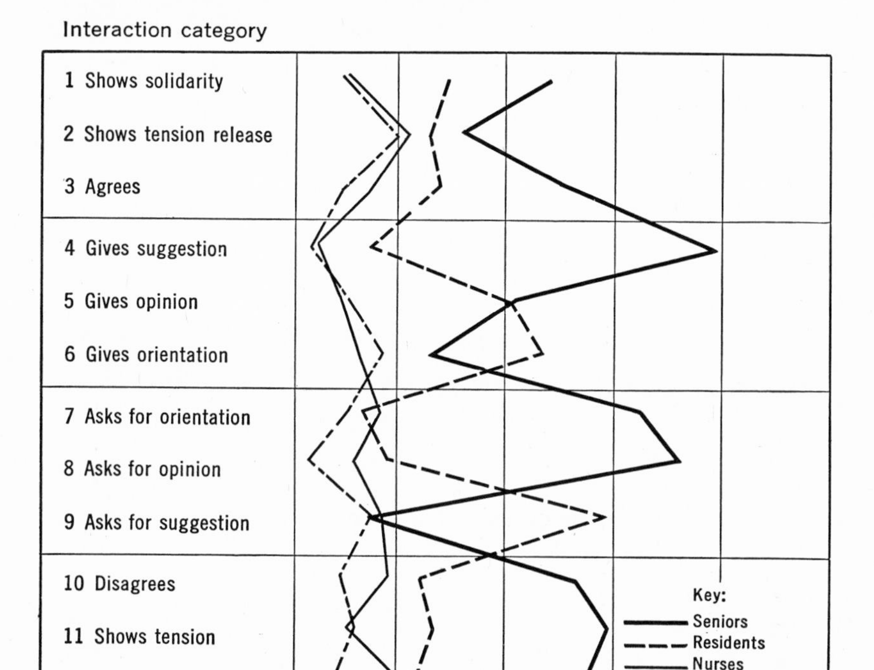

FIGURE 10–3. Profile of the percentage distribution of each role group's average individual participation within each interaction category. Source: Table 10–17

suggestion and asking for orientation and opinion, the residents were low in these categories; but when the residents were high in giving orientation and asking for suggestion, the seniors were low.

When the four role groups are compared in terms of their expression of emotion, it can be seen that by far the highest amount of emotion in both the positive and negative areas was expressed by the seniors, the next most by the residents, with the nurses and other personnel being least. One would conclude that apparently higher status confers greater freedom to express feeling and emotion when the four groups are compared with each other.

A question may have arisen in the reader's mind as to how consistent the patterns appearing in Tables 10–16 and 10–17 and in Figure 10–3 actually were. To test this it is possible to follow the previous procedure of dividing the material into three consecutive periods of twenty-one conferences each, and to make a table identical with Table 10–16 for each of the periods. Thus, the role group participation within a category can

TABLE 10–18. Ranking of role groups according to amount of participation in each interaction category, based on 63 conferences

Role group	Social-emotional area: positive			Task area: attempted answers			Task area: questions			Social-emotional area: negative		
	Categories 1	2	3	Categories 4	5	6	Categories 7	8	9	Categories 10	11	12
Seniors	1	1	1	1	1	2	1	1	4	1	1	1
Residents	2	2	2	2	2	1	3	2	1	2	2	2
Nurses	3.5	3	3	3	4	4	2	3	2.5	3	4	3
Other personnel	3.5	4	4	4	3	3	4	4	2.5	4	3	4

be rank ordered for each of the three periods, and these rank orders can be compared with the rank order obtained from the data on the total sixty-three conferences. For example, in Table 10–16 the rank order in category 1 (shows solidarity) is: 1—seniors, 2—residents, 3.5—nurses, and 3.5—other personnel. Similarly, in Table 10–16 the rank order for category 6 (gives orientation) is: 1—residents, 2—seniors, 3—other personnel, and 4—nurses. The results of such a ranking of the total conference data in Table 10–16 can be seen in Table 10–18. For comparison, the rank order correlations over the three periods can be seen in Table 10–19.

The average participation within categories for each of the three periods has not been given here, as the reader is probably not concerned with such detail; rather the general agreement in rank orders over the three periods is indicated in Table 10–19. It is necessary to note, however,

TABLE 10–19. Ranking of role groups according to amount of participation in each interaction category, based on three periods of 21 conferences each

Role group	Social-emotional area: positive			Task area: attempted answers			Task area: questions			Social-emotional area: negative		
	Categories 1	2	3	Categories 4	5	6	Categories 7	8	9	Categories 10	11	12
Seniors	1	1	1	1	1	2	1	1	4	1	1	1
Residents	2	2	2	2	2	1	3	2	1	2	2	2
Nurses	3	3	3	3.5	4	4	2	3	2	3	4	3
Other personnel	4	4	4	3.5	3	3	4	4	3	4	3	4
Coefficient of concordance	0.37	0.80*	0.88*	0.84*	0.77*	0.94*	0.88*	0.94*	0.48	0.88*	0.85*	0.85*

* Indicates $<.05$ level of significance.

the consistency over time shown in Table 10–19 of the detailed pattern of rank order within separate categories. Such a high degree of consistency in pattern should be of considerable interest to the student of small group dynamics, as these daily conferences were not experimentally created groups but were actual groups concerned with the real problems of running a hospital.

In Table 10–19 it can be seen that it is possible to be confident (at the .05 level) about the consistency in rank order for ten of the twelve categories. The two categories which varied the most in rank order over the three periods were category 1 (shows solidarity) and category 9 (asks for suggestion). A comparison of Tables 10–18 and 10–19 will show that the rank order obtained in terms of the total conference material (Table 10–18) is very similar to the rank order obtained when the conference material was separated into three periods (Table 10–19). Thus, not only was there a consistency over time in the total amount of talking done by the various role groups (see Tables 10–2 and 10–3), but equally there was a high degree of consistency over time in a role group's pattern of talking within the twelve categories.

Following Bales (1950), the relations between the twelve categories can be used to construct indexes of various sorts. Here, only two of these indexes will be given in order to show the possibilities of such analysis. For example, an index of "positive emotion" can be computed by expressing the number of acts in the positive social-emotional area (categories 1, 2, 3) as a percentage of the total acts in both positive and negative social-emotional areas (categories 1, 2, 3, and 10, 11, 12). The formula for this would be:

$$\text{Index of positive emotion} = \frac{(1+2+3)}{(1+2+3) \quad + \quad (10+11+12)}$$

A second sort of index can be computed using the categories of gives opinion (category 5) and gives orientation (category 6). Such an index might be called "willingness to participate" and can be computed by expressing the number of acts in category 5 (gives opinion) as a percentage of the total acts in categories 5 (gives opinion) and 6 (gives orientation). The formula would be:

$$\text{Index of willingness to participate} = \frac{5}{5+6}$$

The rationale behind the computation of this index of willingness to participate rests on the assumption that it takes more effort and involvement to give an act of opinion than it does to give an act of orientation.

By considering first the comparison between these two indexes with-

TABLE 10–20. Indexes of expression of positive emotion and willingness to participate in daily administrative conferences, for all role groups

Index	First 21 conferences	Second 21 conferences	Third 21 conferences	All 63 conferences
Positive emotion	0.53	0.48	0.40	0.48
Willingness to participate	0.50	0.39	0.36	0.42

out regard to role group, and simply treating the entire conference group as a unit, the results can be seen in Table 10–20. This table shows that there was a relation between the amount of positive emotion expressed in the conferences and the willingness to participate. Both indexes were highest in the first period, both decreased in the second period, and both reached their lowest point in the third period. This again reflects the withdrawal of the four groups from each other, which was discussed in Chapter 5.

As one might expect, the expression of positive emotion and willingness to participate varied from one role group to another. The index of positive emotion by role group is given in Table 10–21, while the index of willingness to participate by role group is given in Table 10–22.

There was not a simple and direct relation between willingness to participate and expression of positive emotion when the indexes were computed by role group, as can be seen through a comparison of Table 10–21 with Table 10–22. First of all, in the "all 63 conferences" column in Table 10–21, the expression of positive emotion was highest for the other personnel, the residents and nurses were intermediate, while the seniors were least positive in their expression of emotion. One might speculate that it was easier to express positive emotion the less authority one had in the status system. Almost the reverse order obtains in Table 10–22, where willingness to participate was highest among the seniors, second among the residents, third among the nurses, and least among the other personnel. In general, however, when Tables 10–21 and 10–22 are compared over the three periods within a particular role group, as positive emotion goes down so does willingness to participate. This is

TABLE 10–21. Index of expression of positive emotion in daily administrative conferences, by role group

Role group	First 21 conferences	Second 21 conferences	Third 21 conferences	All 63 conferences
Seniors	0.40	0.42	0.36	0.40
Residents	0.57	0.49	0.47	0.52
Nurses	0.63	0.53	0.27	0.51
Other personnel	0.78	0.53	0.56	0.63

TABLE 10–22. Index of willingness to participate in daily administrative conferences, by role group

Role group	First 21 conferences	Second 21 conferences	Third 21 conferences	All 63 conferences
Seniors	0.63	0.54	0.48	0.56
Residents	0.49	0.34	0.35	0.40
Nurses	0.39	0.37	0.34	0.37
Other personnel	0.36	0.39	0.20	0.32

particularly evident in a comparison between the first and third periods. Thus, the seniors' index of positive emotion in the first period was 0.40 and their willingness to participate was 0.63. In the third period, however, the seniors' expression of positive emotion dropped to 0.36, and willingness to participate dropped to 0.48. Similarly, for the residents, the index of positive emotion during the first period was 0.57, and willingness to participate was 0.49. In the third period, however, the residents' expression of positive emotion dropped to 0.47, and willingness to participate dropped to 0.35.

It is not possible at this point to carry such an analysis by the use of indexes further, as the purpose here was merely to indicate the usefulness of such indexes in evaluating administrative conference data. Other such indexes and their changes over time will be taken up in the discussion of process in Chapter 12.

CHAPTER 11

The Content of Communication

Thus far the administrative conference data have been analyzed largely in terms of the form of the interaction, or "how" things were expressed by the various role groups. In this chapter the discussion turns to an analysis of the content of the interaction, or "what" was expressed.

METHOD OF SCORING CONTENT OF INTERACTION

In order to make a content analysis of the sixty-three daily administrative conferences it was necessary to devise a set of categories which would begin to bring out this information. The first task was simply to number each conference from one to sixty-three so that the material could later be followed from day to day, week to week, and so forth.

The second task was to define the unit to be scored. It was decided to score in terms of topics. A *topic* was defined as any sequence of discussion around an item of communication. The discussion around such an item could follow through until it was completed, or the discussion could be started at one point in the conference, dropped, and then picked up again. In the case of these "broken-up" topics, the several parts were scored as a single topic. Thus, no specific topic could be repeated during a particular daily administrative conference. Another rule was followed in determining what was a topic. When a resident, or one of the other personnel, was reporting a sequence of relatively unrelated facts that had occurred over a period of time, this entire sequence was scored as a single topic. For example, the doctor who was on call the preceding evening might report a number of different events which had happened the preceding evening, and his entire report would be scored as a single topic. If, however, after he had finished making his report, one or more of the events was singled out for discussion, this discussion became a second topic. The same procedure was followed during the Monday conferences when a resident doctor gave a summary of the progress of his various patients during the week. His entire therapeutic summary was scored as a single topic. If, however, one of the patients was singled out by the group for further discussion, this further discussion became a second topic.

The reader should glance again at the sample quotation of parts of a daily administrative conference which was given at the beginning of the preceding chapter as an illustration of scoring within the twelve interaction categories. This same illustrative material will be used to indicate the nature of the content analysis by topics. In the illustrative material there were five topics. These may be designated as topics A through E and summarized as follows.

Topic A:
Dr. Shaw asked who was the doctor on call last night. Dr. Ryan said that he was and that nothing had happened.

Topic B:
Dr. Shaw said that the women's locked ward was full and that no new patients were to be taken in. He mentioned to Dr. Ramsay that no new patients were to be admitted over the week end. Dr. Sears asked what the census was, and Dr. Shaw said that it was quite low but that the women's ward was full.

Topic C:
Miss Nicholas made a joke about Miss Lewis' being the patient voted by the men to come over and occupy the four-bed ward on the open ward. There was laughter, and Dr. Ramsay wondered what sort of recreation tax might be appropriate if Miss Lewis did move to the four-bed ward.

Topic D:
Dr. Reynolds introduced a discussion of what procedures she should follow with reference to a letter that Mr. Innes had written to his parents. She expressed concern over whether she should send the letter because she had not yet established a therapeutic relation with Mr. Innes. There was considerable discussion by various members of the group as to alternative procedures that might be followed. The topic ended with Dr. Shaw's suggesting that Dr. Reynolds either send a personal note along with the letter or else call up the family and explain the situation to them.

Topic E:
Dr. Rolfe made an administrative request that his patient, Mr. Onofrio, be allowed to remain with his relatives outside the hospital over the week end rather than returning each night to sleep in the hospital. Dr. Shaw disagreed with this request and there was a somewhat heated discussion between Dr. Rolfe and Dr. Shaw. The topic ended with Dr. Shaw's refusing the request, and

Dr. Rolfe's agreeing that he would not permit Mr. Onofrio to remain out overnight.

After a decision had been made concerning the procedure to be followed in dividing the material into topics, the next task was to determine how the content of the topics was to be scored. Each topic was scored in terms of two broad questions: How did the topic come up? and What happened to the topic? Five content categories were devised for scoring "how the topic came up," and nine content categories were devised for scoring "what happened to the topic." The manner in which the five sample topics summarized above were scored in the fourteen content categories may be seen in Table 11–1.

Concerning Table 11–1, it should be noted that if a content category was not applicable to a particular topic, this is so indicated by an "x." As can be seen in the table, the scoring of the topic in the fourteen categories should be read down the columns.

A few words of explanation for each of the fourteen categories are necessary.

Category 1: The *number* of the conference in the sequence from one to sixty-three was indicated.

Category 2: The *role group* to which the individual introducing the topic belonged was indicated.

Category 3: The *individual* person who introduced the topic was indicated.

Category 4: The *form* of the topic was indicated. This was scored in one of three subcategories: *routine communication only, questions* which required an answer, and *requests.* The difference between these three subcategories can be indicated very sharply. Routine communication only consisted of descriptive statements—giving orientation and opinion about a topic. Questions consisted of asking for information about a problem. Requests differed from questions in that requests required a decision to be made, whereas questions only involved discussion. If the topic started out as communication only but developed into a question, it was scored as a question. If a topic contained both questions and a request, it was scored as a request. The differences between these three subcategories may be seen in Table 11–1 where topics A, B, and C were communication only, topic D was a question, and topic E was a request.

Category 5: The *area* in which the topic fell was indicated. Similar to the areas of hospital life which have been used throughout this book, and which were specifically developed for scoring the picture interview

TABLE 11–1. Scoring of five sample topics according to fourteen categories used in content analysis

Category	Topic A	Topic B	Topic C	Topic D	Topic E
How topic came up					
1. Serial number of conference	3	3	3	3	3
2. Role group initiating	Seniors	Seniors	Nurses	Residents	Residents
3. Individual initiating	Dr. Shaw	Dr. Shaw	Miss Nicholas	Dr. Reynolds	Dr. Rolfe
4. Form of topic	Communication only	Communication only	Communication only	Question	Request
5. Area of topic	Administration	Administration	Human relations	Administration	Administration
What happened to topic					
6. Specific or general	Specific	Specific	Specific	Specific	Specific
7. Simple or complex	Simple	Simple	Simple	Complex (Adm/Th)	Complex (Adm/Th)
8. Role group complicating	x	x	x	Residents	Seniors
9. Individual complicating	x	x	x	Dr. Reynolds	Dr. Shaw
10. Result conclusive or inconclusive	Conclusive	Conclusive	Conclusive	Conclusive	Conclusive
11. Result of request	x	x	x	x	Decision against
12. Length in acts	3	8	18	50	30
13. Emotional or unemotional	Unemotional	Emotional	Emotional	Emotional	Emotional
14. Balance of emotion	x	Positive	Positive	Negative	Negative

material in Chapter 6, a topic was scored in the administrative conferences according to whether it fell within the areas of *administration, therapy,* or *human relations.* A topic was scored in the area of administration if it began with a reporting of the procedures and details to be followed in the day-to-day operation of the hospital. A topic was scored in the area of therapy if it began with a reporting of the nature of the treatment of a patient; or consisted of an evaluation of the patient's emotional response to an event in the hospital; or concerned the evaluation of the emotional responses of people other than patients to each other.

A topic was scored in the area of human relations if it began by simply reporting an incident of interaction between two or more people without the speaker's introducing any relation of the interaction to administrative or therapeutic matters. As can be seen in Table 11–1, all the sample topics started out in the area of administration except for topic C, which was in the area of human relations. A topic was always scored according to the way it started out. It may have remained in the same area of life throughout the length of the topic, in which case there was no problem. If the topic was complicated by the introduction of references to another area of life, it was then scored as a complex topic and received a separate score under category 7. The details concerning whether a topic was simple or complex will be discussed under category 7, but it may be seen in Table 11–1 that topics A, B, and C were simple, whereas topics D and E were complex.

The five categories discussed above were contained in the broad initial question of "how the topic came up." The second broad question concerned the categories which delineated "what happened to the topic."

Category 6: The question here was threefold: whether the topic was concerned with a specific matter; whether it was a discussion of general policy or procedure; or whether the topic began as a specific matter and then the discussion about it became generalized. Thus, a topic was scored within a threefold classification: *specific, general,* and *specific-to-general.* As may be seen in Table 11–1, all five of the sample topics were specific. Examples of general topics, and of topics which moved from a discussion of the specific-to-general, will be given later in this chapter. Briefly, a general topic might be one in which a senior staff doctor introduced a discussion about changing the general procedure for granting privileges to patients. A specific-to-general topic might be one in which a resident doctor introduced a request for his patient to go to the library, but this request became enmeshed in a general discussion of the policy to be followed in granting privileges to patients.

Category 7: The decision here was whether the topic remained *simple* or became *complex.* As noted under category 5, a topic was always scored in the area in which it started out. It may have been complicated by the introduction of references to another area of life, even by the speaker who introduced the topic. This was the case in topic D in Table 11–1, where Dr. Reynolds introduced an administrative matter concerning whether she should permit a letter written by Mr. Innes to be mailed. Dr. Reynolds immediately went on to complicate this topic herself by introducing therapeutic considerations about her difficulty in being able to form a relationship with Mr. Innes and the bearing this might have on the administrative matter of sending the letter. Thus, this topic was scored as complex (administration-to-therapy), and was complicated by the resident doctor's introducing the topic. A topic may also have been complicated by someone other than the person who introduced the topic. This was the case in topic E in Table 11–1, where an administrative request by Dr. Rolfe that his patient be allowed to remain out of the hospital overnight was complicated by the introduction of therapeutic considerations on the part of Dr. Shaw. Specifically, after some discussion between Dr. Shaw and Dr. Rolfe, which fell solely in the administrative area, Dr. Shaw introduced a therapeutic qualification when he said: "I find it hard to say why I don't feel Mr. Onofrio should do this, but at this stage, with Mr. Onofrio in insulin treatment, it seems best to me that he should not go home now." Thus, the topic was scored as complex (administration-to-therapy), and was complicated by the senior physician, Dr. Shaw. Scoring was always done in the direction of movement of complexity. There were six logical possibilities which were exhaustive of the direction of movement, although the occurrence of some of these was relatively infrequent. The six logical possibilities were: therapy-to-administration, therapy-to-human relations, human relations-to-therapy, human relations-to-administration, administration-to-therapy, and administration-to-human relations.

Category 8: If a topic was simple (see category 7), there was no score in category 8. If a topic was complex, the *role group complicating* the topic was indicated. For example, in Table 11–1, topic D was complicated by the residents (Dr. Reynolds herself), and topic E was complicated by the seniors (Dr. Shaw).

Category 9: If a topic was simple (see category 7), there was no score in category 9. If a topic was complex, the *individual complicating* the topic was indicated. For example, in Table 11–1, topic D was complicated by Dr. Reynolds, and topic E by Dr. Shaw.

Category 10: The decision here was whether a topic ended in a *conclusive* or *inconclusive* manner. All topics were scored in this category—whether they were communication only, questions, or requests. If a topic was concerned with communication only, the person who introduced the topic must have been allowed to finish speaking, and a sense of closure reached, before a score of conclusive could be made. If a topic was a question, the question must have received a specific answer to be conclusive. Equally, a request must have been given a definite yes or no to be conclusive. In Table 11–1, a sense of closure was reached in topics A, B, and C, which were concerned with communication only. In topic D a specific answer was given to Dr. Reynolds' question about whether she should send the letter written by Mr. Innes when Dr. Shaw concluded the topic by saying that she should either send a note along with the letter or call up the family and talk with them. Equally, in topic E a decision was reached in the matter of Dr. Rolfe's request that Mr. Onofrio be permitted to remain out of the hospital overnight. The decision was negative, and the matter was brought to a definite conclusion. The five sample topics do not include an example of an inconclusive topic. Examples of this type of topic will be given later in this chapter; but briefly, if a request such as the one made by Dr. Rolfe in topic E were to have been left up in the air by Dr. Shaw's saying that the matter should be thought about at greater length, then such a topic would be scored as inconclusive. In general, inconclusive topics were those where questions were not given an answer, and requests did not receive a definite decision.

Category 11: This category was scored only if the form of the topic (see category 4) was a *request.* If the topic was a request, it was scored as: *decision for, decision against,* and *undecided.* Again referring to Table 11–1, the decision was against Mr. Onofrio's remaining out of the hospital overnight in topic E. If the matter had been left up in the air, the score would then have been "undecided."

Category 12: The *length of the topic* measured by the *number of acts* contained in it was indicated. As may be seen on Table 11–1, topic A contained 3 acts, topic B contained 8 acts, and so forth. This may be checked by referring to the scoring of these sample topics by the interaction categories in the preceding chapter.

Category 13: The decision here was whether the topic was *emotional* or *unemotional.* For purposes of scoring, a topic was considered to be emotional if it contained any acts falling in the interaction categories 1, 2, 3, 10, 11, and 12. This somewhat arbitrary procedure was necessary for clarity in scoring, and was made somewhat more realistic by the fact that the method used in recording the material in the conferences was such that only gross acts of non-verbal emotion were likely to be recorded. Emotionally laden verbal acts were, of course, recorded as part of the on-going flow of speech. As indicated in the preceding chapter, individual smiles or frowns were not recorded. Actual open laughter or strained silence by either an individual or the group was, however, indicated, as may be seen in the interaction category scoring of the sample topics. Usually an emotional topic contained considerably more than a single act in one of the emotional categories. As may be seen in Table 11–1, all the sample topics were emotional except topic A.

Category 14: This category was concerned with the *balance of emotion,* and a score appears in this category only if the topic was emotional (see category 13). If the topic was unemotional, there was no score in category 14. The topic was scored as *positive emotion* if the sum of acts appearing in the topic in categories 1, 2, and 3 was greater than the sum of acts in categories 10, 11, and 12. Similarly, a topic was scored as *negative emotion* if the sum of acts in categories 10, 11, and 12 was greater than the sum of acts in categories 1, 2, and 3. If there was a tie in the number of positive and negative emotional acts, the topic was then scored as positive emotion. This follows the general logic of the procedure in determining the balance of emotion which was used in developing a scoring system for the picture interview material in Chapter 6.

It is obvious that the scoring procedure for each of the fourteen categories given above was designed so that the material might be placed on IBM cards and the data tabulated by means of machine sorting. In the actual scoring of the material the problems presented were somewhat less formidable than they might seem to the reader looking at Table 11–1. There is an inherent logic in the fourteen categories that follows the two broad questions that were asked: "How did the topic come up?" and "What happened to it?" Summarizing, for any particular topic: interest was first directed toward the role group and the individual who introduced the topic. The next matter of concern was with the form of the topic and the area of life in which it fell. Following this, attention was focused on whether the topic was about a specific matter or was part of a general problem, and whether the discussion remained centered in one area of life or was complicated by the introduction of factors from other areas. If the topic became complicated, the question arose of what role group and individual did the complicating. Moving toward the end of the topic, the interest was on whether the discussion was conclusive or inconclusive; and if a request had been made, what the nature of the decision was. Finally, the focus was on the total length of the topic and whether the discussion had been emotional or not. If the discussion had been emotional, was the balance positive or negative?

The fourteen scoring categories were developed by the writer on administrative conference material other than the sixty-three conferences used in the final analysis. The writer then trained one of his assistants, Miss Nancy Hatch, in the use of the scoring categories. After the writer

TABLE 11–2. Agreement between judges in scoring of topics on every twelfth administrative conference

Conference number	Agree	Disagree	All topics
Twelve	9	2	11
Twenty-four	28	3	31
Thirty-six	9	2	11
Forty-eight	9	1	10
Sixty	6	1	7
All conferences	61	9	70

and his assistant felt that they were sufficiently familiar with the scoring system, they selected every twelfth administrative conference from the sixty-three conferences analyzed here, and independently scored these conferences.

The agreement between the two judges is indicated in Table 11–2. The greater number of topics in the twenty-fourth conference reflects the fact that this was a Monday conference and lasted for forty-five rather than the usual fifteen to twenty minutes. The two judges agreed completely about their division of the material into topics. A disagreement in the scoring of a topic was recorded if there was disagreement on any of the fourteen scoring categories. The extent of agreement on this basis for each of the conferences used in the reliability check can be seen in Table 11–2, as can also the over-all agreement on 61 out of the total 70 topics. The over-all agreement was 87.1 per cent. Since this was considered to be sufficiently high agreement, the assistant, Miss Hatch, then went on to score all the material in the sixty-three conferences. After scoring had been completed, the data were coded, placed on punch cards, and tabulated by machine.

HOW THE TOPICS CAME UP

The answer to the question of how a topic was introduced in the administrative conferences may be seen in Table 11–3, which shows the distribution of the total 745 topics by area of life and form of topic. There were 488 topics in the administrative area, 238 in the therapeutic area, and only 19 in the area of human relations. The low number of human relations topics poses an interesting question with reference to the nature of the on-going work in the conferences. Problems which might have been solved more simply if they had been phrased in terms of human relations were discussed, instead, in terms of administration or therapy. This "masking" of many problems which were essentially ones of human

TABLE 11–3. Total number of topics, by area of life and form of topic

Form of topic	Therapy	Administration	Human relations	All areas
Communication only	184	223	17	424
Questions	40	130	2	172
Requests	14	135	0	149
All forms	238	488	19	745

relations had a definite effect on the adequacy of communication and on the amount of tension in the conferences, as has been indicated in Chapters 3 through 5.

As the conferences were primarily of an administrative nature, it is not surprising to find the number of administrative topics exceeding that of therapeutic topics. Similarly, it is probably to be expected that the number of communication only topics exceeded the number of questions, which in turn exceeded the number of requests.

The nature of administrative topics in the form of communication only consisted of such matters as reports by the doctor on call of the events of the preceding evening, reports by residents and nurses about the day-to-day operation of the administrative structure of the hospital, and reports by seniors and other specialized personnel of routine contacts with the patients and their families. Administrative questions concerned the advisability of moving patients from one ward to another, clarification of specific points of procedure and policy, and so forth. Administrative requests were in the nature of direct requests by residents or nurses for decisions about administrative matters, such as a patient's privileges, whether television could be seen after hours, and so forth.

Therapeutic topics in the form of communication only consisted largely of the reports by residents on the progress of their patients during the week. Therapeutic questions concerned doubts in the minds of residents and nurses about whether a certain procedure was beneficial or harmful in terms of the present condition of the patient. Therapeutic requests were quite low in number and were restricted to such requests as those made by a resident that a nurse attempt to make a more direct relationship with a patient on the ward when the resident felt this would be therapeutically useful to the patient at this point in his progress.

The difference in proportion of the form of topics in the areas of administration and therapy can be seen in Table 11–4. A far greater percentage of therapeutic topics was stated in terms of communication only than was true for administrative topics. Only 22.7 per cent of the therapeutic topics were introduced as questions (16.8 per cent) or re-

TABLE 11–4. Percentage distribution of therapeutic and administrative topics, by area of life and form of topic

Form of topic	Therapy	Administration
Communication only	77.3	45.7
Questions	16.8	26.6
Requests	5.9	27.7
All forms	100.0	100.0

quests (5.9 per cent), as contrasted with 54.3 per cent of the administrative topics which were introduced as questions (26.6 per cent) or requests (27.7 per cent). Part of the meaning of this lies in the indication it gives of the "untouchable" quality of psychotherapy in the hospital. The results of therapy were communicated, *but* many of the actions carried out in therapy were not subject to direct question. Administrative matters, however, were much more open and subject to question. One would therefore expect that administration would be an area of somewhat more open disagreement than therapy. Also, it is probable that many points which were really therapeutic in nature were phrased in terms of administrative questions or requests. This would be particularly true of the topics raised by nurses, who might doubt the efficacy of the therapy being carried out with a particular patient, but would be unable to express this directly because of their feelings about their position in the status hierarchy. They would, thus, indicate their disagreement through administrative questions and requests (see Chapters 3 through 5).

The answers to the question of which role group introduced topics in what areas of life can be seen in Table 11–5. It should be noted that the actual number of topics introduced was influenced by the different numbers of role group representatives, which are indicated by the N's beneath the role group headings in Table 11–5. The simplest way of handling this problem was to express the number of topics introduced in

TABLE 11–5. Number and percentage distribution of all topics, by role group initiating topic and area of life

	Seniors (N=3)		Residents (N=5)		Nurses (N=9)		Other personnel (N=4)	
Area of life	Number	Per cent	Number	Per cent	Number	Per cent	Number	Per cent
Therapy	39	29.5	156	33.9	39	34.5	4	10.0
Administration	91	68.9	296	64.3	68	60.2	33	82.5
Human relations	2	1.5	8	1.7	6	5.3	3	7.5
All areas	132	99.9	460	99.9	113	100.0	40	100.0

an area by a role group as a percentage of that role group's total. On this basis, it can be seen that the seniors, residents, and nurses all had about an equal balance between the percentage of topics introduced in therapy and administration. Roughly, there were about twice as many topics introduced by all three role groups in the administrative area as in the therapeutic area. This seemed to be less the case (though with such a low actual number of topics it was hard to tell) with the other personnel, who restricted their introduction of topics much more to the administrative area (82.5 per cent). This might indicate that the other personnel saw themselves as being farther removed from therapeutic matters than did the other three role groups.

The actual number of topics is important in terms of which role group predominated in the introduction of topics. Here the residents were by far the highest, with a total of 460 topics, and an average of 92 topics per resident. The seniors were next with a total of 132 topics and an average of 44 topics per senior physician. The nurses, with 113 topics, had a larger total than did the other personnel with 40 topics, but both nurses and other personnel had about the same average number of topics —12.6 among the nurses, and 10.0 among the other personnel.

Though the balance in percentage of topics introduced in the various areas was about the same for the seniors, residents, and nurses, the *form* in which these topics were introduced differed considerably from one role group to another. This can be seen in Table 11–6, where the total number of topics introduced by each role group is presented in terms of the form in which these topics were introduced. It is evident that both seniors and nurses were high in introducing their topics in terms of communication only and questions. The residents, on the other hand, tended to phrase their topics in terms of communication only, with a secondary concentration in the form of requests. The other personnel were about

TABLE 11–6. Number and percentage distribution of all topics, by role group initiating topic and form of topic

	Seniors (N=3)		Residents (N=5)		Nurses (N=9)		Other personnel (N=4)	
Form of topic	Number	Per cent	Number	Per cent	Number	Per cent	Number	Per cent
Communication only	68	51.5	289	62.8	52	46.0	15	37.5
Questions	56	42.4	57	12.4	46	40.7	13	32.5
Requests	8	6.1	114	24.8	15	13.3	12	30.0
All forms	132	100.0	460	100.0	113	100.0	40	100.0

TABLE 11–7. Number and percentage distribution of all topics, by subcategories of seniors and nurses initiating topic and form of topic

Form of topic	Head of hospital (N=1) Number	Head of hospital (N=1) Per cent	Chief resident (N=1) Number	Chief resident (N=1) Per cent	Supervisor of nurses (N=1) Number	Supervisor of nurses (N=1) Per cent	Charge nurses (N=5) Number	Charge nurses (N=5) Per cent
Communication only	9	32.1	57	60.6	6	15.8	46	61.3
Questions	19	67.9	34	36.2	25	65.8	21	28.0
Requests	0	0.0	3	3.2	7	18.4	8	10.7
All forms	28	100.0	94	100.0	38	100.0	75	100.0

equally divided between the three categories. Again, as was generally true in the interaction category analysis in the preceding chapter, it is interesting that the seniors and nurses were somewhat more than three times as likely to introduce their topics in the form of questions than were the residents. That is, it was the seniors and nurses who asked for orientation and opinion.

As in the interaction category analysis, so also in the content analysis under discussion, the same tendencies that held true for a role group, also held true for subcategories within a role group. For example, in Table 11–7 it can be seen that the head of the hospital introduced twice as many of his topics in the form of questions as in the form of communication only, whereas this proportion was almost exactly reversed for the chief resident, who introduced twice as many of his topics in the form of communication only as in the form of questions. This same reversal between higher and lower statuses within a role category can also be seen among the nurses; the supervisor of nurses phrased well over half of her topics as questions, whereas the charge nurses phrased over half of theirs as communication only. There was, then, a similarity between the superordinate and subordinate members of a role group in that the top

TABLE 11–8. Number and percentage distribution of all topics, by resident initiating topic and form of topic

Form of topic	Dr. A Number	Dr. A Per cent	Dr. B Number	Dr. B Per cent	Dr. C Number	Dr. C Per cent	Dr. D Number	Dr. D Per cent	Dr. E Number	Dr. E Per cent
Communication only	72	60.5	73	54.1	59	70.2	55	75.3	30	61.2
Questions	10	8.4	22	16.3	16	19.0	1	1.4	8	16.3
Requests	37	31.1	40	29.6	9	10.7	17	23.3	11	22.4
All forms	119	100.0	135	100.0	84	99.9	73	100.0	49	99.9

TABLE 11–9. Number and percentage distribution of all topics, by area of life and length in acts of topic

Length of topic, by number of acts	Therapy		Administration		Human relations	
	Number	Per cent	Number	Per cent	Number	Per cent
1–10	130	54.6	336	68.9	16	84.2
11–20	71	29.8	95	19.5	3	15.8
21–30	26	10.9	29	5.9	0	0.0
31–40	8	3.4	12	2.5	0	0.0
41–50	2	0.8	7	1.4	0	0.0
51–60	1	0.4	5	1.0	0	0.0
Over 60	0	0.0	4	0.8	0	0.0
All lengths	238	99.9	488	100.0	19	100.0

members asked questions, while the bottom members gave communication only.

The point was made in the preceding chapter that the five resident physicians consistently over time kept the same rank order from most to least talking (see Table 10–10), and this point is again borne out in terms of the number of topics introduced. As can be seen in Table 11–8, the ranking of residents according to the number of topics introduced was almost the same as the ranking according to amount of participation. The rank order by number of topics introduced was: 1—Dr. B, 2—Dr. A, 3—Dr. C, 4—Dr. D, and 5—Dr. E.

In general, the relative proportion in terms of the form in which topics were introduced was about the same for the five resident physicians, as indicated in Table 11–8. In this case, the percentages have less meaning than the actual number of topics introduced. Drs. B and C were somewhat higher in the actual number of questions asked, while Drs. A and B were higher in the actual number of requests. Drs. A and B, because of their greater number of topics, were in the forefront of the discussion during the course of the conferences.

The foregoing has shown something of the way in which topics were introduced, and it is now time to turn to questions of what happened to these topics.

WHAT HAPPENED TO THE TOPICS

When the length of the topics is considered, it can be seen in Table 11–9 that therapeutic topics were somewhat longer than administrative topics. As noted earlier, there were about twice as many administrative as therapeutic topics, but it took somewhat longer to discuss the latter.

TABLE 11–10. Number and percentage distribution of all topics, by area of life and balance of emotion of topic

Balance of emotion of topic	Therapy		Administration		Human relations	
	Number	Per cent	Number	Per cent	Number	Per cent
Unemotional	141	59.2	262	53.7	9	47.4
Positive emotion	41	17.2	106	21.7	9	47.4
Negative emotion	56	23.5	120	24.6	1	5.3
Emotional and unemotional	238	99.9	488	100.0	19	100.1

The topics concerned with human relations were very few in number and very short.

As can be seen in Table 11–10, there was little difference between therapeutic and administrative topics regarding the proportions within the several subdivisions of emotion. Over 50 per cent of both therapeutic and administrative topics were unemotional; about 20 per cent showed a balance of positive emotion; while about 25 per cent had a balance of negative emotion. There was some tendency for administrative topics to be slightly more emotional than therapeutic topics, and this is in line with the picture interview material in Chapter 7, which indicated that administration was an area of somewhat greater stress. Further evidence supporting this idea will be presented shortly. The human relations topics were equally balanced between unemotional and positive emotion, and the balance was highly positive in comparison with negative emotion. There were, however, so few human relations topics that one cannot be too confident about these proportions.

Although there was little difference when topics were considered by area and emotion, there was considerable difference when topics were considered by form and emotion. As can be seen in Table 11–11, the highest proportion of unemotional topics occurred in communication only

TABLE 11–11. Number and percentage distribution of all topics, by form and balance of emotion of topic

Balance of emotion of topic	Communication only		Questions		Requests	
	Number	Per cent	Number	Per cent	Number	Per cent
Unemotional	265	62.5	72	41.9	75	50.3
Positive emotion	83	19.6	37	21.5	36	24.2
Negative emotion	76	17.9	63	36.6	38	25.5
Emotional and unemotional	424	100.0	172	100.0	149	100.0

(62.5 per cent), next highest were requests (50.3 per cent), and finally questions (41.9 per cent). The balance between positive and negative emotion was about equal for communication only (19.6 to 17.9 per cent), and for requests (24.2 to 25.5 per cent). The balance of emotion for questions, however, was strongly negative (21.5 per cent positive to 36.6 per cent negative). The probable effect of this on personnel would be to cause them to pause before asking questions and, indeed, residents and nurses said that they did not like to ask questions in the conferences.

It may seem to the reader, having been subjected thus far in this chapter to a great many tables, that the analysis presented has been a matter of "just figures." It is useful, therefore, to begin to introduce a few examples concerning what happened to topics. In this regard, and with reference to Table 11–11, it is easy to show that emotion was not a colorless scoring rubric, but rather that it had a decided effect on the course of discussion in the conferences.

A good deal of the positive emotion (manifested in acts of solidarity, tension release, and agreement) in the conferences occurred in the context of joking about patients and life in the hospital. For example, when Dr. Reynolds was reporting on the progress of her patient, Mr. Earle, she made a "slip" which caused an outburst of laughter:

Dr. Reynolds: Mr. Earle was home this past week end, and this is a matter of considerable ambivalence for him. In many ways he seems to be taking his father's place. He went to visit a former attendant and he recognized that this is a neurotic thing but he felt that he might be helpful with the attendant.

Miss Nugent: Who was the attendant?

Dr. Reynolds: Albert Young. They got in touch and made plans to see each other in the future. . . . Mr. Earle himself is also aware at this time of his mother's sexual interest in him and he is acting out with his mother about—

(At this point there was an outburst of laughter on the part of all personnel in the conference. Dr. Reynolds recovered herself and went on to say): but *not* in those terms with his mother.

Dr. Shaw: The mother is reporting to me that the boy and the father are getting further apart. . . .

Positive emotion also occurred when administrative matters were running smoothly, as can be seen in a request initiated by Miss Nicholas:

Miss Nicholas: The men want to know whether they could see the fight Wednesday night on television?

Dr. Scott: You mean Mr. Erskine said this?

Miss Nicholas (laughing): Yes, I guess that is what I mean.

Dr. Scott: Has the television set been fixed yet, and how late would the fights run?

Miss Nicholas: I believe the set has been fixed, and the fights go on between 10 and 11 p.m.

Dr. Shaw (speaking to Dr. Scott): Do you want to make this a standing order?

Dr. Scott: Yes.

The quality of negative emotion aroused by disagreements can be seen in the following difference of opinion between Dr. Ryan and Dr. Scott:

Dr. Ryan: Mr. Edwards is not much changed in treatment with Dr. Simmons. In my administrative contacts with Mr. Edwards, he has been feeling very strongly about the world situation; he felt that Jesus Christ was responsible for these things and therefore Jesus Christ was failing and religion was failing. I don't think that these kinds of thoughts on Mr. Edwards' part seem to be psychotic.

Dr. Scott (very surprised): What!

Dr. Ryan: No, I don't think they are psychotic. Mr. Edwards says he knows these things are not true, but he'd like to feel that they are true. It's difficult to explain, but I feel that he isn't psychotic.

Dr. Shaw: It is like Dr. Spellman says in conference. You have to be able to distinguish psychotic behavior, and not think that such behavior doesn't really indicate psychosis.

Dr. Ryan (somewhat defensively): Dr. Simmons doesn't feel that the patient is psychotic either.

Dr. Scott (again very surprised): What! It's not a defamatory epithet, this word psychotic, it's just simply that we have to decide whether a person is psychotic or not.

The above exchange between Dr. Ryan and Dr. Scott indicates a rather general point that often became apparent in the administrative conferences. In their contacts with patients, the first-year residents frequently refused to admit the extent of the patient's illness. This is, of course, a complex matter, and it was related, in part, to the feeling of the new resident that if he could establish contact with the patient, then the patient seemed to be less sick than he was previously. It was also undoubtedly related to the resident's own defenses, in that if he could see the patient as not too sick, he would then feel more hopeful of the possibility of helping the patient therapeutically.

A second rather general problem in the administrative conferences was the desire of the new resident to grant a good deal of individual latitude to patients and to chafe under the rules and regulations of the hospital (see Chapter 5). This also often stirred up negative emotions, as can be seen in the exchange between Dr. Reynolds and Dr. Scott over the giving of alcohol to Mr. Owens:

Dr. Reynolds: Mr. Owens is increasingly depressed, and I think he is still hallucinating although he is aware of it. He has not asked for whiskey except for one drink in the evening, a highball, and that sounds reasonable to me.

Dr. Scott: Why is it reasonable!

Dr. Reynolds: He is used to it.

Dr. Scott: What does it do for him?

Dr. Reynolds: I feel it is reassuring. This man has always drunk. The surgeon at the general hospital prescribed it, and I feel that he should have the one drink in the evening.

Dr. Scott: Why don't we give it to all of our patients?

Dr. Reynolds: Well, why not!

Dr. Scott: No, we are not going to give any bourbon out.

Mrs. Netter: This morning at 1 a.m. he took 60 ccs. of bourbon.

Dr. Reynolds: I have changed over to sedation mainly.

Dr. Shaw: We have to have a period of time to evaluate this man. Why do we sedate him?

Dr. Reynolds: I want to know how much anxiety we want to keep a person under.

Dr. Shaw: We don't want to bust him wide open, but we do want to know what he's like.

Dr. Reynolds: Well, we are busting him wide open. He hasn't asked for any liquor on the ward because he feels it's not fair to the other patients and he said this himself. All he wants is his one drink in his room in the evening.

Dr. Scott: We have to assess what the meaning of alcohol in the social context of the hospital is. Mr. Esposito said to me: "I am just as good as Mr. Owens, why can't I get a drink?"

Dr. Reynolds: Mr. Owens said himself he would give it up.

Dr. Scott: Why was it so cavalierly given in the first place?

Dr. Reynolds: It was in the surgeon's orders when he came from the other hospital.

Dr. Scott: We talked of this earlier in its relation to DT's, and I said no bourbon.

Dr. Reynolds: Why didn't we say no in the beginning?

Dr. Scott: I never said I didn't say no.

Dr. Shaw: When the patient was admitted I didn't cut off the liquor because it was in the orders.

Dr. Reynolds: Well anyway, Mr. Owens is upset. . . .

A second aspect of "what happened to a topic" involves the extent of generality. That is, a topic could remain centered on a specific matter, it could be concerned solely with a general matter, or the discussion of a specific topic could turn into a discussion of a general matter of policy. The two categories of general and specific-to-general topics did not bulk very large in the total number of topics, but were nevertheless of extreme importance. One such topic occurring in a single administrative confer-

TABLE 11–12. Number and percentage distribution of all topics, by area of life and extent of generality of topic

Extent of generality of topic	Therapy		Administration		Human relations	
	Number	Per cent	Number	Per cent	Number	Per cent
Specific	230	96.6	439	90.0	18	94.7
General	4	1.7	29	5.9	0	0.0
Specific-to-general	4	1.7	20	4.1	1	5.3
All generalities	238	100.0	488	100.0	19	100.0

ence could result in extended discussion. The number and percentage of topics, by area and extent of generality, can be seen in Table 11–12. By number of topics, general and specific-to-general topics occurred much more frequently in the administrative area (49 topics) than in the therapeutic area (8 topics). These topics represented 10.0 per cent of all topics in the administrative area, as compared with only 3.4 per cent in the area of therapy. Again this is an indication that administrative matters were somewhat more of a problem than were therapeutic matters.

The relation between emotion and extent of generality can be seen in Table 11–13, which shows that from one type of topic to another the percentage of topics with a balance of negative emotion rose precipitously—being 20.8 per cent for specific topics, 42.4 per cent for general topics, and 80.0 per cent for specific-to-general topics. Moreover, the movement here is actually from shorter to longer topics, so that in bulk the general and specific-to-general topics loomed larger than their sheer numbers would indicate.

Perhaps the data in Table 11–13 represent a fairly common attribute of small group interaction in that as the group encounters touchy topics there is a tendency for these to be presented in more general terms.

TABLE 11–13. Number and percentage distribution of all topics, by extent of generality and balance of emotion of topic

Balance of emotion of topic	Specific		General		Specific-to-general	
	Number	Per cent	Number	Per cent	Number	Per cent
Unemotional	397	57.8	13	39.4	2	8.0
Positive emotion	147	21.4	6	18.2	3	12.0
Negative emotion	143	20.8	14	42.4	20	80.0
Emotional and unemotional	687	100.0	33	100.0	25	100.0

Equally, if a specific topic meets with resistance, one way of overcoming this resistance is to generalize the topic. In any case, the fact remains that most of the general and specific-to-general topics occurred in the administrative area (see Table 11–12) and that these topics were very high in negative emotion (see Table 11–13).

The following two examples are of general topics—the first positive and the second negative in emotional balance. Since most of the general topics were rather long, they will not be cited in full, but a sufficient amount of the discussion will be given to indicate the nature of the problem.

The example of a general topic which had a positive emotional balance concerned a plan proposed by Dr. Scott for clarifying the procedures to be followed in granting privileges to patients. This was an area of considerable confusion in the conferences, and this plan was designed to help clear the air. This it did in considerable part, but the matter of privileges still remained a difficult one to solve in day-to-day administrative work:

Dr. Scott: I have a tentative proposal I want to bring up and I want the group to think about. I have been talking this over with a number of people and I feel this is a schedule that might work out in terms of the patients' going-out privileges. First of all, the patients who are at home the most are those on the "day plan," and therefore they can have ad lib permission to go out with only two requirements: first, they must be back by 10 p.m., and second, they have to indicate they are out of the hospital by signing out in the book in the nurses' office. Otherwise, they could be out all day long, and we wouldn't know where they were. The second level of patient privileges concerns the full-time open ward patients. There are two plans here: (a) The first plan includes orders which you write just once, such as: "This patient can be out on Saturday from 10 a.m. to 10 p.m." . . . Next there are blanket orders which you write saying: "The patient can until further notice always be out on Sundays from 10 a.m. to 10 p.m." And, the patient can go out at these times without the nurse's having to call the doctor. (b) An alternate plan at this second level is one in which the patient can be out over the entire week end if you so write the order. So far as the locked wards go, every time the patient goes out you have to write a specific order. . . .

Dr. Rivers: Are these patients who are on the "day plan" to go in and out during the evening freely?

Dr. Scott: Yes, this is in a sense the bait that you get, the sort of goal that you can hold out to the patient. The patients can have more or less total responsibility.

Dr. Reynolds: If the patient was on the alternate "b" plan, could he come back sooner than Sunday night if he felt he wanted to?

Dr. Scott: Of course he could.

Dr. Reynolds: To me the whole plan sounds all right.

Dr. Scott: Let's think about this. I'm going to write out a copy of it. If there aren't any changes by the first of next week, then I don't want any damned deviation from it.

Dr. Rivers (laughing): I think the plan is so broad that there couldn't be any deviations from it.

Dr. Scott (laughing): In this instance I feel that if you can't fight them you can join them.

Dr. Ramsay: I wouldn't want to put Miss Lewis on either of these plans, but can I still go ahead and restrict her privileges to specific things?

Dr. Scott: Yes, that is what the specific orders are for.

Dr. Reynolds: I think the whole plan is just elegant.

Miss Nugent: Even with the high census on the open ward, the majority of patients will still have to be dealt with individually.

Dr. Scott: I want to emphasize that I don't want any exceptions to this plan.

Dr. Rolfe: Who is going to tell the patients about this new plan?

Dr. Scott: Every doctor should tell his patients. I don't feel that this is any hardship.

Dr. Reynolds: I think the plan is very liberal.

Dr. Rivers: I also think the plan is very liberal.

In contrast to the positively oriented topic just presented, many of the general questions that came up resulted in a negative balance of emotion. This was the case in the next example, which concerned Dr. Rivers' feeling that the resident physicians should have the authority to be flexible and creative in the use of ward personnel during the evening. Dr. Rivers introduced this subject, however, in terms of using the ward personnel to take patients out of the hospital, and this met with resistance from Dr. Shaw, who felt that the personnel should be utilized in activities inside the hospital:

Dr. Rivers: I have a problem I want to bring up. Mrs. Nixon (a charge nurse on the locked ward) told me the other night that she had four attendants on duty where usually she only has two. Mrs. Nixon asked me if there wasn't some way we could utilize the attendants for activities for the patients. Mrs. Nixon felt that these attendants were being wasted just sitting around the ward, and couldn't we get them to do something with the patients. I would like to have organized a movie expedition downtown with the patients since the attendants were available and I was the doctor on call that night, but I didn't do this because I didn't have the authority and I knew such things were supposed to be discussed at these administrative conferences. However, the time of the attendants was just wasted that night.

Dr. Reynolds: It's true that these unanticipated things do come up, and we don't know, as residents, whether we can or cannot make these decisions on our own responsibility.

Dr. Shaw: The assumption in this conversation is that the attendants couldn't be used in the hospital for the patients, but rather they would have to take the patients out of the hospital.

Dr. Rolfe: It seems to me that this problem reflects on the competency of the resident and the responsibility that the residents should take. I don't see why Dr. Rivers couldn't have made this decision.

Dr. Shaw: I think she could have too, but just because we have extra attendants doesn't mean we have to use them to invite people to go out of the hospital.

Dr. Rolfe: But if the patients have a chance to profit by the extra attendants, why can't we decide that they can go out?

Dr. Sears: As a general rule in the activities program, one that is a working rule, we have decided that if three or more patients want to go out then the institution will pay for the program, and this sort of rule might apply to the use of the attendants, and might fall into that category. That is, if there were three or more patients then the attendants could go out with them.

Dr. Shaw: It seems to me that there is a greater opportunity for the patients and attendants to work out some sort of organization and recreation within the hospital.

Dr. Rivers: That is true in theory, but practically there is nothing more for them to do beyond what they usually do in the hospital. They can go down to the gym, and that's about all. Actually, if we wanted to use the attendants we would have to let them take the patients out of the hospital.

Dr. Shaw: I expect to have the attendants use their own skills in organizing games and activities for the patients in the hospital.

Dr. Ryan: What skills?

Dr. Shaw: Well, organizing games like canasta, and various other activities they could do.

Dr. Sears: At a later stage Miss Wright (the activities worker) might work along with the attendants in helping them to work out these social activities with the patients.

Dr. Shaw: These things are not mutually exclusive, the inside and outside activities, but I think that things could be worked out in the hospital.

The above are examples of general topics. Turning now to specific-to-general topics, it will be remembered that 80.0 per cent of these had a negative balance of emotion (Table 11–13). This was the case in the following example, where Dr. Ramsay introduced a specific administrative request to allow one of his patients to have certain special privileges and to be permitted to discharge her directly from the locked ward rather than first moving her to the open ward. This request was not given an answer, as the discussion immediately turned to a general problem of the therapeutic use of the physical space of the hospital:

Dr. Ramsay: On Mrs. Paul, she is thinking of leaving within the next week or so but she doesn't want to be transferred to the open ward. However, she would like permission to go out from the locked ward. Since this is a little unusual, I would like to bring this up as a request and get a decision on it.

Dr. Scott: My reaction is that it's a therapeutic problem, and we'd like to know why she is anxious about going to the open ward.

Dr. Ramsay: It's a question of a private room, which she has on the locked ward, versus her having to be on the four-bed ward if she went to the open ward.

Dr. Ryan (generalizing the topic from the specific issue): This raises the very interesting point that the four-bed ward should be the last place a patient occupies before leaving. That is, they learn how to live on the locked ward, then on the open ward in a private room, and then learn how to live with other people on the four-bed ward just before they leave.

Dr. Reynolds: This raises the whole question of the use of rooms. Should rooms just be assigned on a priority basis? This seems to be the case so far. I feel there should be freedom to move patients around. Some patients might do well on the four-bed ward, and others in private rooms. We should feel free to move them around therapeutically rather than on a priority basis.

Dr. Scott: Wait a moment! Look what you said there! Freedom to move them around. Really what you meant to say was freedom to discuss with them about the move. This business of sort of assuming authoritative control over the patients.

Miss Nugent: The patients feel very strongly about the priority.

Dr. Reynolds (almost pleadingly): Could this be then? Could we change the situation around?

Dr. Shaw: It's been that way all along. We have moved people out of single rooms to the four-bed ward for therapeutic reasons.

Dr. Reynolds: All the patients would have to understand this. Miss Packard isn't one who should be in a single room, for example, whereas Mrs. Patterson up on the locked ward is one who probably should.

Dr. Scott: Almost anything is possible in our hospital. I am willing to allow almost anything that is creatively imaginative if we can just keep our tempers and talk about it. If we can do that everything should work out fine.

(At the conclusion of this topic, the conference went on to other matters. Dr. Ramsay's request, which began this topic, was not answered.)

It is interesting that the example of a specific-to-general topic just cited occurred during an administrative conference which actually contained three such topics, a very high number for a single conference. This had additional significance because this particular conference took place precisely at the beginning of the period in which the television petition and the events that led to the collective disturbance were occurring on the ward (see Chapters 4 and 5).

The next problem in analysis concerns simple and complex topics. As mentioned earlier, a simple topic was one in which the discussion remained within the same area. That is, if the topic started out in the administrative area, the discussion remained centered on administrative matters throughout the course of the topic. However, if an administrative

TABLE 11–14. Number and percentage distribution of all topics, by area of life and complexity of topic

Complexity of topic	Therapy		Administration		Human relations	
	Number	Per cent	Number	Per cent	Number	Per cent
Simple	195	81.9	374	76.6	15	78.9
Complex	43	18.1	114	23.4	4	21.1
Simple and complex	238	100.0	488	100.0	19	100.0

topic was subsequently complicated by the introduction of therapeutic or human relations factors, then the topic was scored as complex. The number and percentage distribution of all topics, by area and complexity, can be seen in Table 11–14.

The relative proportion of complex topics was about the same in all three of the areas: therapy—18.1 per cent, administration—23.4 per cent, and human relations—21.1 per cent. Since complex topics tended to be somewhat longer than simple topics, they occupied a fairly large proportion of the over-all discussion. The nature of the complexity in the 161 complex topics, and which role group introduced the complication, can be seen in Table 11–15.

The greatest number of complex topics began as administrative matters (110 topics started out in the area of administration, and 41 in the area of therapy). In terms of the category of person introducing the complication, persons initiating the topics themselves most often also intro-

TABLE 11–15. Number and percentage distribution of complex topics, by nature of complication and category of person responsible for complication

Category of person responsible for complication	Therapeutic complicated by administrative (Th/Adm)		Administrative complicated by therapeutic (Adm/Th)		Other types (Th/HR, Adm/HR, HR/Th, HR/Adm)		All complex topics	
	Number	Per cent	Number	Per cent	Number	Per cent	Number	Per cent
Initiator of topic	20	48.8	47	42.7	2	20.0	69	42.9
Seniors	10	24.4	35	31.8	0	0.0	45	28.0
Residents	3	7.3	18	16.4	4	40.0	25	15.5
Nurses	6	14.6	8	7.3	2	20.0	16	9.9
Other personnel	2	4.9	2	1.8	2	20.0	6	3.7
All categories	41	100.0	110	100.0	10	100.0	161	100.0

duced the complication, and this accounted for 42.9 per cent of the total. Beyond this, if someone other than the initiator complicated the topic, it can be seen that seniors complicated 28.0 per cent of the complex topics, residents 15.5 per cent, nurses 9.9 per cent, and other personnel 3.7 per cent. This is again evidence for the effect of the status hierarchy in the conferences. The higher the status of the role group, the more likely that group was to complicate topics under discussion.

In terms of the nature of the complication, it is interesting that the seniors tended to complicate a greater proportion of administrative topics with therapeutic matters (31.8 per cent) than they did therapeutic topics with administrative matters (24.4 per cent). This was even more the case for the resident doctors, who contributed twice as great a proportion to the complication of administrative topics by the introduction of therapeutic considerations (16.4 per cent), as they did to the complication of therapeutic topics by the introduction of administrative considerations (7.3 per cent). Quite the reverse was true for the nurses, who, proportionately, contributed twice as much to the complication of therapeutic topics with administrative matters (14.6 per cent), as they did to the complication of administrative topics with therapeutic matters (7.3 per cent). This reversal between nurses and residents would seem to reflect the role orientation and duties of the two groups. The other personnel complicated very few topics and mostly remained silent on such matters.

Since the seniors had a roughly equal balance between the two main types of complications, the first examples will be taken from the actions of the seniors. In connection with topics of a therapeutic nature which were complicated by administrative matters, one problem which frequently arose was that the seniors felt they must call attention to financial questions, as these were seldom raised by the residents. For example:

Dr. Reynolds: . . . Miss Packard started out the week quite negativistically in treatment, but she is better now and spontaneously went to occupational therapy. There really is not much going on in treatment at this period.

Dr. Scott: Do you think Miss Packard could handle the open ward?

Dr. Reynolds: No.

Dr. Scott: Well, we have to get somebody off the women's locked ward. Otherwise we'll be turning patients away, and in terms of the business office we simply can't afford to do this.

This example indicates the effect of pressure from the business office on the senior staff, which then was often transmitted to the residents. On the other hand, it was also necessary for the senior doctor to point out to the resident delays in treatment that could be avoided and that were costing the patient or his family money. For example:

Dr. Rolfe: Mrs. Martin shows some small improvement. I use a firm and strict approach and just tears come out. On the ward she is better, and I hope to get x-rays this week and take a look at them.

Dr. Scott: I think one might expedite the x-ray procedure. The delay is costing the family a considerable amount of money.

In the next example another sort of problem arose. The resident spoke briefly about the therapeutic progress of a patient but did not mention current administrative problems. Dr. Shaw and Dr. Scott, however, introduced the relevance of administrative problems for therapy. In addition, Dr. Scott pointed out that his own feelings with reference to some of the senior staff probably had an effect on his feelings with regard to particular patients. This was the type of problem in which the emotional relations between various role groups, and the effect of these on the doctor-patient relationship, were all intimately bound up with the total structure of the hospital, as was also the situation in Chapter 3 in the case of Mr. Esposito. In the following, the reader should be aware that Dr. Saunders was the therapist and Dr. Rivers the administrative physician, for Mr. Isherwood, who was the patient. Dr. Rivers felt there was a lack of communication between herself and Dr. Saunders:

Dr. Rivers: . . . Mr. Isherwood, from what I can observe, seems to be brightening up. I hear from the nurses and attendants that he is more open and easy. He was away on the week end and will be back again today.

Dr. Shaw: No, he won't be back today. He'll be back either tomorrow or Wednesday. A letter came to Dr. Saunders wanting permission for him to come back on Tuesday.

Dr. Rivers: The patient said that he didn't want to miss his hour with Dr. Saunders on Monday.

Dr. Scott: And the family wrote directly to Dr. Saunders instead of to you.

Dr. Rivers: I was not here on Saturday, but the plan was all set for Friday till Monday. But Mr. Isherwood's brother put pressure on him, and he can't stand up to this pressure.

Dr. Scott: If Dr. Saunders got the letter, why didn't we hear about it?

Dr. Rivers: Dr. Saunders has referred the brother to us.

Dr. Shaw: We had to decide on Saturday morning.

Dr. Scott: Why did you give permission?

Dr. Shaw: Well, they were on the steps with the bags and the patient, and were all ready to leave.

Dr. Scott: We had a meeting on Friday of the senior doctors, and it was obvious that Saunders has real ignorance about what the hospital means, and our feelings that we wanted to do something with the patient. Now here I wonder why we didn't hold to our policy.

Dr. Shaw: I didn't know on what basis I could refuse the request.

Dr. Rivers: Dr. Saunders had told Isherwood he could stay till Tuesday, and Isherwood had said he'd rather be back on Monday.

Dr. Scott: Why isn't Isherwood on the open ward if he's going out like this all the time? Well, I suppose it's an irrational feeling, and this probably relates to its being one of Saunders' patients and—well, what the hell!

Dr. Rivers: No, it wasn't that. It was that I felt that there were too few patients on the open ward when we first considered moving him there, but now I feel he should go to the open ward.

Dr. Scott: It may be that the administrative psychiatrist doesn't get as much out of the hospital if he feels that the person he is treating really isn't his patient. It may be that the administrative psychiatrist actually blocks the patient's progress in the hospital. I am asking this in my own mind—why wasn't I more concerned about Isherwood and where he was in the hospital?

Dr. Reynolds: I agree with your feeling.

Dr. Scott: The question is, can you have the feelings if you don't actually have these patients in treatment?

Dr. Reynolds: If you have interest it usually means that you have personal involvement.

Dr. Sears: I think one might give the administrative psychiatrist an entire ward to administer, instead of just a number of patients.

Dr. Scott: Still another answer would be to give more authority to the nurse and let her be the administrative psychiatrist. The whole question is how to use the hospital to help the patient.

Senior doctors did not, as was seen in Table 11–15, confine their complicating remarks to the introduction of administrative matters into therapeutic topics, but also frequently introduced therapeutic matters into administrative topics. This is apparent in the following example, where the resident physicians were trying to decide with Dr. Shaw what the duty schedule should be on the insulin treatment unit; this caused Dr. Scott to raise the problem of the resistance of the residents to performing this duty because it cut down on the number of hours per week they could devote to psychotherapy with their patients. Dr. Scott's position was that it might not be necessary to spend as many hours with a patient per week as the residents felt was required:

Dr. Rolfe: Mrs. Paul will go home tomorrow, and I am wondering what is planned about the organization of the insulin treatment unit?

Dr. Shaw: Dr. Ryan will be on insulin treatment.

Dr. Ryan: Yes, but it takes a great deal of time if there are only two of us on. You get to having to see patients up until 9 o'clock at night if you're working on the insulin unit in the morning. I'm wondering if we couldn't get a third person on the insulin treatment unit?

Dr. Shaw: Well, you start with Dr. Rolfe, and we'll work this out among you.

Dr. Scott: There is another problem here, and that is, as you go along, you as residents have got to come to terms with your interviews. Three times a week is often as good as four, or even two times a week. If you get hostile about your interviews, then they aren't going to be as good with the patient. We don't have any experimental evidence on whether cutting down or increasing the number of interviews has any particular effect. When you have the patient working on his self-scrutiny, you can perhaps get all that he can integrate into three hours.

Dr. Rolfe: Would this apply to psychotics as well as neurotics?

Dr. Scott: Mostly neurotics, schizophrenics are another matter. The point is that you don't have to see the patient every day.

As noted in Table 11–15, the residents were high in the proportion of topics they complicated by introducing therapeutic considerations into administrative problems. A good example of this tendency can be seen in the following discussion, where Miss Nugent, the supervisor of nurses, introduced an administrative matter with reference to Mrs. Matthews, and this was complicated by Dr. Ryan, Mrs. Matthews' doctor, who introduced therapeutic considerations. This is again a specific instance of the general difference of opinion between the nurses, who wanted more orderly routine, and the residents, who desired that flexible procedures be worked out according to the therapeutic progress of each patient:

Miss Nugent: In relation to Mrs. Matthews, we'll have to reconsider carefully whether we want to move her to the open ward. She is so demanding.

Dr. Ryan: I think perhaps we want to re-evaluate some of the old rules on the locked ward and perhaps even publish a little list. This problem is taking up too much therapeutic time. Mrs. Matthews received some flowers in a glass vase and she was told that she couldn't have them. Yet at the same time she had a glass picture frame and a pitcher in her room. She couldn't understand it and neither could I.

Miss Noyes: That's true, we do allow bottles, but they are collected at night. Flowers are not usually collected. Otherwise we would have a huge storeroom full of stuff.

Dr. Shaw: So the bottles that Mrs. Matthews has are only in her room during the day.

Mrs. Wells (a social worker): Maybe she could use papier-maché vases.

Miss Netter: Mrs. Matthews has been getting those up until now. She also told me that her husband was allowed to bring in a day's supply of food for her, that Mrs. Wells said it was okay.

Miss Noyes: Sandwiches and ginger beer have been brought in.

Mrs. Wells: Mr. Matthews is bringing in soup twice a week, and a sandwich each time he comes.

Dr. Ryan: This is his need to make her happier. . . .

In contrast to the residents, the nurses, as seen in Table 11–15, had a greater proportion of their complex topics in the introduction of administrative considerations into therapeutic matters. Such complications were both positive in the sense that they were constructive suggestions about how administrative procedures might serve to further therapeutic considerations, and negative in the sense of introducing administrative matters which would tend to make it impossible to carry out therapeutic suggestions. An example of a constructive suggestion was:

Dr. Ryan: As far as Miss Peters goes, she is still talking in abstract terms. She has violent mood changes, and we've been trying to find out why. The ward routine on the locked ward bothers her. She says she can't smoke on the locked wards. . . .

Miss Newcomb: On the locked ward she is given to fits of walking, and if the locked ward is upsetting, I think that we might arrange the schedule so that someone could be with her, and let her try the open ward.

Dr. Ryan: . . . I would like to try it.

On the other hand, administrative matters were sometimes used as ways of blocking therapeutic suggestions. For example:

Dr. Reynolds: . . . I get worried about Mr. Innes' sitting around on the ward with three attendants, and something needs to be done.

Miss Noyes: The boys have tried, and he just won't respond.

Dr. Ramsay: He brought up the question of wanting to listen to music to me and said that he would like to hear some records. I think that this might be helpful to him, especially as he is not allowed off the ward at present.

Miss Nugent: There is the problem of the current in this building, and the fact that we will need a converter. I do not know that we can get a converter. We have tried to do so before, and it is very complicated. The patients all keep wanting to have electrical appliances in their rooms, and heretofore we have forbidden this because it is not a good thing, and we simply do not have a large supply of converters that we can give out to patients.

A further aspect of what happened to a topic was whether the outcome was conclusive or inconclusive. Table 11–16 gives the conclusiveness of outcome of all topics, by area. The great bulk of topics in all areas ended conclusively. Among the inconclusive topics, the largest proportion (18.4 per cent) as well as the largest number (90 topics) occurred in

TABLE 11–16. Number and percentage distribution of all topics, by area of life and conclusiveness of outcome of topic

Conclusiveness of outcome	Therapy		Administration		Human relations	
	Number	Per cent	Number	Per cent	Number	Per cent
Conclusive	225	94.5	398	81.6	18	94.7
Inconclusive	13	5.5	90	18.4	1	5.3
All outcomes	238	100.0	488	100.0	19	100.0

the area of administration. Thus, roughly one out of every five administrative topics ended on an inconclusive note. This was a far greater proportion than for either therapy (5.5 per cent inconclusive) or human relations (5.3 per cent inconclusive). This lends further credence to the analysis of the interview material in Chapters 7 through 9, where administration was seen as an area of greater confusion in the hospital than was therapy or human relations.

Examples of simple short topics which came to a conclusion can be seen in the following two topics, which followed each other in succession during one of the conferences:

Dr. Rolfe: There is a problem with Mr. Erskine and the football games he wishes to go to. He would like to see several games. His father can't go, and he's putting pressure on me to allow him to go anyway. He's asking if Mrs. Nixon can't go with him.

Dr. Sears: Couldn't we get an escort?

Dr. Shaw: It depends upon the availability of the escort and his quality. It would have to be a very responsible escort.

Miss Nicholas: How about the graduate nurse that's been assigned to Mr. Erskine? I think that he would be good.

Dr. Shaw: I think he probably would be good also. Let's try to do that, and use Mr. Erskine's nurse.

Dr. Rolfe: I want to know if we could give Mr. Onofrio three tablets of dilantin to take with him on his week end trips home?

Dr. Shaw: Yes.

The above examples were quite unequivocal in their conclusiveness. Things did not always work out so clearly, however, as in the topic cited earlier as an example of specific-to-general topics, where Dr. Ramsay requested certain privileges for his patient, Mrs. Paul. In that example, the request was lost sight of in the ensuing general discussion, and since no decision was reached, the topic was scored as inconclusive.

The number and proportion of conclusive and inconclusive topics by *area* have been given in Table 11–16. The question now arises of which *role group* received the lowest proportion of inconclusive outcomes to the topics that it introduced? From Table 11–17 it can be seen that the seniors had the lowest proportion of inconclusive topics with 8.3 per cent, the residents were second with 13.5 per cent, the other personnel third with 17.5 per cent, and the nurses fourth with the highest proportion, 21.2 per cent, of inconclusive topics. Again, in a general way, this rank order represents the status hierarchy at work, in that the higher the status of a role group, the lower the proportion of inconclusive topics for that group. This is particularly important with reference to the nurses as,

TABLE 11–17. Number and percentage distribution of all topics, by role group initiating topic and conclusiveness of outcome of topic

Conclusiveness of outcome	Seniors Number	Seniors Per cent	Residents Number	Residents Per cent	Nurses Number	Nurses Per cent	Other personnel Number	Other personnel Per cent
Conclusive	121	91.7	398	86.5	89	78.8	33	82.5
Inconclusive	11	8.3	62	13.5	24	21.2	7	17.5
All outcomes	132	100.0	460	100.0	113	100.0	40	100.0

on this basis, they would be the group most often left with a sense of frustration. That is, one out of every five topics that were introduced by the nurses ended on an inconclusive note, and they were quite right in their feelings, at least as these applied to themselves, that "nothing gets decided at the conference" (see Chapter 9). This once more serves to highlight the difficult position occupied by the nurses in the structure of the hospital hierarchy.

The following example is of a topic introduced by the nurses that ended conclusively:

Miss Newcomb: I would like to know if Mrs. Lasswell has permission to go to the open ward.

Dr. Ramsay: Mrs. Lasswell was very good over the week end.

Dr. Ryan: She might be sent to the open ward during the locked door period on the open ward.

Dr. Shaw: I agree, I think that is a good idea.

A good example of a topic introduced by the nurses which ended inconclusively was cited in Chapter 5 and will not be repeated verbatim. The topic concerned the question raised by the nurse, Miss Noyes, about the problem of Mrs. Matthews' going out unaccompanied from the locked ward. Miss Noyes' question was not answered because the discussion became generalized about whether or not any patient should leave the locked ward unaccompanied, and no agreement was reached.

A special aspect of the conclusive-inconclusive topics is what happened to those topics which were *specific requests* requiring a decision. There were 149 such topics, and they provide a sensitive index of the state of affairs in the administrative conferences. What happened to these requests will be discussed in terms of Tables 11–18 through 11–21.

Table 11–18 shows the distribution of the 149 specific requests by area and nature of decision. As to the actual number of requests, they were almost entirely concentrated in the area of administration (135 requests), with very few in the area of therapy (14 requests), and none in

TABLE 11–18. Number and percentage distribution of request topics, by area of life and nature of decision on topic

Nature of decision	Therapy		Administration		Human relations	
	Number	Per cent	Number	Per cent	Number	Per cent
For	5	35.7	72	53.3	0	0
Against	3	21.4	13	9.6	0	0
Undecided	6	42.9	50	37.0	0	0
All decisions	14	100.0	135	99.9	0	0

the area of human relations. Perhaps the most interesting feature of Table 11–18 is the large proportion of undecided requests in the areas of therapy (42.9 per cent) and administration (37.0 per cent). This means that well over one third of the requests in either area were likely to be left undecided. This would indicate that there was a lack of clarity in the work of the administrative conferences.

A further aspect of what happened to requests is given in Table 11–19, where it can be seen that the residents initiated many more requests than any other role group—114 of the 149 requests were made by the residents. A point of particular interest in Table 11–19 is that a resident doctor's request had slightly less than a 50 per cent chance of being granted (49.1 per cent decisions for). When a request by a resident doctor was not granted, it was three times more likely to be left up in the air (38.6 per cent undecided) than to receive a clear-cut negative decision (12.3 per cent against). It is, therefore, understandable that the residents did not like to bring up requests in conference and felt they might do better to go ahead and make decisions covertly on their own initiative (see Chapters 5 and 9). But, as was noted in Chapter 5, this tendency to make decisions but not to report them at the administrative conference created a breakdown of the flow of communication which resulted in much confusion.

TABLE 11–19. Number and percentage distribution of request topics, by role group initiating topic and nature of decision on topic

Nature of decision	Seniors		Residents		Nurses		Other personnel	
	Number	Per cent	Number	Per cent	Number	Per cent	Number	Per cent
For	4	50.0	56	49.1	10	66.7	7	58.3
Against	0	00.0	14	12.3	1	6.7	1	8.3
Undecided	4	50.0	44	38.6	4	26.7	4	33.3
All decisions	8	100.0	114	100.0	15	100.1	12	99.9

TABLE 11–20. Number and percentage distribution of request topics, by balance of emotion and nature of decision on topic

Nature of decision	Unemotional		Positive emotion		Negative emotion	
	Number	Per cent	Number	Per cent	Number	Per cent
For	50	66.7	20	55.6	7	18.4
Against	2	2.7	7	19.4	7	18.4
Undecided	23	30.7	9	25.0	24	63.2
All decisions	75	100.1	36	100.0	38	100.0

The analysis of requests is continued in Table 11–20, which shows the nature of decisions by the balance of emotion in request topics. An important aspect of the data is slightly hidden by the form of the table. If decisions for and against are added together to obtain the number of *clear-cut* decisions as opposed to those left undecided, then clear-cut decisions were reached on 69.4 per cent of the unemotional topics, on 75.0 per cent of the positive emotion topics, and on only 36.8 per cent of the negative emotion topics. In other words, when a topic had a negative balance of emotion the chances of its being decided in a clear-cut fashion were only 1 in 3, whereas when a topic was unemotional or positive in balance its chances were 2 out of 3 for a clear-cut decision.

There was a direct progression in the decreasing proportion of decisions for a request from unemotional topics with 66.7 per cent for, to positive emotion topics with 55.6 per cent for, to negative emotion topics with only 18.4 per cent for. When the nature of a decision was against a request, the topic was much more likely to have been emotional—whether positive or negative—than unemotional. Thus, only 2.7 per cent of the unemotional topics were decided against, as compared with 19.4 per cent of the topics with a balance of positive emotion, and 18.4 per cent of the topics with a balance of negative emotion. A request was most likely to be left undecided when the balance of emotion was negative (63.2 per cent), and about equally likely to be left undecided when the emotion was either positive (25.0 per cent) or unemotional (30.7 per cent).

The next question concerns what happened to requests in terms of whether the discussion around them remained within the area of life in which the request was introduced, or whether the discussion was complicated by the introduction of factors from another area of life. As defined earlier, the former were called simple topics and the latter complex topics. As can be seen in Table 11–21, when a topic was simple in form it was

TABLE 11–21. Number and percentage of request topics, by complexity of topic and nature of decision on topic

Nature of decision	Simple		Complex	
	Number	Per cent	Number	Per cent
For	63	64.3	14	27.5
Against	6	6.1	10	19.6
Undecided	29	29.6	27	52.9
All decisions	98	100.0	51	100.0

much more likely to receive a clear-cut decision than when it was complex. That is, adding together the for and against requests as indicative of clear-cut decision, 70.4 per cent of the simple topics received clear-cut decisions, compared with 47.1 per cent of the complex topics. A further aspect of Table 11–21 is that a topic was more than twice as likely to result in a decision for when it was simple (64.3 per cent for) as when it was complex (27.5 per cent for). Similarly, a topic was three times as likely to result in a decision against when it was complex (19.6 per cent against) as when it was simple (6.1 per cent against).

With the data in Tables 11–18 through 11–21 in mind, it is useful to look at some examples of simple and complex requests where the decisions were for, against, or undecided. Simple requests which were granted were mostly routine administrative matters which were handled in a direct unemotional manner. The following three examples are of this type:

Dr. Rolfe: I'd like to have permission for Miss Fellows to go out this afternoon.
Dr. Shaw: Okay.

Dr. Rolfe: Also, Mr. Erskine would like to go to dinner with his father this evening.
Dr. Shaw: Okay.

Dr. Rivers: Miss Farrell . . . has asked for permission to go to the theater tonight, and I would like a decision on this.
Dr. Shaw: Is she going to go to the theater alone?
Dr. Rivers: She is going alone.
Dr. Shaw: Okay.

The simple requests which were decided against were also handled rather directly. Often these decisions against were on the basis of legal considerations, which were not clearly understood or evaluated as such by the patients or personnel. In the following example, Mr. Oliver had requested permission to go to a ball game, and Dr. Shaw refused this because of legal considerations in the face of considerable feeling on the part of the activities worker, Miss Wright, and the nurse, Miss Nicholas, that it might be useful for Mr. Oliver to go to the ball game. This conflict between legal consideration and what might be useful for the individual patient was an area of considerable misunderstanding in the hospital, and hospital personnel who were involved in the situation often found it difficult to see why a certain procedure should be followed:

Dr. Ramsay: Ray Oliver has a man coming down to see him, and he wants to know if he can go out to the ball game with him.

Dr. Shaw: This person coming to see him is just a friend and can't legally sign him out.

Miss Wright: He's looking forward to this and wants to go. I think it's a real question of whether we can keep him in here unless we can provide activities.

Dr. Shaw: Well, we'll have to deal with this.

Miss Nicholas: He very much wants—

Dr. Shaw (cutting off Miss Nicholas): I asked Dr. Sutton and Dr. Scott about that. He is a minor and he can't go.

The simple requests which were left undecided were those requests in the administrative area which aroused emotion and, at the same time, involved judgments about matters on which there was no clear-cut policy; hence decisions on such requests were avoided by the senior staff. For example:

Dr. Ramsay: Miss Patterson, Mrs. Fox, and Miss Murdock want to go and hear a talk by Professor Brighton on Wednesday. This is what comes of putting up those calendars of events on the bulletin board.

Dr. Shaw: I expect not. I don't think they should go.

Mrs. Wells: The lecture has to do with the rearing of children, and I don't think they would get anything out of it.

Dr. Reynolds: Why not! Who's to decide this matter?

Dr. Shaw: I expect that their interest in this is probably introspective.

Dr. Rivers: If they were interested in this matter, they could read a book about it.

Dr. Ramsay: Well, if we put up the calendar of events, this sort of thing is going to happen.

Dr. Shaw: When does the lecture come off?

Dr. Ramsay: Wednesday night.

Dr. Shaw: Well, I guess we can talk about this further at some other time.

As was seen in Table 11–21, a much greater percentage of simple than of complex requests was granted. However, about one fourth of the complex requests did result in a decision for, and these were usually concerned with a rather clear-cut matter, even though it might be complicated by the introduction of considerations from another area of life. For example, in the following topic, one of the nurses, Miss Newcomb, asked if Mrs. Lasswell could be moved from one room to another on the locked ward. Dr. Ryan complicated this administrative request by introducing some therapeutic considerations about Mrs. Lasswell, but these tended to be in line with the request made by Miss Newcomb. Dr. Shaw, therefore, was not presented with any conflicting statements, and it was fairly easy for him to grant the request:

Miss Newcomb: Mrs. Martin's room is empty. Could we move Mrs. Lasswell into that?

Dr. Ryan: After Mrs. Lasswell has finished her shock treatment I would like to move her to the open ward. But at present I think your request would be in line with her behavior. In occupational therapy the other day she made a speech from the table top, so perhaps we should keep her on the locked ward for a week after the shock treatment is finished.

Dr. Shaw: Well, let's move her into Mrs. Martin's old room.

Complex requests which eventuated in decisions against usually contained a good deal of emotion, as was true in the following example, where an administrative request was made by Dr. Rolfe about whether Mr. Ashton could be moved to the open ward or, alternatively, could be provided with a quiet place to study on the locked ward. This request raised a fairly heated discussion in which various feelings about Mr. Ashton were expressed. The topic was further complicated by Dr. Scott's introducing the fact that Mr. Ashton was being treated by a senior therapist, Dr. Salton, who had little contact with the day-to-day operation of the hospital. The result was that Dr. Shaw denied the request to move Mr. Ashton to the open ward:

Dr. Rolfe: There is a problem of studies with Ashton. It is just impossible, Ashton says, for him to study with Innes' radio going all the time and Mr. Esposito making noise. I feel that Mr. Ashton has done very well on the locked ward, and I would like to move him to the open ward.

Dr. Ramsay: We might fix up one of the seclusion rooms as a place for him to study.

Miss Nugent: Well, in that case we would have to lock him in. We can't use ward personnel for a couple of hours just to watch him, so we would have to lock him in.

Dr. Shaw: He would have the free run of the entire seclusion area if he wished, in such a case.

Miss Nugent: We would have to lock that outside door, or he would also have free run of the kitchen.

Dr. Scott: He doesn't want to study.

Miss Nugent: I have never seen him study!

Dr. Scott: The conflict here is between the therapist and the hospital. The therapist says he is well enough to study and go to college, and we say that he isn't. I don't think Dr. Salton as the therapist knows our position well enough.

Dr. Shaw: Ashton sure is in a rage.

Dr. Scott: The issue should not be whether there are attendants that are available or not, but the issue should be whether he is well enough or not.

Dr. Shaw: If he is really serious about an attempt to study, he can do it in a locked seclusion room. He was in a rage over not being allowed to go to college, and wanted me and Dr. Scott to talk to Dr. Salton. I feel in this case I must decide that he cannot be moved to the open ward.

Dr. Scott: Tell Innes to turn his radio down.

Miss Nicholas: He will turn it down if he is asked.

Dr. Scott: The trouble with Innes is that we are all afraid of him.

The complex requests which remained undecided, and which made up 52.9 per cent of all complex requests, were very indicative of the more sensitive areas of problem in the administrative conferences. In the following example, Dr. Ryan introduced an administrative request for Mr. Edwards to go into town unaccompanied, and Dr. Ryan himself complicated this by therapeutic considerations. In this case, Dr. Ryan was the administrative psychiatrist for Mr. Edwards, and Dr. Simmons was Mr. Edwards' therapist. As in the preceding example, this request was also complicated by Dr. Scott's introducing the problem of difficulties in communication between senior therapists and other members of the staff. The result was that Dr. Shaw tabled Dr. Ryan's request for further discussion at a later date:

Dr. Ryan: Mr. Edwards had an interview with Dr. Simmons yesterday, and Dr. Simmons introduced the question of Mr. Edwards' going out unaccompanied. Mr. Edwards then brought this question to me, and asked for my decision. I talked to Harold about going to the library, and we talked also about his use of alcohol. Harold feels that he can't give up alcohol, but that he won't do very much more than have an occasional beer in a restaurant, which is about what any of us would do. Harold says that he is willing to be searched when he comes back into the hospital, and I would rather like to see him go out in order to see if he can handle this sort of situation.

Dr. Shaw: What would you expect would happen?

Dr. Ryan: Nothing, or perhaps at most a glass of beer.

Dr. Reynolds: Wouldn't it be hair tonic?

Dr. Ryan: Hair tonic seems to be a solution for not being able to get beer, and if we were to let Mr. Edwards do this, we would probably cut down our worries with him on the ward.

Dr. Shaw: Well, we can't decide this here. We'll have to talk more about it. We'll have to talk with Dr. Simmons. Harold's behavior, according to the nurses, is getting to be more bizarre.

Dr. Ryan: Well! How is it getting more bizarre? You mean when he's out on the terrace?

Dr. Shaw: I mean when he's running around the ward.

Dr. Ryan: I agree that the running around the ward is a little more bizarre, but if you spent time with him, you'd find he was quite a different person. He would also like to go to the dentist, as well as to go to the library.

Dr. Shaw: Well, let's not decide now.

Dr. Scott: Again, this seems to raise the problem of communication. I know less about Edwards than any other patient in the hospital, when we should know most about these patients who are in intensive treatment with other therapists. We've got to solve this problem of communication some way.

The preceding two examples illustrate a type of problem that arose frequently when the therapy was carried out by a senior doctor who had little contact with the daily operation of the hospital, while the administrative doctor had to take into account the procedures used in the hospital (see Chapter 9 and Stanton and Schwartz, 1954). Often this resulted in quite divergent views on the part of the hospital staff and the senior therapist about what was correct for a patient. Out of this sort of situation there arose attempts by the hospital staff to change the therapist, and attempts by the therapist to circumvent the hospital.

The fourteen content categories that have been utilized in this chapter to discuss some of the aspects of "how topics came up" and "what happened to topics" have proved to be quite revealing. Through these content categories it has been possible to see many of the underlying factors at work in the daily administrative conferences. It is not, however, the intention of such an analysis to leave the reader with the idea that the fourteen content categories used here are the only ones which might be devised for analyzing such material. They proved useful and were easily handled in terms of scoring, but this chapter represents only a beginning in the content analysis of the kind of material represented by the administrative conferences. Other content categories could easily be developed to show further properties of such group interaction.

In this chapter, the analysis of the topical content of the material has been made largely in a structural, or static, sense. It is possible to utilize the same 745 topics, but to treat them more dynamically, and in terms of process, by seeing the variations in the material over time. The following chapter turns to a brief discussion of these problems of process.

CHAPTER 12

Indexes of Process

In order to work out some of the dynamics over time in the administrative conferences, it is first necessary to give an indication of the material available for analysis by weekly periods. It will be remembered that the conferences were held each morning, Monday through Saturday. The maximum amount of material available, therefore, for any one week would consist of the records on all six of these daily conferences. It will also be remembered that the Monday conferences were somewhat longer than the others and included reports by the residents of the therapeutic progress of their patients, as well as the usual discussion of day-to-day administrative matters. It is for this reason that the materials available on the Monday conferences, and on the Tuesday through Saturday conferences, are indicated separately in Table 12–1. It is evident that the amount of material is satisfactory for the period from the second through the fourteenth week. During none of these weeks are there less than four conferences available for analysis, and in most of the weeks five, or all of the six, daily conferences are available. It will be noted that there are no data available for the eighth week. This is because the writer was out of town attending an annual professional meeting. He has since lived to regret being out of town during this week, but at the particular time that this occurred, he was not aware that he was going to analyze the data in the fashion indicated in this chapter. Indeed, the kind of analysis about to be presented is more in the nature of a finding of the study and an area suggested for further research.

The total 745 topics analyzed in the preceding chapter by means of the fourteen scoring categories can be divided into their occurrence during each week. The scoring of the topics for each week can then be analyzed in terms of a number of indexes constructed by combining

Table 12–1. Distribution of 63 daily administrative conferences over 15 weeks of observation

Conference data available for:	Fifteen-week period: 1	2	3	4	5	6	7	8[1]	9	10	11	12	13	14	15	Total
Monday conferences	0	1	1	1	1	1	1	–	1	1	1	1	1	1	0	12
Tuesday through Saturday conferences	1	5	5	5	4	3	3	–	3	5	5	3	4	4	1	51
All conferences for which data available	1	6	6	6	5	4	4	–	4	6	6	4	5	5	1	63

[1] No data as writer was away from hospital during eighth week.

Table 12–2. Indexes of various aspects of topic discussion in daily administrative conferences, by weeks

Indexes	Weeks: 2	3	4	5	6	7	8[1]	9	10	11	12	13	14
1. Withdrawal	51	45	47	54	44	74	–	*76*	64	74	76	57	44
2. Total emotion	42	48	36	44	54	40	–	*61*	42	41	37	45	41
3. Negative emotion	24	26	22	17	26	21	–	*39*	28	20	18	13	28
4. Complexity	17	32	31	14	24	10	–	*27*	19	13	25	11	22
5. Administrative difficulty	69	68	69	70	70	50	–	49	*71*	41	55	81	87
6. Control by seniors	20	13	14	9	32	21	–	14	*26*	9	20	13	25
7. Confusion	13	8	6	6	8	0	–	6	*17*	6	2	2	9
8. Inconclusiveness	12	23	15	14	10	2	–	10	*14*	11	12	15	22

[1] No data as writer was away from hospital during eighth week.

certain of the fourteen categories in various ways. Eight indexes were developed in the hope that they would show something of the dynamics of the conferences over the period from the second through the fourteenth week. These indexes were constructed as follows:

1. *Index of withdrawal.* This index might also be called "willingness to participate," in that it is similar to the one used at the end of Chapter 10. The index used here was constructed by expressing the sum of topics per week introduced in the category of communication only as a percentage of total topics for the week. Thus, the formula would be:

$$\text{Index of withdrawal} = \frac{\text{Sum topics: (communication only)}}{\text{Sum topics: (communication only)} + \text{(questions)} + \text{(requests)}}$$

The assumption underlying this index is that it took more "push" to make a request or to raise a question than it did to confine oneself to communication only. Thus, if members of the various role groups restricted themselves to the bare reporting of descriptive material which was scored as communication only, it was felt that they were tending to withdraw from active participation in the conference.

2. *Index of total emotion.* This index was constructed by expressing the sum of emotional (both positive and negative) topics for the week as a percentage of total topics. The formula for this would be:

$$\text{Index of total emotion} = \frac{\text{Sum topics: (positive emotion)} + \text{(negative emotion)}}{\text{Sum topics: (unemotional)} + \text{(positive emotion)} + \text{(negative emotion)}}$$

3. *Index of negative emotion.* This index was constructed by expressing the sum of the negative emotion topics for the week as a percentage of total topics. The formula for this would be:

$$\text{Index of negative emotion} = \frac{\text{Sum topics: (negative emotion)}}{\text{Sum topics: (unemotional)} + \text{(positive emotion)} + \text{(negative emotion)}}$$

One simple result of first constructing an index of *total emotion* and then an index of *negative emotion* is that when these two indexes are plotted graphically, as will be seen later in Figure 12–1, the distance between the negative emotion curve and the total emotion curve is, of necessity, a measure of the proportion of *positive emotion.*

4. *Index of complexity.* This index was constructed by expressing the sum of the complex topics during a week as a percentage of total topics. The formula for this would be:

$$\text{Index of complexity} = \frac{\text{Sum topics: (complex)}}{\text{Sum topics: (simple)} + \text{(complex)}}$$

5. *Index of administrative difficulty.* This index was based on the assumption that the greater the proportion of administrative topics during a week, the more likely it was that administrative matters were of

greater importance, and more of a problem, during that week. The formula for such an index would, therefore, be:

$$\text{Index of administrative difficulty} = \frac{\text{Sum topics: (administration)}}{\text{Sum topics: (administration)} + \text{(therapy)} + \text{(human relations)}}$$

6. *Index of control by seniors.* It has been noted several times in previous chapters that, proportionately, the senior doctors tended to speak most, the residents second, the other personnel third, and the nurses least. Therefore, it was felt that the proportion of topics introduced by seniors, relative to total topics, would give an index of the amount of direct control exercised by the senior staff over the work of the conference. That is, the greater the proportion of topics introduced during a week by seniors, the more directive was the nature of the conference, and the more passive were the other three role groups in their participation. The formula for such an index would be:

$$\text{Index of control by seniors} = \frac{\text{Sum topics: (seniors)}}{\text{Sum topics: (seniors)} + \text{(residents)} + \text{(nurses)} + \text{(other personnel)}}$$

7. *Index of confusion.* As noted in the preceding chapter, general and specific-to-general topics were much more likely to have a balance of negative emotion. It was also felt that the frequency of these two types of topics provided a rather sensitive indication of confusion in that when ambiguities began to arise in the work of the hospital, these were likely to be reflected in increased discussion of general policy in the conferences. The formula for such an index, therefore, would be:

$$\text{Index of confusion} = \frac{\text{Sum topics: (specific-to-general)} + \text{(general)}}{\text{Sum topics: (specific)} + \text{(specific-to-general)} + \text{(general)}}$$

8. *Index of inconclusiveness.* On the basis of the discussion in the preceding chapter, it can be said that inconclusive topics were more likely to cause difficulty and confusion than were conclusive topics. Therefore, the proportion of inconclusive topics during a week would provide one way for getting at the equilibrium of the daily administrative conferences. The formula for this index would be:

$$\text{Index of inconclusiveness} = \frac{\text{Sum topics: (inconclusive)}}{\text{Sum topics: (inconclusive)} + \text{(conclusive)}}$$

It is, of course, quite apparent that all eight of the indexes are interrelated and are not independent of each other—being simply various facets of the on-going interaction during the conferences. Nevertheless, when these eight indexes are plotted graphically they show some interesting relations. Table 12–2 gives the result of the numerical computation of the indexes over the period from the second through the fourteenth week.

The focus of attention in Table 12–2 is on the period from the sixth through the twelfth week. Interest in this seven-week period stems from the fact that the open manifestation of the collective disturbance on the ward, described in Chapter 5, occurred mainly during the eleventh week. In Chapters 4 and 5 a qualitative analysis has already been made of what was happening during this particular week, as well as the events prior and subsequent to it. Here, by means of the indexes, quantitative evidence is given to complement the more qualitative analysis presented earlier and to show the possibility of *predicting* such occurrences as the collective disturbance.

During the period from the sixth through the twelfth week, the first four indexes reached a high point in the ninth week. Similarly, the last four indexes reached a high point in the tenth week. These high points are indicated by italics in Table 12–2. Seven of the eight indexes dropped off sharply during the eleventh week, but the index of withdrawal remained high during the eleventh and twelfth weeks. Thus, the general disturbance in the hospital system would seem to have shown itself at the administrative conference level in the two-week period *prior* to the collective disturbance on the ward, and to have worked its way down to the patient level by the eleventh week.

The implication of this sort of analysis is not that when a rise occurred in the eight indexes used here the result would inevitably be a collective disturbance on the ward. The type of response to a disequilibrium in the hospital system of the kind indicated by a rise in the indexes might take a number of other forms. It should, however, be possible to predict that if there was a rise in the indexes at the administrative level, the expectation would be for some sort of disturbing response at the patient level, and at other places in the hospital system, within a short time. This would be true unless, of course, some action was taken by the staff to change the course of events on the basis of a conscious recognition and understanding of the behavior underlying the indexes.

The eight indexes presented in Table 12–2 are shown graphically in Figures 12–1 and 12–2. Figure 12–1 shows the four indexes which reached their high point during the ninth week, while Figure 12–2 shows the four which reached their high point during the tenth week. The only reason for separating these two groups of indexes on different figures is one of visual simplicity, as logically the eight indexes should be plotted together. As mentioned earlier, these eight indexes are not independent of each other, but rather all of them represent related aspects of the interaction in the conferences.

Certain events occurring at various times during the period of greatest

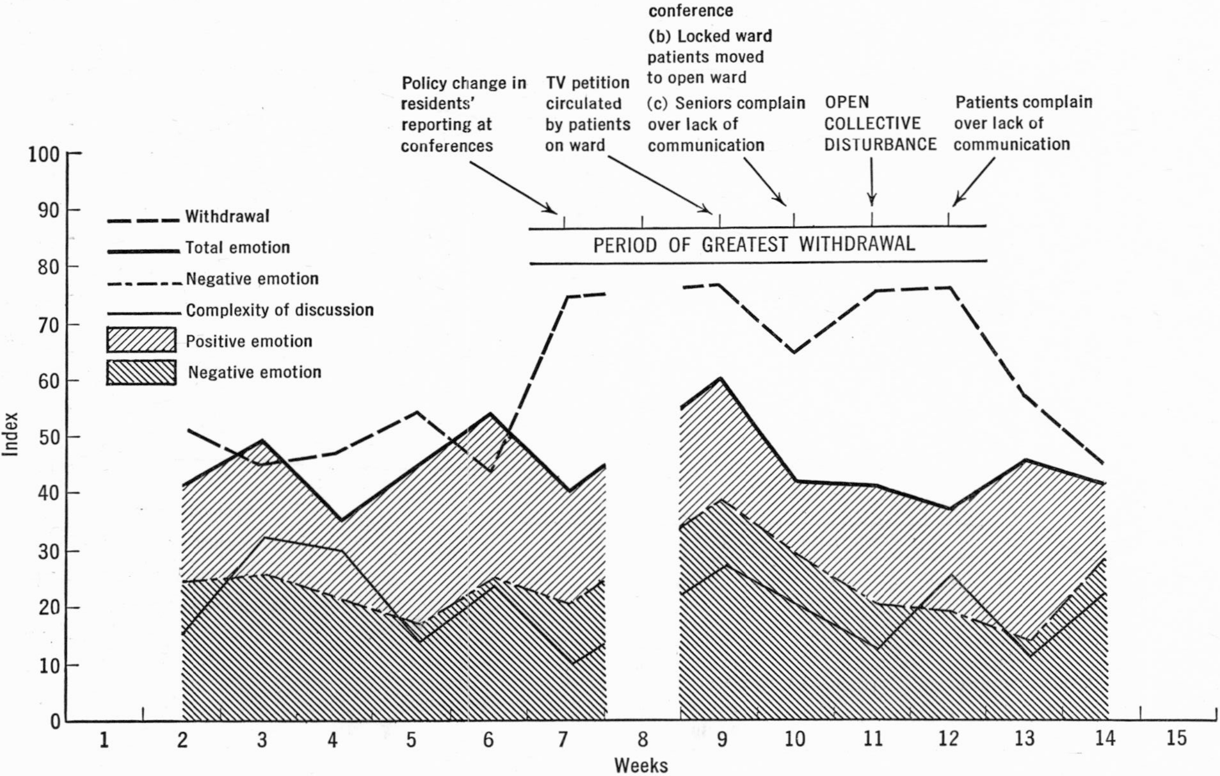

Figure 12–1. Indexes of withdrawal, total emotion, positive and negative emotion, and complexity of discussion in administrative conferences, by weeks. Source: Table 12–2

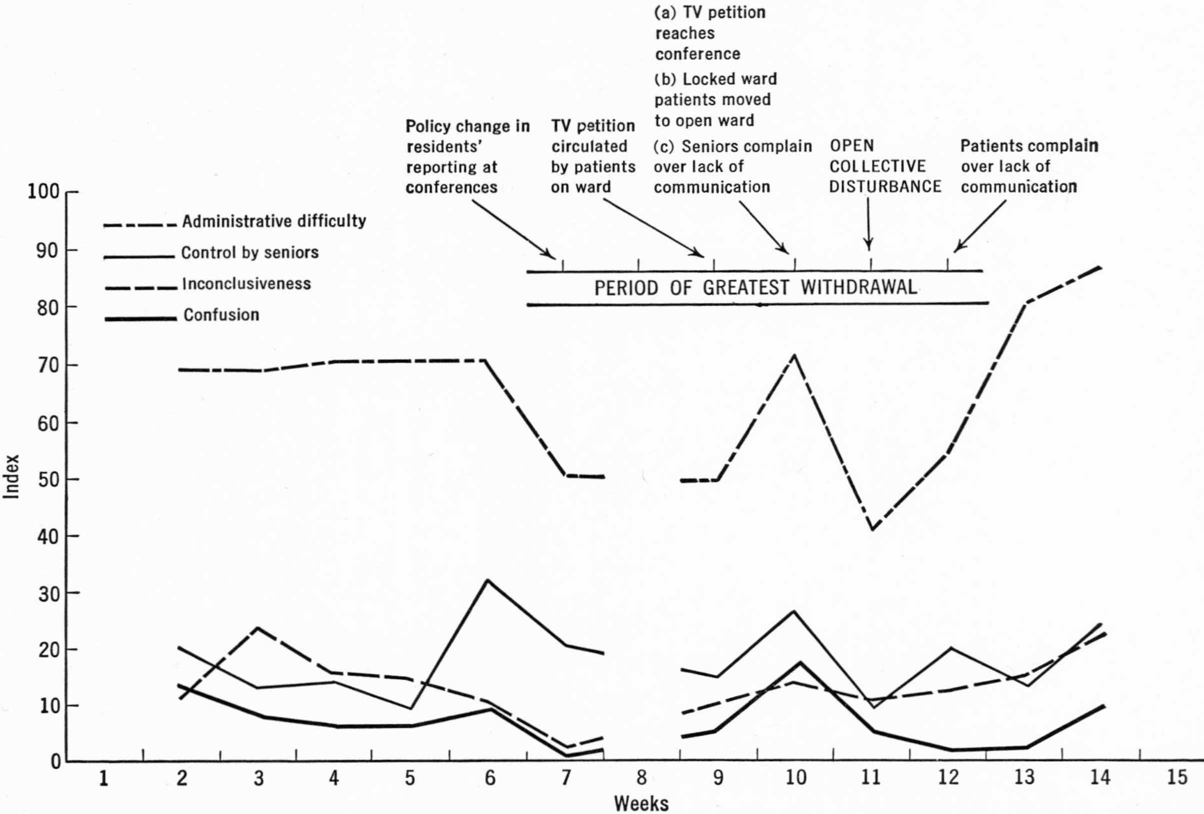

FIGURE 12–2. Indexes of administrative difficulty, control by seniors, confusion, and inconclusiveness in administrative conferences, by weeks. Source: Table 12–2

withdrawal are indicated by arrows in Figures 12–1 and 12–2. Many of these events have already been referred to in Chapters 4 and 5. It is useful at this point, however, to review briefly the observational data on these events, keeping in mind the changes in the indexes in Figures 12–1 and 12–2.

The period of greatest withdrawal indicated on the two figures began in the seventh week, with a change in policy regarding the residents' reporting at the administrative conferences. This is seen as an important event in the beginning of withdrawal because the result of this decision was to place a greater apparent, more than real, authority in the hands of the residents to make administrative decisions. In a sense, the senior staff were withdrawing from control of the situation. As a result, the proportion of communication only topics took a considerable upswing in the seventh week, as indicated by the withdrawal index, which meant the residents were bringing fewer problems for discussion to the administrative conference. The legitimacy for choosing this point as the beginning of the withdrawal period can be indicated by the discussion at the conference during which the policy change was introduced:

Dr. Shaw: I want to shift the purpose of these morning conferences, and instead of bringing up things for approval, we want you to bring up problems that you have doubts about. Not all the problems that confront you, but those which involve the use of the hospital and seem to be major problems. Instead of bringing up picayune details, we want you to state the problem of what you want to do, the problems surrounding the actual decision. We want to change it from a matter of my arbitrarily deciding yes or no. This is in concurrence with the idea that we all should take responsibility in using the hospital for the patients' benefit. The decisions for your patients lie now with you.

Dr. Scott: I'd like to add a few remarks to what Dr. Shaw said. And I hope that you understand we are shifting these conferences from being controversial to being communicative, so that this shifts the burden to you. The decisions which involve all of us should be brought up here. I have a feeling that we are all harassed and stressed, and hell, it ought to be fun running this hospital. I'd like to get rid of the controversial issues between nurses, residents, and patients. On evenings that involve rearrangements on the ward, such as some of the locked ward patients coming to the open ward to see TV, the nurse should take the responsibility, and does not have to communicate with the doctor about this. She should make the decision and should do whatever she feels comfortable with. . . .

(There was no comment from the conference personnel on what Dr. Shaw and Dr. Scott said, and, after a rather long silence, Dr. Scott went on to another matter.)

In terms of the topic just cited, it is interesting that while the policy of allowing the residents to make certain decisions never was officially changed, the withdrawal index remained high only until the twelfth week, and then returned to the level which existed during the period from the second to the sixth week. In other words, the proportion of communication only topics remained high only during the period of withdrawal.

The shift in policy accentuated the breakdown in communication that took place during the ninth week. It was during the ninth week that, as noted in Chapter 5, the senior staff were unaware that individual patients had been moved from one ward to another until some days after the movement had taken place. It was also in the ninth week that the TV petition, as described in Chapter 4, was circulated by the patients on the ward, although it did not actually reach the attention of the administrative conference until the tenth week because Mr. Ashton kept the petition in his room for a week before giving it to his doctor. As indicated in Chapter 4, this series of events seemed to be more than an isolated difficulty in communication, and to represent a symptom of a wider disequilibrium in the hospital system. As evidence for this, it was also during the tenth week that, as discussed in Chapter 5, the male locked ward patients were moved to the open ward on a semi-permanent basis because of a misunderstanding in communication between the head of the hospital and the supervisor of nurses. At the end of the tenth week Dr. Scott expressed his dissatisfaction in the administrative conference over the lack of adequate communication:

Dr. Scott: I have two comments I want to make. First of all, frequently we hear as the night report that nothing happened on the ward. Obviously this is not true. Is it that you feel that only negative things are worth reporting? . . . I feel it is just as important to know that Mr. Osgood did talk to someone as that he was isolated. Secondly, the little defensiveness that seems to come up about one's patients. When the nurse says something about the patient, the doctor feels it is necessary to say: "But he isn't like that." We should accept what the nurse says, and shouldn't defend ourselves by saying it's not true. The nurse sees the patient from one point of view, the doctor from another. . . . She is not fabricating what she says. We should get more accepting of remarks such as when the nurse says the patient is more seclusive. The doctor feels that this is disturbing, and the doctor frequently says: "Well, he talks to me." It's obvious that we should hear various people's opinions, as the patient must behave differently with different people.

There was a sharp rise in the tenth week in the number of specific-to-general and general topics, which is reflected in the rise of the index of confusion in Figure 12–2. As reported in Chapter 5, it was during the tenth week, for example, that the question was raised by Miss Noyes of Mrs. Matthews' going out unaccompanied from the locked ward, which turned into a general discussion of the privileges and possession of physical objects appropriate for patients on the locked wards.

Also in the conferences of the tenth week there was a temporary reversion by the residents to the older pattern, not in line with the newer policy of their making their own decisions, of bringing specific requests to the conferences for decisions. This tendency accounts for the dip in the index of withdrawal during the tenth week, and probably indicates that the residents were not feeling very secure in their authority at this point. In addition, the senior doctors did not turn these requests back to the residents, but gave decisions on them; in this way the seniors also were responding to a feeling of confusion in the conferences and attempting to mitigate it.

As can be seen from the foregoing highlights, the period from the seventh to the tenth week was a rather difficult one. It was during the latter part of the eleventh week that the open collective disturbance, as described in Chapter 5, occurred on the ward and caused the staff to be somewhat taken aback, as they had not anticipated the disturbance. During the first part of the eleventh week there was a paucity of information in the administrative conferences about events on the ward. For example, as indicated in Chapter 5, a quite successful going-away party was given by the patients for Miss Lindsey and Mr. Onofrio. This party involved almost all the patients in the hospital, occupied most of the day in planning, and was given in the evening. It, however, received almost no notice at the following morning's administrative conference.

On the evening following the party the collective disturbance manifested itself on the ward when the patients who had privileges were allowed to leave the hospital to go into town. As discussed in Chapter 5, the patients left the hospital either individually or in pairs, whereas during previous weeks they had gone out in groups of four or five. All patients returned to the hospital in an upset state, and all patients who went out in pairs returned singly. These events were noted the following morning at the administrative conference, but the discussion centered largely around the individual psychopathology of several patients who were diagnosed as having character disorders. The openly disturbed situation among the patients continued for about a week and was especially to be noted over the week end between the eleventh and twelfth week.

Finally, with relation to the last event indicated by arrows in Figures 12–1 and 12–2, the twelfth week was highlighted by the patients' dissatisfaction over what they felt was a lack of communication in the hospital. As described in Chapter 5, Dr. Ryan had a meeting with most of the male patients on the open ward during his rounds one evening. At this meeting the patients had an extended discussion with Dr. Ryan and expressed their desires for a better channel of communication to the staff.

Dr. Ryan brought up his discussion with the patients at the administrative conference during the twelfth week. However, as indicated in Chapter 5, his attempt to bring this matter to the attention of the staff met with little success.

As noted in Chapter 5, at the end of the fourteenth week the whole issue of the difficulty in communication and the differences in goals among the various role groups finally came to a head in an open discussion at the administrative conferences. This discussion is reflected in the indexes in Figures 12–1 and 12–2 by a sharp drop in the index of withdrawal and an equally sharp increase in the index of administrative difficulty—this latter because the issues were being openly examined.

The reader should not be left with the impression that it was possible during the course of the study to predict events in the total hospital system. The writer was busy gathering material and was no more aware of the phenomena revealed by the indexes than were the staff. It was only after analysis of all the data—the observations on the wards and at the administrative conferences, the interviews, the hospital records, and so on—that it was possible to see clearly the patterns that emerged. Such an analysis, however, sets the stage for prediction in future study and for the adaptation of the research methods for practical use.

The data from the administrative conferences were such that it was possible to make a quantitative analysis of certain processes over time. As the interrelated nature of group processes at various levels in the hospital became apparent, other types of data were assessed to see if an analysis similar to that presented in this chapter could be made in other areas of hospital life. Unfortunately, as indicated in Chapter 2, the material on psychotherapy, as represented by the daily progress notes of the residents for the entire group of patients, was not adequate enough to make possible any sort of quantitative analysis over time. The daily progress notes were good in isolated cases, such as those for Mr. Esposito which were used in Chapter 3, but were totally inadequate in other cases. It was not possible, therefore, to make a summary statement of how the patients as a group seemed to be progressing during any particular week. Equally, it was not possible to analyze the data at the senior staff level or at the ward observational level in a quantitative manner.

In future research it should be possible to develop indexes for other areas of hospital life similar to those developed here for the administrative conferences. Such indexes would be of considerable help in gaining further understanding, in operational terms, of what is meant when the psychiatric hospital is characterized as a therapeutic community.

Section V

IMPLICATIONS

CHAPTER 13

Conclusions from the Hospital Study

The chapters in this final section of the book draw together some of the conclusions and implications of the hospital study in the areas of content, method, and theory. Thus, this chapter summarizes the main findings from the study of one small psychiatric hospital and tries to relate these findings to those from studies of other psychiatric hospitals. Chapter 14 is focused on method in the sense that if the materials that have been presented have seemed useful, then there is the question of who is to gather such materials and put them to use in a clinical manner in the work of the hospital. Chapter 14 also contains a beginning attempt to see how the ideas arising from this study might be placed within a broader theoretical framework concerning the relation of disease and its treatment to cultural and social processes.

In the course of the preceding sections of this book, the data from three studies, each using a different approach, have been brought to bear on the question of the nature of the hospital as a social system. Thus, the second section was concerned with tracing the interrelations in the hospital by means of daily observations at various levels: the influence of the hospital on the doctor-patient relationship was examined first; then problems of communication in administrative processes were discussed; and finally the operation of the entire hospital over time was seen in terms of the development of a collective disturbance. The third section turned to an analysis of the perceptions of the hospital among patients and staff as these were indicated in the material collected through use of the picture interview. Lastly, the fourth section consisted of a small group analysis of the daily administrative conferences, in which it was possible to see the interplay between individual personality, social role, and the general social structure of the hospital. Throughout the presentation of these three studies, the attempt has been made to throw into bold relief the effect of the overt formal and informal structure, and of the covert emotional structure, in the operation of the hospital. It is hoped that by this time the reader is reasonably convinced that a psychiatric hospital is indeed a social system, and that the properties of such a system constitute a set of significant variables which affect the quality of behavior in all areas of hospital life. This is the main conclusion of the present book, and the following discussion will review some of the consequences that seem to evolve from such a state of affairs.

One possible consequence of the social system of the hospital centers around the question which has been raised in several chapters of whether or not there is a "ground swell" affecting psychotherapy in a hospital so that a majority of patients might be doing well or poorly at a particular time. As indicated in Chapter 2, it was not possible in the studies reported here to make any very extensive use of material from psychotherapeutic hours because of the inadequacy of the records kept by the residents. In the closing section of this book, however, it is well to refer to the "ground swell" question again, as the observational data on interrelations in the hospital lend credence to such a hypothesis and suggest the need for a more thorough testing of it. A serious consideration of this matter might well lead to the opening up of an additional approach to the development of a truly therapeutic community.

One aspect of the social structure of the hospital which would be important in the investigation of the occurrence of a "ground swell" in psychotherapy is the "mobility blocked" nature of roles at various levels in the hospital. The data from the observations, picture interview material, and administrative conference analysis, have all shown how such a structure influenced communication between the different role groups. The difficulties in communication in this sort of system would increase the likelihood of disturbances in three-person groups, as in the disagreements between several staff members concerning the treatment of a patient which have been reported by Stanton and Schwartz (1954).

The interaction processes in these hierarchically structured small groups in the hospital are related to the more general processes that appear to characterize three-person groups wherever they are found. Mills (1953, 1954, 1956), in his experimental work, has shown the inherent instability of three-person groups, in that interaction usually results in the coalition of two persons against the other. Since this seems to be a general property of any meaningful group of three persons, it is tantalizing to speculate whether the Oedipal conflict is intensified because it is basically a case of conflict between three persons, or whether later triangular situations always involve a residue of early familial problems. In any case, triangular situations are continually occurring among various combinations of patients and staff in a psychiatric hospital, and it might be possible to develop a predictive measure of disturbance on the ward by taking into account the numbers of patients who were involved in such three-person groups at any particular time. Interest is expressed in this because it might provide a method of arriving at an index of the state of the ward similar in function to the indexes developed from the data on the administrative conferences in Chapter 12.

Along these lines, it was noted in Chapter 5 that the number of heterosexual pairs among patients on the ward increased during the period of mutual withdrawal of the various role groups. A hypothesis concerning these heterosexual pairs is that they are really triangles involving the two patients and their individual therapists. When difficulties arise between the therapist and the patient, the patient may attempt to solve them by pairing off with another patient. The obverse of this is also possible—the therapist may respond to difficulties with his patient by developing a paired relationship with another therapist, or with a nurse. Beyond this, it seems likely that the number of such triangles would increase when the over-all system of the hospital is in a state of disequilibrium, as during the period of mutual withdrawal in the collective disturbance.

A further interesting question is suggested by the observational material in Chapters 4 and 5. Triangular relations seemed to occur in which the structure of the triangle involved entire role groups rather than merely individuals. For example, in Chapter 4, Dr. Scott seemed to be identifying himself with the patient group in his difference of opinion with the nurses. Similarly, in Chapter 5 the period of paired role groups can be thought of as including two triangles composed of role groups rather than individuals: one triangle came into being through the identification of the residents with the patients against the senior staff, while a second triangle was apparent in the coalition of the nurses with the senior staff against the residents. The dynamics of these triangular relations among role groups would seem to be akin to those among individuals, but to be even more complicated by the general state of the social system of the hospital at a particular time.

Such triangular relations, among both individuals and role groups, would seem to offer a further opportunity for the development of indexes which might prove to be sufficiently sensitive to changing processes on the ward or throughout the hospital so that they could be used for predictive purposes in a way similar to the indexes suggested in Chapter 12. If these measures could be worked out, they would provide yet another approach in the effort to make explicit the meaning of a therapeutic community.

The question of the effect on the patients of certain combinations of staff who were on duty is related to the foregoing discussion of triangular relations. This question was raised in Chapters 1 and 5, where it was pointed out that the particular combination of persons on duty was a purely chance occurrence because the scheduling of doctors and nurses on duty was carried out independently by the chief resident and the nursing supervisor. Observations on the wards indicated that different combinations of staff on duty seemed to produce different effects on diagnostic or social groupings of patients. This is a matter for further research in which it will be necessary to study combinations of specific individuals who occupy different roles in the hospital system. Moreover, it will be necessary to know the state of integration or equilibrium of the hospital system at the time of observation: no matter how compatible or antagonistic the resident and nurse on duty may be, the chances of their forming a harmonious couple will be increased if the general relations between residents and nurses are good at the time, and conversely, their chances for harmony will be decreased if there are difficulties between the various staff role groups.

Most of the general consequences of the hospital as a social system that have been mentioned above have received illustration throughout this book, and it is useful to turn to a summary and review of specific chapters as a means of bringing together further implications and conclusions. In Chapter 3 the focus of interest was upon the doctor-patient relationship as represented by Dr. Ryan and Mr. Esposito. As will be remembered, the eight weeks of Mr. Esposito's stay were divided into three periods. During the first period attention was drawn to the several sources of satisfaction to which a patient who entered the hospital might turn in an effort to obtain help with his immediate needs. These sources were: the patient's physician, the nurses and aides, the use of the physical space of the ward in ways the patient found comfortable, the other patients, and the patient himself—in terms of his psychological and physical resources. It seemed clear from the observations on Mr. Esposito that the hospital took account of only a few of these sources in the initial effort to understand and help the patient. This was apparent in the almost exclusive attention that Dr. Ryan gave to the patient's past history without turning to advantage what the patient repeatedly brought to the psychotherapeutic sessions concerning his relations with the nurses, the other patients, and the use of the physical space of the ward. In general, it is probably true that much significant information about the patient is lost because of such a lack of awareness on the part of the staff during the crucial period of the patient's first few days in the hospital.

In the second period of Mr. Esposito's hospitalization, Dr. Ryan became more active in his efforts to help the patient with the result that the therapeutic relationship became entangled in the covert disagreements over policy between the residents and the senior staff and nurses. Most of the things that Dr. Ryan tried to do were criticized by the senior staff and obstructed by the nurses, and this led to increased defensiveness on Dr. Ryan's part. At this point, Dr. Ryan, as a first-year resident, felt threatened by the staff on the one hand, and insecure in his ability to handle the more open expression of emotion by the patient on the other hand. The latter point, for example, was evident when, just prior to his withdrawal from the attempt to work intensively with the patient, Dr. Ryan dictated: "He expressed very strong feelings in the things he said, the ideas he had on how his illness got started, and certainly it is useless to push him on these points. He will just have to air his feelings as he can." In this situation Dr. Ryan was backing away from the emotion of the patient, just as earlier he had made little direct use of the patient's other attempts at reintegration, and it is difficult to see how Dr. Ryan could have done otherwise when he was receiving so little support from the staff.

The difficulties in which Dr. Ryan found himself raise the more general question of the problems faced by residents when they are asked to do psychotherapy with disturbed patients who, as often happens, have been referred to the hospital by more experienced psychiatrists because the latter have been unable to manage the treatment of the patient in the community. There would not appear to be any practical way to avoid such problems since, under present conditions, residents will continue to do the bulk of the treatment of patients in psychiatric hospitals. It should be possible, however, to so order the organization and work of the hospital that a resident would feel supported in his efforts rather than finding himself thwarted by the types of conflicts among the staff which have been described in this book.

Such problems of the residents are related to the point made at the end of Chapter 3 concerning the "reverberations" of events within the relatively closed system of the hospital. Psychotherapy carried out inside the hospital, in distinction to that carried out in the community, is systematically subject to pressures from many sources because the doctor and patient are part of the same network of interpersonal relations. Any action of the doctor or patient stemming from their therapeutic relations quickly impinges on the actions and feelings of other residents, nurses, and patients. As mentioned in Chapter 3, the effect of this in a hospital is analogous to the effect of a rock tossed into a bathtub of water, whereas the effect of psychotherapy in a community is more that of a pebble thrown into a lake. In connection with this, the distinction made in psychodynamic theory between talking and acting is overdrawn when applied within a psychiatric hospital. In much of the psychodynamic literature the point is made that a patient is less accessible to psychotherapy if he is primarily acting out his problems rather than talking them out with the therapist. Yet, talking is a type of acting, and even unverbalized thinking can create emotional interplay between persons. Emotional acts of this sort certainly tend to reverberate through the hospital to a greater extent than is true in the community. Such phenomena complicate the problem of the transference and countertransference between patient and therapist. As indicated in Chapter 3, it would appear that within the hospital the course of events in psychotherapy is influenced not only by the more narrowly defined aspects of transference and countertransference behavior based on the past learning of the patient and therapist, but also upon the use of the psychotherapeutic relationship to obtain relief from tension arising out of the participation of therapist and patient in other areas of their life in the hospital.

The observations in Chapter 4 centered on the confusion between administrative and psychotherapeutic processes, and the distortions in communication that stemmed from the paucity of information concerning the events that led to the television petition. This confusion and paucity of information served to increase the covert tensions among the staff and helped to precipitate a considerable overreaction to a relatively simple request from the patients. In this way the patients became heir to many of the tensions which more properly belonged to the staff. This was true, for example, for Mr. Esposito in Chapter 3 and for Mr. Erskine in Chapter 4, both of whom were unwittingly caught up in conflicts between the senior physicians, residents, and nurses.

The tendency to focus on a particular patient as the source of a problem, rather than also utilizing knowledge about the wider context in which the problem occurs, seems to be a very general phenomenon in a psychiatric hospital, and it can be illustrated by two theater parties in which Mrs. Lasker participated. Mrs. Lasker returned from the first party after having had a very successful evening, and the discussion in the administrative conference the next morning centered on how much progress Mrs. Lasker had made in the integration of her defenses. A few weeks later Mrs. Lasker returned from a second theater party in a state of confusion, and the discussion the following morning at the administrative conference concerned the difficulty Mrs. Lasker was having in handling her defenses and her regression to a psychologically less integrated state. Now, the composition of the group of patients who attended both theater parties was the same except for the inclusion in the second party of an additional patient whose presence proved to be very disturbing. It is undoubtedly true that it was easier for Mrs. Lasker to maintain her equilibrium in the first party than in the second, yet, at the same time, the social structure of the two parties was different, and this should have been considered in the discussion. In the first party Mrs. Lasker was with a group of people who were congenial, while in the second party the addition of the disturbing patient made it impossible for the group to have a successful evening.

The above situation is similar in nature to the previously mentioned problem about the effect of certain combinations of staff on duty together. Just as the combinations of staff were a matter of chance, so similarly the way in which most group activities were formed resulted in a chance collection, or "aggregate," of patients. The procedure followed in arranging an activity was for the group worker first to bring a request for an activity to the attention of the staff at the administrative conference. The group worker would then ask the residents for a list of their patients who were considered ready to participate in such an activity. Upon receiving the list, the group worker would go to the ward and ask each approved patient individually if he would like to attend the activity. In this way an aggregate of ten or twelve persons was obtained whose congeniality with one another was largely fortuitous. Yet, the success of the activity, and the resulting feelings of achievement or failure on the part of individual patients, depended to a great extent on how well these people were able to get along together. It seems fairly clear that a theater party is not likely to succeed if it is made up of people with widely divergent backgrounds and interests, coming from several social class strata, choosing very different clothing as appropriate for the occasion, and having conflicting desires about what to do after the theater—ranging from having a chocolate soda at the drugstore to having shrimp

Arnaud at a supper club. Such an aggregate of people would be very unlikely to have a pleasant evening together in normal social relations in the community, and would be far less likely to do so if, as is so often true for psychiatric patients, they felt they were wearing the label of the hospital on their backs.

At the end of Chapter 4 the question was raised of whether there was a reversal in the sequence of phases in administrative and therapeutic processes, and the further question of whether such functions could, therefore, be handled by the same person at roughly the same time. The work of Fiedler (1957) and Bales (1956) was cited as indicating that adaptive and expressive functions seem to require different attitudes and roles which usually are taken by separate individuals during interaction in small groups. In the experiments carried out by Bales and Slater (1955), two types of "leaders" tended to appear in the course of interaction in any single small group. One was the "task specialist," and the other was the "sociometric star." Originally, Bales felt that these two functions were mutually exclusive. In later work, he came to feel that while the abilities to carry out these two functions did not very often occur in a single leader, there was no necessary incompatibility between them. Thus, concerning the abilities necessary to perform adaptive and expressive functions, Bales (1956) recently said: ". . . [they] are not opposites which *preclude* each other, but are rather approximately *orthogonal* to each other. That is the traits to which the factors refer are . . . uncorrelated; at least they are not linearly correlated." It is interesting that similar findings have begun to emerge from the study of the family. For example, Papanek (1957) found, in her study of patterns of authority and the quality of interpersonal relations in a series of urban families, that the type of parental control over the children varied independently of the expression of parental warmth toward the children.

The findings of such studies of experimental small groups and of families are pertinent for the study of the psychiatric hospital, since the usefulness of small group analysis has already been shown in the treatment of the administrative conferences in Chapters 10 through 12, and the similarity of the role structure of the hospital to that of the family emerged from the picture interview data given in Chapter 7. Moreover, studies of small groups and families have relevance for the question of whether administrative and therapeutic functions should be separated in the work of the psychiatric hospital. The conclusion that there was no necessary incompatibility between the exercise of control and the expression of warmth would suggest that it was possible, though perhaps difficult, to allow both administrative and therapeutic functions to remain in the hands of a single person. Such a procedure would probably help to avoid the types of disagreements discussed by Stanton and Schwartz (1954) between persons with power over a patient, and would serve to reduce the number of triangular conflicts mentioned earlier in this chapter. At the same time, the interesting suggestion by Parsons, Bales, and Shils (1953) that the sequence of phases in administrative and therapeutic processes is reversed would point to the need for a clear awareness on the part of the doctor (or other staff member) of which process he was participating in. Such a clarity of purpose was lacking in the handling of the television petition as outlined in Chapter 4. In general, there would not yet seem to be an unequivocal answer regarding whether the attempt should be made to separate administrative and therapeutic functions, and this is a matter for further research. It is apparent, however, that whatever procedure is followed, it should not confound the two functions.

The discussion of the collective disturbance in Chapter 5 provided the opportunity to introduce the idea of a covert emotional structure underlying the overt formal and informal structure of the hospital. During the course of the collective disturbance it was possible to identify four periods, or phases, during each of which there was a different balance in the relations between the covert and overt structures in the hospital. The four phases used in the analysis of the observations were those of mutual withdrawal, open collective disturbance, paired role groups, and restitution. These phases were also reflected in the quantitative analysis of the administrative conference material presented in Chapter 12.

Since Chapter 5 was written as an attempt to show the operation of the entire hospital over time, there was little opportunity to go into detail concerning the social organization among patients on the ward, although this received some attention. For example, one positive use the patients made of each other was indicated when Mrs. Lasker made a joke out of the visit to her room of the psychiatrist-in-chief, the head of the hospital, and the chief resident. During the visit the question was raised in her presence about the possibility of a court commitment, and this aroused her anxiety, which later she was able to discharge to some extent by joking with the other patients about the visit she had had from the three bears. This function of the patient group as an outlet for anxiety was also noted by the writer (Caudill, *et al.*, 1952) as one aspect of a previous study of the social organization and values of patients on a ward. The observations in this previous study have been confirmed repeatedly in subsequent work by others such as Jones (1953), Stanton and Schwartz (1954), Greenblatt, York, and Brown (1955), and most recently in a study by Fonseca (1956) where there is almost a point-for-point similarity in the findings.

In general, the observations of patients on the ward, presented in Chapter 5, could have been amplified and reorganized to bring out more sharply the social groupings and human relations on the ward, and it is worth while to consider this topic briefly since it is tied so closely to the major theme of this book—that the psychiatric hospital is a small society.

The individual who enters a psychiatric hospital finds himself placed in a number of new social situations all of which, as has been seen throughout this book, influence his behavior and affect his therapeutic progress. In line with this, it is possible to conceive of day-to-day life on the ward as a therapeutic experience in its own right, and somewhat apart from such specific measures as psychotherapy, group therapy, occupational therapy, and so on. In order to apply such a concept, however, much further detailed study is needed of the interaction between patients on the wards. One thing is certain, and that is that patients on a ward are much more than an aggregate of individuals; rather, they form a social group whose behavior is governed to a considerable extent by an implicit set of values that the patients have built up among themselves and which they impose upon new arrivals. Some of these values are verbalized as such, while others must be inferred from the patterns of behavior on the ward.

The content and organization of the values held by patients would vary with the type of hospital and the nature of the patients, but in the small psychodynamically oriented hospital in this study, such a set of values might partially be stated as follows. (1) In his attitudes toward himself: a patient should not deny the reality of being in the hospital for therapeutic purposes, should try to give up what the other patients consider his "defenses," and should try to bring himself to a middle ground where he neither engages in extreme regressive behavior nor attempts to carry on life as if the hospital did not exist. (2) In his actions toward other patients: a patient should suspend judgment and make an effort to see all sides of a person, should support others, and if requested, should try actively to help other patients by providing a sympathetic sounding board for their problems. (3) Toward psychotherapy and the therapist: a patient should believe in the ability of his doctor, cooperate in working with him, and feel that, for the time being, it is better to receive treatment in the hospital than in the outside world. (4) Toward nurses and other personnel: a patient should try to be thoughtful and pleasant, and abide by the rules of the hospital up to the point where either the demands of the nurses become unreasonable or the rules conflict with a more important value toward other patients. Some aspects of such a value system were inherent in what the patients said in their picture interviews as reported in Chapters 8 and 9, and were evident in the observations of ward life in Chapters 3 through 5.

The value system of the patients as sketched above tended to be put into action by ascribing to each new arrival what might be called the *role of a patient.* This role required that the patient act in accordance with the foregoing expectations concerning behavior. In addition, it was anticipated by the patients that each individual would take a *personal role* which was rooted in his background outside the hospital. A new patient, then, had the task of integrating his personal role with the role of a patient; or, at least, seeing to it that the values and behavior characteristic of his personal role did not conflict directly with those of the patient role.

The distinction between the patient role and the personal role is similar to the distinction made by Parsons (1951) between the sick role and the patient role as mentioned in Chapter 1. These three roles—the sick role, the patient role, and the personal role—form an interlocking continuum of expectations from the more general to the more specific with which every patient must contend. This continuum of roles must be taken into account at the time of entrance of a patient, throughout his life in the hospital, and during the period transitional to leaving. In the course of the four months in which the observations used in this book were made on the wards, it was possible to follow the entrance of twenty-three patients (ten men, thirteen women) into the hospital, and the leaving of twenty-two patients (twelve men, ten women).

In the observational and interview material reference was made to the entrance of several patients and the pressures placed upon them to take on the role of a patient. This was true for Mrs. Lasker, who initially denied the reality of the hospital and insisted that she would be leaving shortly. It was also true for Mr. Ulrich, who tried to treat the hospital as a "country club" and attempted to initiate dances, iceskating, and so on. The patients quickly moved to bring both Mrs. Lasker and Mr. Ulrich into line by pointing out to them that their behavior was not in accord with the fact that they were patients in a psychiatric hospital. The effect on a new patient of such pressure is considerable, and usually results in the patient's making an effort to conform to the expectations of the group.

It is not possible to explore this matter at great length here, but the reader may want to review Chapters 3 through 5 and Chapters 8 and 9 with the idea of entrance into the hospital in mind.

If a patient would accept the ascribed role of a patient, then the group would, in turn, support the patient in his personal role. Particularly this was true if the personal role of the patient served some positive function in the group. For example, Mrs. Lasker's role of "hostess" was most useful to the patients, as was Mr. Erskine's ability to organize acceptable activities and to take responsibility for seeing that requests were correctly channeled through administrative red tape. Even the explosive actions of patients who were otherwise unacceptable to the group provided vicarious satisfactions, and thus these patients became enmeshed in the role system of the ward. This was the case when Miss Miller refused to obey her doctor's orders, and when Mr. Ulrich smashed his hand into a door on his way to the locked ward. As mentioned in Chapter 1, much of what would be considered instinctual, "antisocial" behavior in the outer world became "social" behavior in the hospital because of the suspension of judgment and wider range of acceptable actions that were part of the value system of the patients. Seen in this way, a psychiatric hospital ward is not only, in the traditional sense, a place where a patient should be free, if need be, to regress with some degree of comfort, but it is also a place where primitive, instinctual behavior is often directly utilized in, and reinforced by, the subculture and role system of the patient group.

The degree of success achieved by a patient in the integration of his personal role with the role of a patient had a great deal to do with the place he came to occupy in the total structure of the group. For example, Mr. Onofrio's personal role corresponded almost completely with what was expected of him in the role of a patient. He was sensitive to group approval and pressure, and had good social techniques for relating to others. He was always willing to sustain group activities and was receptive when others came to him with their personal problems. As a result Mr. Onofrio was a highly pivotal person on the ward, with whom all of the patients acknowledged some ties. The other extreme could be represented by Mr. Ulrich, whose personal role conflicted in almost all respects with what was expected of him in the role of a patient. He attempted to assert his leadership on the ward in an aggressive way and raised the anxieties of the patients by treating the hospital as if it were a sporting fraternity. Eventually, Mr. Ulrich was isolated by the patients because he would not conform, but his isolation was very different from the self-imposed withdrawal of Mr. Edwards, which was respected by the patients. Though physically present on the ward, Mr. Edwards only infrequently entered the social field of the patients, who held a neutral attitude toward him and scarcely recognized his existence. Most of the patients fell somewhere between the extremes just sketched. Their personal roles neither completely corresponded nor drastically conflicted with the role of a patient, but they did accept the group's values, and in turn received support.

It cannot be said that the place occupied by a patient in the group structure was entirely what might have been expected from his previous psychodynamic history. Mr. Onofrio was more highly rewarded for his type of behavior in the patient group than he probably would have been in the outer world, where he would have been considered too passive a person. On the other hand, Mr. Ulrich would probably not have been so strictly censored for his nonsupportive and often hostile behavior by the outer world. What seems to be indicated is that the nature of a patient's social integration on the ward will affect his therapeutic progress, and that patients who are either overdependent on, or undersupported by, the patient group may experience more than ordinary difficulty in ultimately leaving the protection of the hospital environment.

Often the integration of a patient into the group was less a matter of his ability to reconcile his personal and patient roles and more a question of whether the structure of the group could provide a place for him within the balance existing between the various personal roles of the other patients at the time. For example, as noted at the end of Chapter 3, Mr. Eggan had a difficult time finding a personal role in the hospital because he was an adolescent, and there were not sufficient other patients of his age group with whom he could interact. Equally, the strong, silent, personal role which Mr. Innes chose to play had the misfortune to be coupled in the eyes of the other patients and staff with the physically violent personal characteristics of the patient who had previously occupied Mr. Innes' room. A somewhat more complicated example was referred to in passing in Chapter 5, when Mr. Edwards' introduction into the patient group was sponsored by Mr. Erskine as a means of bolstering his own position of leadership which was threatened by Mr. Ulrich. Thus, the shift from Mr. Edwards' previous isolation to his temporary participation in the active life of the ward was not solely a matter of his "coming out of his shell," but was more owing to the state of the social field and the balance of the roles within it at the particular time.

The preceding discussion has been mainly in terms of the issues confronting individuals in their relations with the patient group as a whole.

Actually, matters are more complicated. The patient group "as a whole" is real enough, but individuals are not distributed evenly throughout it in a network of relations; rather, its structure consists largely of a clustering of patients into a number of friendship, or clique, groups. In the hospital reported on here, one function of the clique was to increase the opportunities among its members for social interaction. A second function was to act as a sort of "mutual therapy" group within which patients could talk over their problems and test out new ways of relating to others that they may have arrived at as a result of psychotherapy. On the other hand, of course, the clique provided a convenient setting for acting out personal conflicts, but the combined effect of the other members of the clique on an individual who was obviously acting out was to dampen and restrict such behavior instead of increasing it. If an individual persisted in acting out his problems, this usually resulted in a temporary withdrawal from the clique and a pairing off with another patient. Beyond this, if the acting out of the individual became more extreme, the paired relationship would break up, and the troubled patient would find himself isolated. A third function of the clique was to provide an opportunity for letting off steam, and thus act as a safety valve, since it was not always easy for a patient to maintain a constant attitude of toleration and support toward all other patients. In connection with this, a fourth function became operative when a patient felt oppressed by the closeness of ward life and wished to draw away from the patient group, but did not want to isolate himself completely. At such times, a patient could, for a few days, restrict his participation in ward life solely to his clique members, thereby gaining a certain degree of intimacy and privacy without necessarily arousing the feelings of depression and loneliness that usually accompanied isolation.

The problem of leaving the hospital is a very real one for patients. Although most of the patients expressed dissatisfaction at times over their life in the hospital, they became quite dependent upon such a mode of existence and were often thrown into an ambivalent state over the problem of leaving. This was well phrased by Mrs. Lasker when she said: "I feel like I am stepping off into quicksand. I don't know how a person can hate a place so and still feel so squeamish about leaving."

The defenses most frequently used by a patient to help himself meet the problem of leaving were a mobilization of energy and aggression for the purpose of making himself feel more competent and independent of the hospital; a verbal review of his therapeutic progress with his clique members in order to convince himself that he was better; a withdrawal from the patient group and its activities; and, a taking of control of actions back into his own hands, as, for example, by no longer feeling accountable to the nurses for his movements in and out of the hospital. If a patient was unable to bring himself to the point of actually leaving by such defenses, he usually went through a period of regression when he would feel completely inadequate, indulge in fantasy, fall back upon physical symptomatology, or rationalize his position by saying that he must be sensible and stay in the hospital until he was completely cured.

The hospital tried to help the patient with his problem of leaving by providing, for those patients who could avail themselves of it, a plan whereby the patient left the ward for the community during the day, but returned at night. Alternatively, a patient could spend the day in the hospital, but be in the community during the night. Both Mr. Onofrio and Miss Lindsey, who figured so prominently in the events at the beginning of Chapter 5, were on the first of these plans and had jobs in town but returned to the hospital at night.

The patient group tried to help its members with their problems of leaving by encouraging a patient in the realistic consequences of his efforts, as in the matter of getting a job. The patients knew that it was necessary to mobilize aggression in the attempt to leave, and the group absorbed and supported the actions of a patient directed to that end. Patients were not censured if they became authoritative or vociferous because they were worried over leaving.

The need to withdraw from ward life during the period transitional to leaving was recognized by the patient group. To make this process easier, the patients often, just prior to the time of departure, once again drew around the patient who was about to leave and gave him a small party at which reassurances and goodbyes were said. This sort of going-away party, given for Mr. Onofrio and Miss Lindsey, was described in Chapter 5.

After a patient had gone, his clique members often felt the loss sharply, as among those patients who had been close to Mr. Onofrio and Miss Lindsey. Patients were both threatened and encouraged by departures—threatened because they were left behind, encouraged because it showed that people actually did leave. Soon, however, new relations were formed, and life on the ward went on as before.

The preceding remarks about the social organization and values on a ward suggest the need for a knowledge of the social dynamics among patients in somewhat the same degree of detail as is usually given for individual psychodynamics. This need was stated by Dr. Rolfe in the discussion among the staff during the period of restitution as cited at the end of Chapter 5. Dr. Rolfe said: "The trouble is, we make our decision on psychodynamic reasons, but we have nothing more than really just a few ideas about this. You take the case of Miss Fellows. Her psychodynamics are that she hates her father, yet in the last week or so we have let her go home, and she gets along very well. . . ." The important point here is that in the hospital there was reasonably good information about the individual patient *per se,* but there was insufficient information about the quality of his relations to others. In psychodynamic terms, this means that the residents tried to concentrate too much on determining the underlying conflicts of their patients and gave too little attention to the adequacy of the patient's defenses. The types of observations presented in this book were simply not available through the usual communication channels of the hospital.

The making of administrative decisions would seem to require that details of both the social dynamics of the situation and the individual psychodynamics of the patients in it should be taken into consideration. This raises the problem of the confidentiality of the psychotherapeutic relationship to which Dr. Reynolds referred during the period of restitution following the collective disturbance, when she said: "Patients will only talk about the present and do this freely if they feel it is not going to be used as a basis of further restriction and punishment, and I think there is a very general feeling among the patients of insecurity. . . ." Attempts to solve this issue have usually been along the lines of the separation of administrative and therapeutic functions, but, as indicated earlier in this chapter, this is likely to be a difficult, if not impossible, task. It would seem more appropriate, in view of the special problems presented by treatment in a psychiatric hospital, that some matters which would be confidential in psychotherapy carried on in the community be examined more freely in the hospital. If this is to be done, a creative rather than a punitive use must be made of such confidential material whether it concerns administrative or therapeutic action. This is not an issue that concerns only the patient's life. As has been noted throughout this book, the conflicts between individual staff members, or between role groups in the staff, are often as important for the understanding of the nature of a problem in the hospital as are the actions of particular patients. If the goal of a therapeutic community is to be reached, there must be a greater openness among staff members than is usually the case at present, and a willingness on the part of the staff to examine their own motivations rather than to project problems onto the patients. This is, perhaps, asking for a good deal, but if it is expected of disturbed patients, it is possibly not too much to ask of those who are better integrated. In order to achieve such a state of affairs, however, changes in the organization and atmosphere of the hospital must be made so that neither staff nor patients are punished for their efforts at greater openness and understanding. Changes in this direction are necessary, since it was concluded at the end of Chapter 5 that it is not possible or desirable to do away with the processes that underlay the collective disturbance; rather, the attempt must be made to learn more about them.

Stressing the value of a conscious awareness of the interrelation between social dynamics and psychodynamics raises once again a question which was mentioned in passing at the end of Chapter 5 and explicitly stated by a number of the patients in their discussion of human relations in Chapter 9. This question concerns the invasion of the privacy of both staff and patients who work and live within the hospital. Life in a psychiatric hospital is often a difficult business at best, and the question is bound to arise of whether the type of analysis that has been presented in this book should be made a conscious part of the on-going work of the hospital. For the writer, there seems to be no conclusion but that it should. It is necessary, but frequently painful, in psychotherapy to examine processes of which one is usually unaware in order to come to deeper understanding. It would seem to be equally necessary to examine the social dynamics of life in a psychiatric hospital in order to work satisfactorily toward a therapeutic community. A psychiatric hospital may be thought of as a setting which provides the opportunity not only for the reorganization of some aspects of individual personality, but also the opportunity to achieve a better understanding of relations between people. The potential advantages in such a setting are sometimes minimized by emphasizing the artificiality or unreality of the hospital in contrast to the outer world. There is nothing unreal about life in a hospital except as the present-day internal social structure of many psychiatric hospitals and their insulation from the community fosters the wishes of staff and patients to comfort themselves with a world of make-believe.

Many of the points which have been made in summarizing the conclusions to be drawn from the observational material presented in the second section of this book are to be encountered again in the analysis of another type of data in the third section, where the perceptions of the hospital among staff and patients were discussed by means of the picture interviews. One of the more striking findings from the picture interviews was that, in a general way, the senior staff and the patients shared the same pattern of perceptions about life in the hospital, and this shared pattern differed from that found among the residents or among the nurses —each of these latter two role groups having a distinctive pattern of perceptions. It was suggested that perhaps the intriguing similarity between the seniors and patients was related to the tendency found in many types of social systems for extremes, or alternate levels, to share certain ways of looking at things, as for example, the patterns of mutual indulgence and affection between grandparents and grandchildren in a family.

At the end of Chapter 9 a general hypothesis concerning interaction in the hospital was formulated in an attempt to account for the discrepancy between the considerable amount of optimism expressed in the interviews, and the difficulties and frustrations that so frequently occurred in the actual work of the hospital. A clue to the meaning of this seeming discrepancy could be gained from the opinions about interactions given by the particular role groups who were actually engaged in these interactions each day. For example, when the material from the area of therapy was considered, the majority of both residents and patients were found to be optimistic about their therapeutic interaction. In contrast to this, while nurses were, on the whole, optimistic about their therapeutic efforts with patients, the patients were pessimistic in speaking of therapeutic contacts with nurses. On the other hand, patients saw their administrative interaction with nurses optimistically, while the nurses were pessimistic about administrative work with patients. The point is that when an analysis was made of the congruence of opinion between role groups in regard to the emotional tone of the interaction in which they were directly involved, there was underlying disagreement in the great majority of cases. Moreover, the nature of the hierarchical structure of the hospital and the formality of relations across status lines served to impede people in differing roles from becoming aware of the discrepancies in the emotional evaluations of their interaction. The main exception to these difficulties in communication was in the specific area of psychotherapy, where the process is such that attempts are usually made to iron out these sorts of difficulties. Given such a situation, it might be anticipated that more problems would arise from administrative than from therapeutic tasks in the hospital, and such indeed seemed to be the case from the analysis of the administrative conference data in the fourth section of this book.

The recent work of Spiegel and Kluckhohn and their coworkers with sick and well families is in line with the analogy of the hospital to a family which was developed from the picture interviews. Spiegel (1957) points out that in the disturbed families, the children inevitably became involved in a conflict or disequilibrium situation which existed between the parents. Most frequently neither the child nor the parents were aware of this fact, nor were they aware of the way in which it came about. Spiegel discusses these conflicts in terms of discrepancies in role expectations, about which he says: "Ego and alter have conflicting or incompatible notions of how to play their reciprocal roles. The conflict is not over which of several possible roles to take, but rather how to enact the role each has decided to take." Such a view of role conflict would seem to be directly applicable to the hypothesis resulting from an analysis of the picture interviews concerning the incompatible notions between two parties to an interaction about how they should play their roles. In indicating some of the ways in which these processes came about in the families being studied, Spiegel concurs with the findings of Johnson and Szurek (1952) to the effect that there seemed to be an identification with the unconscious wishes of the parent so that the child was acting out the parent's unconscious emotional conflict. Stated in this manner, in psychodynamic terms, the process would seem to be the same as that suggested for the period of paired role groups, when the patients appeared to be acting out the forbidden wishes of the residents. Spiegel also notes what has been pointed out frequently in this book, that while it is possible to describe these processes in psychodynamic terms, such a description is not entirely satisfactory. As he says:

> Even with the qualification of the term "unconscious," the description sounds too planned, and too much under the control of one or more persons. A constant observer of the family—or of any other persistent group process—has a somewhat contrary impression that much of what occurs in the way of behavior is not under the control of any one person or even a set of persons, but is rather the upshot of complicated processes beyond the ken of anyone involved.

The struggle here is with the same problem that has been met with throughout the foregoing chapters of trying to find a way to describe the interrelated nature of phenomena in a social field over time. By themselves, the concepts of psychoanalysis, sociology, and anthropology are not really sufficient. And as yet there is not an adequate terminology available.

In addition to the general patterns that emerged from the analysis of the picture interviews, there were many detailed points of interest related to the various areas of work in the hospital. For example, the interviews indicated that among the senior doctors and nurses there was a real lack of familiarity with many of the physical aspects of the hospital. This was so because the seniors seldom came onto the wards, and nurses who worked on one ward did not very often find occasion to visit on others. These findings led to the suggestion that, among the various role groups, the patients were in touch with the greatest number of situations involving contact with persons on different levels during the course of the day. This circumstance would help to explain the seemingly mysterious process by which patients often sensed or even knew what was happening in the hospital before this information was available to other role groups.

In the area of therapy, an important point was the confusion of the nurse about which aspects of her behavior and role were to be considered therapeutic. The nurse was fairly clear about how she was to act toward psychotic patients, but she felt uncomfortable and unsure of herself in her contacts with neurotic patients. Coupled with this was the feeling that warmth expressed toward a patient was in some way "unprofessional," and therapy was considered more as a "thing" which was to be given to a patient, similar to a dose of medicine. This line of thought would seem to be related to the greater number of times that electric shock treatment was introduced into the interview material by the nurses than by the other role groups. On the other hand, the separate analysis of Picture 17 indicated that the nurses did want an emotional relationship with the patient, but were not sure how to go about getting it. They were most able to express their desire for such a relationship within the highly traditional situation of nighttime medication shown in Picture 17. A further difficulty was the resentment the nurses expressed over the inclusion of domestic tasks as part of their work. These tasks were seen as outside their professional role, and this again raises the question of the need for a different type of training for the psychiatric nurse, particularly in her contact with neurotic patients. Ideally, it should be possible for a nurse to be both creative and therapeutic in carrying out domestic activities on the ward, just as a mother may find this possible in her work within the home. A few of the nurses did find satisfaction in such a domestically structured role, as indicated in the interview material given by Miss Nash. These nurses, however, as did Miss Nash, usually left the hospital shortly to be married and to create their own families.

The fourth section of this book turned to an analysis of sixty-three daily administrative conferences. One of the major findings was the effect of status and role on the amount of participation. It was perhaps not surprising to find that, when corrected for differing numbers of persons present in a role group, the senior staff talked most, the residents next, and the other personnel and nurses least. When this matter was pursued further, however, it was found that within the senior staff the head of the hospital talked more than the chief resident; at the same time, the supervisor of nurses talked more than the charge nurses, who, in turn, talked more than those few staff nurses who occasionally attended the conferences. The effect of status both between and within a role group could be seen very clearly from these results.

The data on the residents were used to bring out a somewhat different phenomenon. When the sixty-three conferences were divided into three consecutive periods of twenty-one conferences each, the five residents consistently maintained the same rank order from most to least talking resident. The effect of individual personality within a role group was evident here in that Dr. A, who talked the most, was an assertive, mature man who was much involved in his work, while Dr. E, who talked the least, was a passive woman who tended to withdraw from many situations. Nevertheless, over the three twenty-one conference periods, Dr. E always talked more than the supervisor of nurses *despite* the fact that the supervisor was, like Dr. A, a forceful and outspoken individual. This latter finding brings out rather sharply the interplay of individual personality and social role in administrative interaction. Dr. E's role as resident served to increase her participation over what it might have been, but for the supervisor of nurses, her role acted as a brake on the amount of participation she was motivated to engage in because of her personality.

As indicated in Chapter 10, the consistency over time in the rank ordering of most to least talking residents was not anticipated. After analysis of the data, the writer was struck with the correspondence between the rank order of the residents and what he predicted would be the senior staff's ranking of the five residents according to their general clinical competence during their year on the inpatient service. To test this hypothesis he wrote to each of the six senior physicians giving the names of the residents in alphabetical order, and requested the senior men to put these names in rank order. The results showed that the six seniors agreed among themselves very closely regarding the rank order of residents. Moreover, there was a high degree of consistency between the rank order of most to least talking resident and the degree of competence of a resident in the opinions of the six senior physicians.

As pointed out in Chapter 10, it is difficult to know exactly what these results may mean. In general, it is felt that the residents who talked the most were more personally involved and more serious in their work with patients, and that this both made them talk more and drew the attention of the senior staff to them. As a consequence, there was more disagreement between the residents who talked the most and the senior staff; yet, as noted in Chapter 10, the senior staff tended to evaluate these people more highly, and Dr. A became the chief resident in the year following the study.

In Chapter 11 attention was shifted to the content of the administrative conferences, and a special set of categories used in the analysis was developed around the questions of how a topic came up in the conferences and what happened to it. The effect of status between role groups was again evident in this content analysis as it had been in the analysis of the form of the administrative conferences. For example, the seniors had the lowest proportion of inconclusive topics of any of the role groups, relative to the number of topics introduced by a group. The residents had the second lowest proportion, the other personnel were third, and the nurses were fourth. Among the nurses, one out of every five topics they introduced ended inconclusively.

Finally, in Chapter 12 the 745 topics that were scored in the analysis of the content of the conferences were combined into a series of indexes in order to show the effect of certain processes over time. To do this the data were divided into twelve one-week periods, and eight indexes were constructed in the attempt to follow such matters as the extent of control exercised by the senior staff, the level of confusion in discussion, and the degree of withdrawal from active participation with each other on the part of the several role groups. When these eight indexes were plotted, it was found that four of them reached a peak in the ninth week, and the other four in the tenth week. The period of the open collective disturbance on the ward, which has been reported in Chapter 5, took place during the eleventh week.

The processes which were shown to be in operation by means of the indexes, when considered with the observational analysis of the collective disturbance, serve to point up the interrelatedness of all the data presented in this book. In a way, Chapter 12 represents a condensed summary of the patterning of events in the hospital. This patterning became clear from the observations of the behavior of staff and patients, it was influenced by the attitudes appearing in the picture interviews, and it was re-enacted in miniature each day in the administrative conference. The analysis in Chapter 12, through use of the indexes, was, of course, after the fact. The writer himself did not know at the time he was gathering these data, nor were the staff aware, that changes were taking place at the administrative level prior to the time that similar changes would take place among the patients on the ward. It is to be hoped that in the future such indexes could be further refined for use at the administrative level, and that additional indexes, perhaps based on the occurrence of triangular relations as discussed earlier, could be developed to mark changes on the wards.

At the close of a review of the study of one small private psychiatric hospital, it is necessary to raise again the question of how representative of other hospitals is the material presented here. Fortunately, a fair number of other studies have been made of both private and public psychiatric hospitals, and, in general terms, many of the same phenomena have been reported. Reference has been made repeatedly to the study by Stanton and Schwartz (1954) of a small private hospital, and to the work of Jones (1953) in England. The similarities between the findings of these two studies and the findings of this one are close. This is also true for the small state hospital reported on by Greenblatt, York, and Brown (1955). It might seem as if the large state hospital presented such a different situation that comparison would be fruitless. Yet, the pioneer studies of Rowland (1938, 1939), and the later work of the Cummings (1956) and Belknap (1956), all show many of the same phenomena as have been noted in this book. One important difference from the small hospital, however, concerns the locus of power in large state hospitals, which is often in fact, if not in theory, in the hands of the ward personnel, such as the hard core of senior attendants described by Belknap, or the nonprofessional administrative personnel discussed by the Cummings.

The psychiatric hospital today still retains many aspects that have been borrowed, perhaps unfortunately, from the organization of the general hospital, and the results of studies of general hospitals will sound familiar to the reader of this book. To mention several, recent studies of the general hospital include those of Smith (1949), Wessen (1951), Burling, Lentz, and Wilson (1956), and Argyris (1956).

Beyond the specific study of hospitals, it would seem that many of the problems of a psychiatric hospital are shared with any hierarchically structured organization for work whether it be a factory, a school, an army unit, and so on (see Goffman, 1957). Parsons (1957) has recently considered the psychiatric hospital in relation to a general sociological theory of organizations, and a very direct parallel to some of the unrecognized processes which occurred during the collective disturbance described in this book were observed by Rice (1951) in a factory.

The social structure of a hospital is, however, unique in the extent to which it consists of mobility-blocked levels. A good many of the problems of the psychiatric hospital may be related to this system of organization, but the way to overcome these problems is by devising a better organization, not by doing away with it entirely. It would be most unrealistic, and probably unwise, to attempt to circumvent the hierarchical arrangement that is characteristic of most psychiatric hospitals. This is too deeply embedded in the already existing institutional system and in medical practice. Nevertheless, while working in terms of present realities, some changes must be made.

One of the most discouraging obstacles to be found in psychiatric hospitals is the tremendous weight of apathy and inertia. Attempts to improve specific therapeutic techniques or administrative procedures tend to work well for a time, but after the novelty wears off, things are much as they were before. One of the reasons for the failure of such attempts at improvement is that they usually are constructed as additions to the content of the over-all program of the hospital, while carefully staying within the already existing form of the hospital. Thus, the usual emphasis is on providing more therapy, more training, and more buildings, rather than at the same time thinking creatively about shifts in the functions of the doctor, the nurse, and the patient. On the whole, the specific therapeutic techniques and the details of administrative procedures in a hospital are often satisfactory enough, but the way in which these are integrated into a system, and the manner in which responsibility for them is delegated, is most unsatisfactory. As has been mentioned frequently throughout this book, such an unsatisfactory state of affairs is related to the extent to which the formal structure of the psychiatric hospital contains what Henry (1954, 1957) refers to as systems of multiple subordination, where one worker is under the authority of several independent chiefs.

In line with the foregoing points, a practical problem that must be faced is the lack of job satisfaction among personnel in hospitals, particularly on the lower levels. In this regard, the results of Schoenfeld's (1952) questionnaire survey are interesting concerning the question, "Why do people work in hospitals?" The main reason for taking the job was that it was the only job available; the main reason for keeping the job was that it was close to home; and the main reason for leaving the job concerned the poor attitudes of supervisors and coworkers. While these may be similar to the attitudes toward work in some industrial situations, they do not, at the very least, indicate a strong motivation for employment in hospitals.

There are few studies of turnover and its costs in hospitals, but one was made by Hamilton (1955) in a general hospital which had an average work force of 507 employees. In this hospital the annual turnover rate was just over 63 per cent. The nursing service accounted for well over half of the turnover costs. This was a study of a general hospital, and the greater difficulties in holding psychiatric nursing personnel are well known. This was borne out in the study by Belknap (1956) of a state hospital in which there was an appalling turnover among all levels of personnel. The annual rate was approximately 67 per cent for the doctors and nurses, and was 80 per cent for the attendants. This latter figure, however, hides a further significant fact which was that the hard core of senior attendants had the lowest turnover rate of any group in the hospital. As Belknap (1956, pp. 150–151) says:

> The informal organization of the wards is maintained and transmitted in its essentials by a core of about 18 per cent of the attendants. The annual turnover rate of this group is less than 1 per cent, as compared with 83 per cent for the remaining 82 per cent of the attendants. Seven out of ten of this core live on the hospital grounds, and six out of ten are married to other attendants employed in the hospital. Two out of each ten men in the core had fathers or mothers who had been employed in Southern State Hospital or other state hospitals. The median length of hospital employment for this core is 12 years, as compared with the median length of employment for ward physicians of 1.5 years, and a median tenure for the hospital superintendents of 2.6 years. . . . In the direct work of Southern State Hospital with its patients, these core attendants are almost the only career employees in the medical part of the hospital.

There are many ways in which turnover rates can be utilized to obtain significant information, but one in particular concerns the attempt to answer the question, "Who provides continuity in the hospital?" In a sense, the answer to this may be that the chronically ill patients provide the continuity, since they often remain in the hospital longer than any other group. In the hospital reported on in this book, the nurses provided the continuity, while in the state hospital studied by Belknap, the senior attendants did so. But in both cases the nurses and attendants were insulated from free communication with other role groups by the nature of the social structure and the separateness of their attitudes and values. In situations of such deeply entrenched personnel, some combination of heroic measures involving removal, drastic retraining, and thorough reorganization would first seem to be necessary before any new therapeutic program would have a hope of succeeding.

It is in part the frustrations of having to try to work under conditions such as those referred to above that account for the high turnover of the more strongly motivated psychiatrists and ward personnel. Somewhere along the line, these compelling problems of job dissatisfaction must be faced.[1] One possible way out of this might be the open delegation of greater responsibility and commensurate power to the junior medical staff and nursing personnel. This is a different matter from the assumption of power through unspoken agreement, and in a somewhat surreptitious manner, by the attendants in Belknap's study. It is also a different matter from the shifting of responsibility for decisions to the residents during the period of mutual withdrawal as noted in Chapter 5 without truly giving the residents the power necessary to take on such added responsibility. The open delegation of control over certain matters to personnel lower in the hierarchy of the hospital would have to be accompanied by changes in the training program and in the definition and integration of roles in the hospital structure.

Implied in the foregoing discussion is the need for increased attention to the development of what might be called "lateral echeloning."[2] Essentially, this is an attempt to work within the reality of the tight vertical structure of the hospital by providing lateral opportunities at all levels for individuals to develop activities in which they are interested. Simultaneously, it is the job of the chief to see that such individuals are provided with the funds, opportunity, authority, and responsibility to carry out their interests, and also to see that such special interests become part of the on-going activities of the hospital. An example of this would be the case of a young psychiatrist who was about to leave for full-time private practice. Effort would be made to find him a university appointment and to allow him to expand his practice and research within the framework of the hospital in order that he would have the opportunity for growth while at the same time the hospital retained the benefits of his service. Such "lateral development" could apply at any of the levels in the hospital, including that of the patients. The hospital system, of course, has to be flexible enough to encompass such changes and has to have a chief who is seriously committed to such a program.

In view of the amount of research that has now been published on psychiatric hospitals, it is time to go beyond the types of criticisms that have often been made of such institutions, as, for example, the frequency

[1] In part, such job dissatisfaction is related to the basic financial question of salaries and wages. The discussion of this question would quickly involve matters beyond the scope of this book, such as the comparative study of occupations, the relations between hospitals and the state and federal governments, the standards set by professional associations, and so on.

[2] This concept was suggested by Dr. George E. Gardner, director of the Judge Baker Guidance Center, in the course of discussion with the writer.

with which a large state hospital creates the impression of a poorhouse or a jail, owing partly to the shortage of funds and the apathy of personnel. There is little of value, however, to be gained any longer by simple indignation over such conditions. Large state hospitals are overburdened, in addition to the care for patients with strictly psychiatric illnesses, with the responsibility for large numbers of patients who are suffering from mental deficiencies associated with organic factors and from physical disabilities of old age. The gross anomalies and inadequacies of such institutions must be rectified before the kinds of research or suggestions for change which form the central interest of this book can be carried out.

It is also probably time to go beyond suggestions for making life pleasant for patients on a ward by providing such activities as reading, entertainment, and congenial occupational tasks. It would seem obvious that a certain amount of friendly human contact between patients, and between patients and staff, is necessary before clinical use can be made of a more sophisticated understanding of group dynamics. In general, the writer agrees with Stanton (1956) when he points out that in some not very precise way it has been known for a long time that respectful treatment of patients favored their recovery. Consistently, over the past one hundred and fifty years concerted efforts to bring about improvement in patients—whether by moral, chemical, electrical, or environmental means—have met with success in that more patients were discharged. Yet, as Stanton (1956, pp. 144–145) says:

> The statistics were interesting and important but there was little that could be done once one had the general finding; we were in the position of being against sin. . . . The discharge rates seem again to be mounting. If they are, perhaps the outstanding clinical responsibility of our generation is to try, while we are succeeding for reasons we are not clear about, to seize the chance to identify what we can, and to hold fast in the network of scientific theory the means of effective institutional treatment. If this is to be done, the generalities which have surrounded the notion of social or milieu or institutional treatment must be replaced by more clearly analyzed understanding. . . . It would follow that research in milieu therapy should be directed toward the increasingly accurate and specific identification of special patterns of interaction or transaction with other people, which characterize various types of disorder. Milieu therapy would be differentiated sharply from good custody; therapy from uninstructed humanitarian efforts.

The study presented in this book has tried to do just this—to direct attention to the specific identification of special patterns of interaction or transaction among people within one small psychiatric hospital. Equally, a major implication of the conclusions from this study would seem to be the reasonable, albeit radical, notion that the present form of the psychiatric hospital has been largely determined by historical circumstances, and that psychiatric hospitals in the future might be structured very differently depending upon the specific therapeutic goals which were in mind. It is likely that the most effective use of modern knowledge in the treatment of patients is being impeded by outmoded administrative procedures, and that some thoroughgoing changes in the physical and organizational structure of psychiatric hospitals are long overdue.

CHAPTER 14

The Possibility of a Clinical Anthropology

The role of the anthropologist, or other social scientist, in a hospital is usually confined to research or, in a more general setting as a medical school, to research and teaching. The other extreme of hiring a person to do only clinical work, as is often the case with clinical psychologists or social workers, would not be likely to be acceptable to the anthropologist whose training has not prepared him directly for this type of work, and even if he had the capabilities for it, he would see such a concentration in a service function as a threat to his professional identity.

There seems to be a need, however, as indicated in much of the literature cited in this book, for a professional person from the fields of anthropology or sociology who would combine some clinical responsibility with the teaching and training of residents and nurses, and would, in addition, carry out his own research. Perhaps the most important clinical job that such a person could do, as suggested in Chapters 5 and 13, would be to keep track of the entire system of the hospital over time and to communicate his observations and suggestions concerning the state of the system at the appropriate regular staff meetings and conferences. In general, the term "clinical anthropology" that is introduced here denotes both a practical taking of serious responsibility in the work of the hospital or other medical setting and an approach to research through observation and interviewing in which the emphasis is on day-to-day contacts with people in meaningful situations.[1]

The stress laid on a direct approach to people through observation

[1] The idea of a clinical anthropology in a medical setting is similar to the idea of "the clinical study of society" set forth by Lee (1955) for sociologists in their work on practical problems with executives and specialists in business, labor, and government.

and interviewing in the clinical and research work of the anthropologist does not entail a lowering of scientific standards in the collection and analysis of data. It is quite possible to engage in what is called clinical anthropology here and be very scientific indeed with the appropriate use of hypotheses and quantitative as well as qualitative analysis. It is hoped that examples of this have been indicated in this book in the quantitative small group analysis of the administrative conferences in Chapters 10 through 12 and in the analysis of observations made in Chapters 3 through 5.

If there is to be a greater formalization than exists at present of an approach which might be called clinical anthropology, then it is necessary that the interests of a person in this kind of work have firm roots in his own discipline. Here the reference is mainly to anthropology, since the writer is an anthropologist. If he is to suggest seriously, as he is, that some members of his profession might identify themselves with such an approach, then they need to have the feeling that what they can receive from this specialization will be of general benefit to them in their profession, as well as a contribution to the work of a psychiatric hospital or other medical setting. Along these lines, the discussion in this chapter will be divided into three parts: (1) the background and roots of clinical anthropology in general anthropology, and a comparison of some of the relations between anthropology and psychiatry; (2) what the anthropologist can contribute to the psychiatric hospital; and (3) what the anthropologist can receive from the psychiatric hospital which will be of use in his understanding of his own and other cultures.

SOME RELATIONS BETWEEN ANTHROPOLOGY AND PSYCHIATRY

Over the past twenty-five years, anthropologists and other social scientists have increasingly come to work in medical settings. The general state of this field has been reviewed for anthropology by the writer (Caudill, 1953a), and for sociology by Freeman and Reeder (1957) and Straus (1957). Within the last few years the beginning results of this work have appeared in such books as Saunders (1954) on cultural difference and medical care, Simmons and Wolff (1954) on social science in medicine, and in a volume edited by Paul (1955) of case studies of public reactions to health programs in many cultures. Even more recently, there have begun to be discussions of how some social science content might be introduced into a medical curriculum (Eaton, 1956; Stainbrook and Wexler, 1956).

The cooperation between anthropologists and psychiatrists has a fairly long history in studies of culture and personality (Kluckhohn, Murray, and Schneider, 1953; Honingmann, 1954), and through the work of members of the Society for Applied Anthropology (see the journal, *Human Organization*).

The more directly clinical aspects of anthropology which are the focus of this chapter probably had their first mention in the articles published in the early thirties by Sapir (1949). Subsequently, the relations between anthropology and psychiatry have been reviewed by Kluckhohn (1944), Henry (1948a, 1948b), Mead (1952), and Devereux (1952, 1956). Most recently, Opler (1956) has written a general discussion of culture and psychiatry. More extensive clinical use of anthropological materials has emerged from the work of such psychoanalysts as Erikson (1950), and such anthropologists as Devereux (1951).

In line with the above work, one needs to think about the question, why anthropologists and psychiatrists have been able to work well together. Members of both disciplines share an interest in attempting to follow over time the history of an individual or a group as a whole. They are more concerned with matters of configuration and pattern than with the statistical manipulation of data. Both anthropology and psychiatry tend to retain the uniqueness of the individuals or groups they study and to interpret their data by referring it to an ever-widening context. As Kroeber and Kluckhohn (1952) have pointed out, just as the psychiatrist, beginning with Freud, was saying that the most trivial event and the most bizarre behavior of the patient had meaning, so the anthropologist was saying that other cultures were not simply outlandish, but made sense in terms of an integrated way of life. Neither psychiatrist nor anthropologist, in his actual work, can use an experimental method very satisfactorily. The psychiatrist cannot experiment with his patients, nor can the anthropologist create a culture—both psychiatrist and anthropologist must participate with the individual or the group that they are studying, and it is from such a close interpersonal experience that much of the data of both disciplines comes.

Such "clinical" procedures in the collection and analysis of data have their own hazards, and anthropologists have been less articulate and conscious about these than have psychiatrists. One of the anthropologist's most valuable tools lies in the understanding to be gained from the direct relationship with another human being. There is a real need in anthropology for further development of methods of interviewing and observation in order more accurately to apprehend the meaning of an individual's actions (the regularities of which often may be attributed either to his "personality" or to his manifestation of "culture," depending on the focus of interest). This concern with the process of what happens between two or more people in a relationship is related to what Sapir (1949) meant when he spoke of "a distinctive kind of imaginative participation by the observer in the life around him," to what Kroeber (1952) was getting at in his discussion of "empathy," and to what Mead (1949) was referring when she stressed that "the surest and most perfect instrument of understanding is our own emotional response, provided that we can make a disciplined use of it."

Although the method of observation by living within a small community for a period of one or more years in close contact with the people and their life is a major one in anthropology, as yet there have been very few accounts of what goes on during it—what the processes are by which the anthropologist comes to an intellectual and emotional understanding of the culture, and how his presence affects the lives of the people he is studying. Recently Bowen (1954) has given a detailed account of her participation with an African group. Her story, written in fictional form, is presented in a frank and personal manner, but it does not attempt to discuss the matter from the point of view of anthropological method or psychoanalytic insight, and much more work in this area is needed. Redfield (1953a, pp. 151–152) puts the problem well when he says: "It is that disturbing fellow, the living human individual, who makes trouble for the scientist's stern principle of perfect objectivity. Whenever the anthropologist looks at him, something human inside the anthropologist stirs and responds. It is easy enough to be objective toward objects; but the human individual refuses to be only an object." Thus, in his interviewing and observation the anthropologist is always forming relationships with the people he is studying and must also draw back from these relationships to examine the meaning of them. This is one way of stating the "clinical" problem in research that confronts the anthropologist.

In some ways, then, what the anthropologist does is similar to what the psychiatrist does. Although there are important differences in the psychiatrist's procedure, such as the presence of a therapeutic goal, there is much the anthropologist can learn from him concerning an awareness of emotional interaction that goes on during observation, and the processes of transference and countertransference. This has led Henry to suggest that the training of the anthropologist include some familiarity with clinical psychiatry and especially with psychiatric case material. As he says (Henry, *et al.*, 1955): "You cannot train a student in geographical distribution, social organization, and general theory, and expect him to perceive the difference in anxiety between men and women." The writer, in his published discussion with Henry about this question (see Henry, *et al.*, 1955), tends both to agree and to disagree with this position. It would be unfortunate if the need for familiarity with psychiatric case material was interpreted to mean only patients and not persons in a somewhat wider range of situations. It is the method and insights of the psychiatrist that should be emphasized, more than contact with various kinds of unhappy and distraught people, although a certain amount of this kind of contact is all to the good because of the sharpness with which various problems stand out in such cases.

This is an area, indeed, where the anthropologist and psychiatrist could learn from one another. It is valuable for the anthropologist to recognize something of the meaning of his own feelings as these influence his data, and it would be equally valuable for psychiatric residents to participate in a wider range of cultural experiences than is usually included in their own backgrounds. Ideally, this latter should mean more than engaging in therapy with persons from various cultural backgrounds; it should also include participation in a training program which provided some actual field work in another culture, whether this is carried out in the ethnic areas of cities in this country or involves going to another culture outside of the United States. An anthropologist could be of much help in planning such a program and could give to the psychiatrist as well as receive from him in the mutual process of learning.

The writer feels strongly that social anthropologists, particularly those interested in studying culture and personality, should have more training than they usually now receive in psychoanalytic thinking and supervised "clinical" experience in interviewing and observation as preparation for field work. In addition, more formal training in psychoanalysis is certainly advantageous for some advanced students. This is not to say that all anthropologists should go through a full course of psychoanalytic training, and the selection of candidates for such training should still be a matter of finding those individuals who would derive special benefit from such a learning experience because of a combination of ability, motivation, and personality characteristics. In either case, however, whether the anthropologist received this part of his training as a candidate at a psychoanalytic institute, or in courses in anthropological method which might be developed in the university curriculum, he needs to become sensitized to details in his own and others' behavior that most often go on out of awareness.[2] This sensitivity is helpful for many reasons—to avoid some of the distortion that comes from projecting one's own feelings onto the subject matter, to become partially aware of the process by which the observer inevitably influences what he observes, and to aid in realizing the importance of many small details of behavior which otherwise would not become part of the recorded material.

For an anthropologist gathering data through observation and interviewing, there would probably be a place for a type of supervision similar to that provided for the psychiatrist. This does not mean only while the anthropologist is learning his trade; it equally means that just as the mature psychiatrist frequently makes use of supervision for his cases in order to obtain a greater degree of understanding of the participation between himself and his patient, so also might the anthropologist make use of a colleague having little to do directly with his research as a person who could act as a supervisor in this clinical sense. As for the psychiatrist, supervision for the anthropologist should be a confidential matter. Under usual anthropological field conditions, it might not be possible to have direct supervision, but a real use could be made of a truly confidential correspondence; for anthropological work done under modern urban or rural conditions, however, and particularly in psychiatric hospitals, a direct sort of supervision would be quite feasible. For example, the writer has recently had the experience of being a consultant in a confidential relationship between himself and a social scientist who is carrying out a study of a medical center. This type of consulting relationship has gone on for more than a year now, and it is the writer's belief that both he and the social scientist have been able to work more creatively as a result of it.

It has been mentioned earlier that both anthropology and psychiatry share an interest in data which is interpreted by being placed in an ever-widening context. Firth has called such an approach "contextualization," about which he says (Firth, 1951, pp. 22–23):

Social anthropologists are usually said to study a society, a community, or a culture. But this is not what they *observe*. The material for their observation is human activity. They do not even *observe* social relationships; they infer them from physical acts. The anthropologist as observer is a moving point in a flow of activity. At any one time he has

[2] The writer's own course work in psychoanalytic theory, which he received from Dr. Charlotte Babcock through a tutorial arrangement at the University of Chicago, and his later nonmedical candidacy at the Boston Psychoanalytic Institute, have been of tremendous value to him.

only a limited field of social observation—the people whose acts he can see or hear, or about whose acts he can get description by others who have observed. . . . In his study of behavior the anthropologist works by contextualization. He assumes that if he grasps the context adequately, he can apprehend the meaning of the behavior . . . almost more than for any other field scientist, research means a process of learning and practising new modes of personal behavior.

Firth goes on to illustrate this approach with a beautiful example of the meaning to be found in a vermilion paint-mark smeared on the timbers that supported the roof of a house in Tikopia. At first it did not seem that the mark had any relevance, but inquiry revealed that it was to signal the end of turmeric-making. Still later a deeper significance was found—the mark was a notification not to men but to spirits. Moreover, the mark was not an isolated example but was part of a series spaced out in time and place which served to mark the approach to further ceremonial events. Thus, something as seemingly irrelevant as a smear of paint came, by ever-widening interpretation, to be involved significantly with almost all the activities and feelings in a small society.

This analysis of the contextual meaning of an event in Tikopia is similar to the analysis used in this book. Mr. Esposito's painting, for example, as discussed in Chapter 3, gains in meaning as it is seen within the same sort of widening context as the vermilion mark described by Firth.

Such examples, from a group of Pacific Islanders or from a psychiatric hospital, tell something about contextualization, but do not tell *what* the context is. For the anthropologist, the context is usually what he calls culture—a concept singularly hard to define (see Kroeber and Kluckhohn, 1952). Anthropologists, at one time or another, have included within the concept of culture almost all aspects of human life—social structure as a part of culture, personality as a part of culture, and practically everything that man ever did or made. And, anthropologists are almost mulishly resistant to the dissolution of this concept by breaking it down and subsuming parts of it under other concepts. There is a valid reason for this which lies in the anthropologist's approach to his subject matter. When one asks the anthropologist what indeed is he interested in, the answer that comes from such varied sources as Kroeber, Firth, and Sapir, is: "I am interested in man and his patterned behavior." Kroeber (1948, pp. 1 and 12) says:

Could it be that the specific subject matter of anthropology is the interrelation of what is biological in man and what is social and historical in him? The answer is Yes. Or, more broadly, anthropology does at least concern itself with both organic and social factors in man, whereas nearly all other sciences and studies deal with one or the other. . . . The other social sciences recognized culture in its specific manifestations as they became aware of this or that fragment or aspect of it—economic or juridical or political or social. Anthropologists became aware of culture as such. From that they went on to try to understand its generic features and processes and their results. This is one of the few points that sets off from anthropology a science which in the main is almost a twin sister; sociology. . . . One other distinction is that sociology has been more concerned with strictly social problems: the relations of classes, the organization of family and society, the competitions of individuals within a group. The names are indeed significant here: sociology tends to be concerned with society, anthropology with *anthropos,* man, and his specifically human product, culture.

Kroeber's position in the above would at least seem to be in line with Firth's emphasis on real people in contexts as the subject matter of anthropology. This would also be true for Sapir who, in addition, perhaps more than any other anthropologist of his generation, was acutely sensitive to the place of the individual in his culture. In this regard, Sapir (1949, pp. 578 and 585) says:

Any one who deals habitually with what man makes and thinks, not because he is interested in man directly but because he wishes to find law and order in what man makes and thinks, slips, by insensible degrees, into the assumption that such regularities of form and process as he finds in selected categories of man's behavior are fundamentally due to a peculiar quality of self-determination in those categories rather than to the ceaseless, eternally shifting, balancing of concretely definable motivations of particular people at particular times and in particular places. . . . Through the sheer weight of cultural detail and, more than that, through the far-reaching personality-conditioning implications of variations in the forms of socialized behavior, the cultural anthropologist may, if he chooses, advance from his relatively technical problems of cultural definition, distribution, organization, and history to more intimate problems of cultural meaning, both for individuals and for significantly definable groups of individuals. And the psychiatrist may, if he chooses, advance from theories of personality disorganization to theories of personality organization, which, in the long run, have little meaning unless they are buttressed by a comprehension of the cultural setting in which the individual ceaselessly struggles to express himself.

It would be possible in similar fashion to go through the literature of anthropology, but as can be seen from the foregoing, many anthropologists do not seem to want to let go either of *man* as a whole person or of his culturally patterned *context.* One solution to this problem of interrelatedness is to move in the direction of the humanities (Redfield, 1953b), and a large proportion of anthropologists would classify themselves as culture historians. A second group of anthropologists, concentrated in Great Britain, has chosen to emphasize social structure and might be classified as comparative sociologists. A third group, particularly in the United States, has come in the past generation under the influence of the general development of the social or behavioral sciences and usually identify themselves as social anthropologists. Kroeber (1955) has recently discussed some of these stresses and strains in present-day anthropology and has called for a reintegration of the subspecialties in anthropology (physical anthropology, linguistics, archeology, ethnography, and social anthropology) which have tended to draw apart. There are some compelling reasons for this in terms, for example, of a renewed interest in the relation between biological and cultural phenomena which is bringing the physical anthropologist and cultural anthropologist together again after a long separation.

This renewal of interest in anthropology in the interrelations of what is biological, psychological, and cultural in man has drawn the attention of the biologist Huxley, and the physical anthropologist Howells. Huxley (1955) is impressed by the fact that "man differs radically from all preceding successful types in not having diverged into numerous biologically separate species or lineages . . . [but] has remained one species, a single interbreeding group." Huxley believes, therefore, that the changes taking place in man are more in the psychosocial sphere than in the biological, and he suggests that anthropology should increase its study of the processes of cultural evolution and go beyond a comparison of the structural details of specific cultures. In making this suggestion, Huxley is drawing an analogy with biology, which originally used a descriptive approach, then went through a period of typological comparison, and now is concerned with the causes of the differences exhibited within a particular population. Howells (1955), writing on universality and variation in human nature, expresses a similar idea in the need for anthropology to move away from racial or cultural typologies and into the study of the biological and cultural processes going on in a group of significantly varying individuals.

These ideas are in accord with the emphasis in this book on the importance of keeping track of combinations of particular individuals in roles within the social structure of the hospital over time. Much the same point must be made for more general studies of interpersonal relations where culture is a variable (F. Kluckhohn, 1953). No individual knows all aspects of his society's culture, and what he does know and is affected by, is first learned in the specific (and in some respects unique) setting of his own parental family. Culture, as well as personality and genetic inheritance, descends in "family lines" (Spiro, 1951). It is important to know what particular version of a culture the person under study received from his family, how he later expanded or changed this, and what version is currently represented in his own family life and is being passed on to his children.

This way of speaking of culture is very close to what is often said in approaching personality, and in this regard it is difficult to distinguish the two concepts except in the sense that anthropologists arrive at this point by working from the outside in, while psychiatrists work from the inside out. Further, such "culture-family-personality" variation is complicated by (or perhaps integrated with, and this is a major research question) individual genetic variation. One wonders, with reference to the suggestive studies of Benedek (1949, 1952) on the mother-child relationship, to what extent the emotional balance between mother and child tends to affect the developing physiological patterns in the child. Does the child, according to the quality of the relationship to the mother, develop patterns of physiological response that are similar (or even attuned) to hers, or that are in counter directions? Does such a patterning, if it exists or persists, have anything to do with the emotional and perhaps physiological resonance that the individual experiences with some persons later in life and not with others? And is there a shift in the types and range of such patterns from one culture to another?

In teaching and discussion the writer has upon occasion attempted to relate the results of his work in psychiatric hospitals in the United States and Japan to a set of more general ideas concerning the context of illness and its treatment. Most recently (Caudill, 1953b, 1955) he has tried to express these general ideas in terms of the disturbances that can occur at different points in the linked systems that are to be found in the psychiatric hospital or in ordinary life. As indicated at the end of Chapter 1, these systems might be thought of as: (1) physiology, (2) personality, (3) relatively permanent meaningful small groups—e.g., the family or friendships, and (4) wider social structures—e.g., the hospital or community. Such systems are open rather than closed in that what happens in one can have effects in another, and this process tends to be of a self-regulating nature (von Bertalanffy, 1950). Moreover, the particular characteristics of any of these systems are, in differing degrees, influenced by the culture of the society in which they occur.

Stripped of its abstractedness, this may seem a simple, perhaps obvious, idea, but it is hard to find studies illustrating the idea in which more than two of the possible system variables have been built concretely into the design of the research. Physicians have shown relations between physiological phenomena and what have been conceived of as psychological (fear, rage), psychodynamic (unresolved dependency, anxiety), and environmental (cold, imprisonment) conditions. Social scientists have shown relations between the structure of the family and its position in the social class system, or have worked with a concept of basic or modal personality in relation to the patterns of child rearing in a culture. To date, however, there have been only a few studies (see Lindemann, 1950; Coleman, Greenblatt, and Solomon, 1956; and Hill, *et al.,* 1956) where, as more than static background phenomena, three such variables have been truly included in the research so that, for example (1) the structure of the on-going life in a family was related to both the personalities and physical health of the family members, or (2) physiological processes in patients were related to their types of personalities as these were integrated into the social dynamics of the ward within the over-all structure of the hospital. It is perhaps easy to understand why such studies have not been frequent—they encompass a wide range of knowledge and must have a high level of professional and technical competence throughout to be more than suggestive, if not downright misleading.

In thinking about the linking of systems, it is particularly pertinent to conceive of examples where the disturbance in one system is sufficient to call forth adaptive or maladaptive defenses from other systems. For example, an individual under great psychological stress which the integrative capacity of his personality cannot handle, may be able to shift some of the load to his family, but if the family is itself disrupted and he has no other sustaining small group to which to turn, the strain is likely to be shifted to the body and he may develop such symptoms as ulcerative colitis (Lindemann, 1950). If the body is under stress, and the individual cannot find added support from his psychological resources, or aid from some small group system, then death may result as in cases of schizophrenic exhaustion or "voodoo death" (Cannon, 1942). Equally, if the family is fractionated by the loss of one or more of its members, this puts a heavier load on the personality structures of the survivors and probably also on community resources such as social service and financial aid. Buell's (1952) concept of the "problem family" is relevant here, as he found that about 6 per cent of the families in St. Paul were utilizing well over half of the combined health services. Finally, conditions of disaster (see Wolfenstein, 1957) such as floods and war may disrupt the community and national systems so that a greater load is placed on individual families.

In thinking of examples of the alternative lines of defense that are available when the disturbance cannot be handled within a single system, it is necessary to think not only of the differences in the patterning of the availability of such defenses from one culture to another, but also of the differences confronting individuals at various age levels. A child under stress is in a somewhat different situation both physiologically and socially from an adult. The same sort of precipitating event may have more drastic psychological and physiological consequences for a child: he is in a dependent position, he has fewer social roles and less differentiated behavior patterns to help him meet a problem, and his life is not so sharply divided in as many spheres (occupation, recreation, religion, family and kinship) as is true for the adult. Much of this may also be said of the old person: physical and psychological stresses may produce more drastic effects, there are problems of a greater dependency on others, and many of the roles of adult life are no longer available.

This classic pairing of early childhood and old age—of birth and death—where similar problems occur with an intensity they do not have in the years between, suggests a further pairing of the period during which the child learns to control and enjoy basic biological oral, anal, and kinesthetic needs with the period of late adulthood when occupational and procreative tasks are less urgent and there is often a turning to greater participation in avocational and recreational interests. Finally, the period of late childhood most concerned with the mastery of genital needs and the maturation of interpersonal relations would seem to be linked, through an adolescent transition, with the period of young adulthood with its problems of the creation of a family and the establishment of a place in the world. Thus, the varying emphases to be found in the stages of psychosexual development may, in reverse order, reoccur in the movement through adulthood to old age.

If some such sequence of development is to be found, it is likely that significant differences from one culture to another will also be found in the patterns of biological-cultural integration in and between individuals at any one stage, and in the relations of one stage to another (see Mead and Macgregor, 1951). It would seem fair to say that quite a good deal is known already in the various areas of the systems that have been linked together here. There is considerable knowledge about the physiology of the stomach, the psychodynamics of neuroses, the working of the family in various cultures, and the integration of social systems. It should be possible in future work to make use of these variables in studies designed to explore new patterns of relations among them.

Such a concern with the patterned interrelations of the linked systems in human behavior is one of the central problems of anthropology, which tends to be lost sight of when, for practical purposes, studies are compartmentalized as culture and personality, social structure, primitive economics, and so on. A similar situation has recently obtained in medicine, so that psychosomatic medicine, with an attendant array of psychosomatic diseases, is sometimes seen as a special branch of medicine, contrasted with other specialties such as internal medicine, pediatrics, and so on. This point of view is wrong, as it does violence to the fact that the term psychosomatic denotes a fresh conceptual approach to the interrelation of many factors in any sort of disease (Grinker, 1953).

In all of the above, an important question relates to what might be called the universals of culture and psychodynamics. These are the kinds of problems in growing up that human beings, as human beings, have to meet in any culture throughout the world. In a sense that there is not space to go into here, such universals are as much cultural (in the generic meaning of the term) as they are biological or psychological (see Kluckhohn, 1953). In part this arises out of the fact that man is the only truly symbol-using animal, and that language and other behavior are learned by the small and immature child while he is being cared for by large and more or less mature adults of both sexes in some sort of family situation in any culture. This is related to the more universal characteristics of man seen in the perspective of evolution referred to earlier (Huxley, 1955) and to phenomena of common interest to physical and cultural anthropology. Such universal aspects of culture provide an opportunity for closer work between anthropologists and psychiatrists on the question of the basic nature of man.

As has been suggested, one advantageous place to work on comparative or universal questions concerning the linked systems of human behavior is a psychiatric hospital. For a social anthropologist, a psychiatric hospital—thought of as a small society—can be an exciting place, since it provides an easily accessible, sharply defined, and often dramatic setting for exploring practical and theoretical questions. In his work, it is important for the anthropologist that the hospital setting is such that, first of all, interaction and communication between people can be followed over time in great detail and, secondly, that those actions have real consequences. Anthropological work in a hospital seems to the writer to stand somewhere between a field study of a small community—in which motivations and feelings about actions are real enough but hard to follow because there are few boundaries regarding where actions may take place—and observation on experimentally created small groups in a laboratory where accuracy in recording of data and refinement of method are possible but one is never certain how meaningful the experimental tasks are to the participants.

By work in a hospital or other medical setting in cooperation with physicians, an anthropologist, as indicated by the foregoing discussion, is not necessarily going off to the fringes of his discipline, but is, in a real sense, remaining at the center of it. And this question concerning the extent to which the anthropologist feels he is contributing to his own discipline by work in a clinical setting is a matter of some strategic importance in the practical problems of motivation and personal identity that influence the availability of such persons for employment.

WHAT THE ANTHROPOLOGIST CAN CONTRIBUTE TO THE PSYCHIATRIC HOSPITAL

Many of the ways in which an anthropologist may be of use in a psychiatric hospital have been summarized in Chapter 13 and need not be repeated here. In general, as stated earlier, perhaps the most important clinical job an anthropologist could do would be to make available to the staff information about the on-going integration of the component parts of the hospital system. A second function of an anthropologist could be to participate in the development of training and teaching programs, while a third would be to assist in plans for both the physical and social restructuring of the hospital and the creation of new roles for staff and patients.

By conscious intent, as mentioned in Chapter 1, little has been said in this book concerning the relations of the hospital to the community. It is, however, necessary in closing to point out the importance of such relations and to suggest some of the ways in which an anthropologist could be of help in clinical and research work in this area. The following discussion will, therefore, elaborate a bit on some of the aspects of the role of an anthropologist within the hospital, and the role he might take in the relations of the hospital with the community.

Within the Hospital

Numerous times throughout this book attention has been called to the relative lack of awareness among one role group of the nature of another role group's activities. In a teaching and training program an anthropologist could be particularly helpful in increasing the awareness of staff and patients concerning the over-all structure and social dynamics of the hospital system. Along these lines, a valuable procedure in training might well be to require any entering staff member to spend a certain amount of time in becoming familiar with each of the major services and role groups in the hospital before assuming his own particular duties. For example, as part of such a "rotating study of the hospital," a first-year psychiatric resident might well have as his sole responsibility the living on a ward on a twenty-four-hour-a-day basis for several weeks. At the beginning of this period he could frankly tell the patients that his goal was to achieve some real feeling for the round of life on the ward. During this time he could also explore what he was learning in supervisory hours with a senior psychiatrist in order to consolidate his experience. Following this, a resident might profit from several more weeks of intensive work with the nurses on their activities. An additional week spent under the direction of the senior staff on problems of policy, administration, and finance would help to bring further realistic awareness of the hospital setting to the resident's major task of working therapeutically with patients.

A similar training program might be worked out for other types of personnel. It would be of great benefit to the nurse if, like the resident, she was relieved of other duties to spend several weeks living on the ward. The nurse should also be provided with the opportunity to increase her understanding of the process of psychotherapy. Each nurse might be assigned to a particular resident who would act as her supervisor for a month. During this time, where facilities were available and there was research going on in psychotherapy, she could watch through a one-way screen the actual interaction between doctor and patient and could participate in discussions around sound-recorded interviews. Equally, an incoming senior staff psychiatrist would be well advised to spend a month getting acquainted with life among the various role groups and in the several parts of the hospital. The patients themselves, as they came to improve, would gain satisfaction and knowledge if they were to assist the resident and nurse in the routine aspects of their jobs. This might help to remove some of the threat and mystery felt by patients concerning some areas of the hospital and to decrease the dependency and apathy often brought on by ward life.

In general, if people are to work and live together, it is better for them to know something about the details of each other's jobs and responsibilities, and for this sharing of knowledge to come about not in a capricious manner but as a part of a specific training program designed to make people on various levels more realistically aware of the problems of others and to open avenues of communication.

Related to the foregoing questions of familiarity with the physical and social structure of the hospital is the effect of inadequate knowledge in these areas on the perceptions of staff and patients, such as the varying concepts of "time" indicated for patients and staff in Chapter 9. This problem was rather forcefully brought home to the writer at one point in his research when a senior psychiatrist told him that during therapy a patient had said that the men's locked ward was in terrible condition—the furniture was broken, there were cracks in the wall, and that he could not stay there. The psychiatrist was concerned over this report, and, coming down to the ward, walked through it noting its physical characteristics. After this, the psychiatrist told the writer at lunch that he could see little the matter with the ward—it was not elegant, but it was satisfactory; he then went on to explain the patient's criticism in terms of psychodynamic factors. While this explanation certainly had much truth in it, a more direct explanation of what had happened was that the patient had had to live in the physical space of the ward for twenty-four hours a day, whereas the therapist had only been on the ward for fifteen minutes. Indeed, he preferred not to come on the ward at all in accordance with the philosophy that it is better for the therapist not to enter the patient's personal life in any way, and it was with some irritation that the psychiatrist descended to the ward to pick up the patient when ward personnel were not available to bring the patient to his office. In this example there is a linking of the concepts of "time" and the perception of "physical reality." Time is a very different thing for the patient who spends hour after hour on a ward than it is for the busy nurse on an eight-hour shift, or for the resident whose rounds bring him to the ward for half an hour each day. For the patient, subject to the slow drag of time, the walls in the ward become an unpleasant green, the cracks in the furniture appear wider and the light more glaring. There is here a subtle relation between social structure, the emotion involved in the perception of physical objects, and the physical objects themselves. This is a type of problem which some anthropologists have worked with in their attempts to understand the art and material culture of another people, and it is a kind of problem which could be explored by a clinical anthropologist in a psychiatric hospital.

This matter of the physical structure of a hospital is one to which much thought must be given in the future, as the situation today is most unsatisfactory. Following the example of the general hospital, the psychiatric hospital continues to be referred to as a so-many-bed unit—with all the procedural, emotional, and architectural factors that the term implies—when only a handful of patients under the age of sixty are likely to remain in bed. The ambulatory psychiatric patient, usually in possession of many of his social interaction techniques, requires a very different type of physical space from the general hospital patient. This factor of physical construction is all the more important when related to the psychiatric patient's much longer stay in a hospital. It has been suggested that psychiatric hospitals in the future might be modeled upon a small village (World Health Organization, 1953). It would seem likely that the anthropologist, given his professional concern with village life and organization, might be of use in the analysis of the social dynamics of such a psychiatric hospital community.

An anthropologist, in line with his own area of specialization, could also contribute to a clarification of the ethnic or social class differences which enter into therapeutic or administrative processes to blur the understanding between people in the hospital. For example, in the case of Mr. Esposito in Chapter 3, his lack of shaving and his reporting of his previous drinking patterns with cronies at night were received with a more middle-class tinge of disapproval by the nurses and Dr. Ryan than was called for by the realities of that segment of Italian culture from which Mr. Esposito came and within which such activities were normal. In this regard, the effects of ethnic differences on behavior and psychopathology have been neatly presented by Opler and Singer (1956) in a comparison of Italian and Irish schizophrenics. Equally, the effects of social class on the kinds of patients who come into contact with psychiatrists and the types of treatment they receive have been shown by Hollingshead and Redlich (1953), and Schaffer and Myers (1954).

Such studies on the relations between ethnic and social class variables in the treatment of psychiatric illness are extremely interesting. Yet, in the actual day-to-day clinical work of the hospital they provide information that is more in the nature of background data than of material directly applicable to particular cases. This was demonstrated for the writer during his own experience in teaching anthropology to psychiatric residents and in his participation in clinical case conferences. There is as yet little in the literature that is satisfactory as a discussion of the details of interpersonal relations in families at various class levels in our own society or in other societies. Research along these lines is very much needed, and one approach to the collection of these data would be to begin with the patient in the hospital and move out to the family. Some systematic research in this area is now being carried out by Ackerman and Behrens (1956), by Spiegel and F. Kluckhohn (see Spiegel, 1957), and by others.

Relations of the Hospital to the Community

The contribution to be made by an anthropologist working in the area of the relation of the psychiatric hospital to the community involves a general philosophy concerning the use of the hospital. All too frequently, particularly in Western culture, hospitals are isolated both physically and psychologically from the community. In the analysis of the links between a hospital and the surrounding world, the anthropologist has a particularly pertinent function because his discipline is so much concerned with a detailed knowledge of the community—its social structure, ethnic and class composition, and so on. These links between the hospital and the community include questions of: (1) paths to the hospital, (2) relations with the family and community while the patient is in the hospital, and (3) the discharge of the patient from the hospital and his return to the community.

There is really very little knowledge concerning the events that lead to the arrival of the patient at the hospital. It seems to the writer that, all too frequently, the arrival is an emergency. As mentioned in Chapter 3, this was true for Mr. Esposito, who was admitted in the early morning hours, and for Mr. Innes, who was brought by the police. Although some people are escorted fairly calmly to the hospital by their families, and others are able to walk in by themselves, the more usual state of affairs is clouded by anxiety and a lack of information on the part of everyone—the patient, his family, and the hospital. This impression is in line with the findings of Clausen and Yarrow (1955), who say: "The hospitalization of the mentally ill persons whom we have studied was seldom accomplished efficiently." One of the real difficulties for the family members is in knowing what persons in the community are the "gate-keepers" to psychiatric care. As Clausen and Yarrow (1955) point out: "We have seen that families experiencing emotional troubles tend to turn to certain professional groups before seeking psychiatric aid—namely to the clergy, doctors, lawyers, and the police." The anthropologist in a hospital could be of help in evaluating the effects of these various kinds of help on the families of patients and in assisting in the clinical job of extending the channels of communication and services of the hospital into the community.

In some situations it might also be possible to bring in the members of the patient's family to participate actively in the life of the hospital. This has been described by Cote, Dancey, and Saucier (1954) for a sanatorium in Montreal where, some twenty years ago, arrangements were made to have a close member of the family live with the patient because of the financial inability of many patients to secure the services of private nurses. This idea was the basis for a research program carried out in 1951 during which time 230 patients were admitted with selected relatives to care for them.

In a way, this use of family members is similar to the practice which obtained in Japan until fairly recently. To take the place of family members in the hospital there then developed a category of nursing personnel called *tsukisoi*. These are women, below the level of the graduate nurse and more in the category of aides in American hospitals, who act as motherly servants. They are with the patient twenty-four hours a day, seven days a week. They sleep in the same room as the patient and serve as housekeeper and companion. Although hospitals in Japan consider these women in terms of their housekeeping functions, a very close relationship often develops within the limits set by the relative positions of *tsukisoi* and patient. More about this and other aspects of the comparative organization of hospitals in the United States and Japan will be considered in the final section of this chapter.

It seems reasonable to the writer that from the very moment of his entrance into a hospital, a patient's attention should be gently and positively turned back to the community. It should be possible to plan experiences for groups of patients in the community which would bring them into contact with the kinds of situations they were unable to handle prior to their admission, but would bring them into contact with these situations under such controlled conditions that little by little they would be able to build up the ability to participate successfully in areas of life where they previously had experienced much difficulty. The anthropologist working in the hospital would be of importance here because of his knowledge about the on-going nature of the network of relations in the hospital, coupled with those aspects of his job that involved knowing about resources in the community.

Concerning the question of discharge and the transition back to the community very little is known. All too frequently, the hospital loses track, for practical purposes, of the patient once he is discharged. This is particularly true in large state hospitals, despite the "parole" system, because the hospital actually has little knowledge of where the patient goes, or what kind of situation he goes into (see Williams, 1953). In a therapeutic hospital community linked with the outer world, it should be possible to get to know the community thoroughly, and this could be one of the tasks of an anthropologist. In such a way it would be possible to tailor a situation for a patient. If a patient was comfortable in artistic or academic circles, then a room or an apartment for him should be found in surroundings suitable to his interests. Equally, if a patient was more comfortable in ordinary middle-class life, he should be so placed. It might be advantageous to return a patient to such a familiar setting; on the other hand, it might be just as advantageous to know beforehand that one was not returning him to such a setting by simply discharging him into a community to find his way as best he could. All this would involve a more thoroughgoing interrelation between the hospital and the community than is generally achieved today. In any case, one of the major clinical and research problems in which an anthropologist could assist concerns the question of what happens to a psychiatric patient once he returns to the community.

One of the very few research projects concerned with what happens to the patient after discharge is being carried out by Simmons and his group in the Boston area. Recently, Simmons, Davis, and Spencer (1956) have pointed to an interesting dilemma faced by the large state hospital in particular at the present time. Under the impact of current thinking about the effects of institutionalization, psychiatric personnel frequently believe, in the case of those patients whose behavior makes it at all possible, that almost any kind of community setting is preferable to remaining in the hospital. At the same time, the influence of psychodynamic theory often has been such as to create suspicion of the patient's family, which is viewed as a "pathogenic milieu." Thus, there is doubt about the patient's staying in the hospital, and also about the patient's returning home.

Out of such dilemmas as the one just sketched, has come a renewal of interest in family care for the patient and in the creation of "half-way houses" to act as bridges between inpatient and outpatient care (see Schwartz, 1953). Also, there is much to be said for keeping the hospital open as a temporary avenue of retreat for a patient. If a patient, after living in a community, feels he would like to return to the hospital for a week end or longer, it might well be therapeutically useful for him to do so, and this should be made an easy rather than a difficult matter in terms of administrative procedures. In such a way the hospital would be drawn further into participation in the life of the community.

There is perhaps a further reason why "half-way houses" are assuming increased importance. This became apparent in the studies made by the Cummings (1957) of community attitudes toward mental illness. An educational program was conducted in an attempt to change for the better the attitudes of the community toward such illness, but the unfortunate results of this program were to increase anxiety and hostility in the community and to cause people to hold more firmly to their ideas concerning mental illness. Such findings are perhaps discouraging in that the major focus of the foregoing chapters has been on the possibility of developing within the hospital a more adequate therapeutic milieu which would help patients to become better so that they might return to the community. If, however, the community refuses to accept these people, then they often have little choice but to return to the hospital. There is much need for further investigation of the whole complex area of rehabilitation and of the relations between the hospital and the community, as well as for more research into what goes on within a hospital—which has been the subject matter of this book.

WHAT THE ANTHROPOLOGIST CAN RECEIVE FROM THE PSYCHIATRIC HOSPITAL

The term "receive" in the above heading is something of a misnomer, since by carrying out the kinds of clinical work that have been suggested in the preceding section of this chapter, the anthropologist receives much. However, the focus of this concluding section is on work which is somewhat distant from the day-to-day clinical operations of the hospital. It concerns what the anthropologist can gain by comparative research on hospitals in various cultures.

Out of the writer's experiences in research in the United States and Japan over the past ten years has come a central interest in what might be called the comparative study of the "natural history" of psychiatric illness in different cultures. Phrased in another way, this is a concern with the meaning for the patient of the cultural and social processes in which he participates before, during, and after hospitalization. Such a concern rests on the assumption that the structure of the situation for the patient in the family and other social groups, and the structure of the situation in the hospital, is highly important in influencing the course of the illness. Since the structure both of the family and of the psychiatric hospital is strongly influenced by the general culture, there should be meaningful differences in some aspects of the types and dynamics of psychiatric illnesses from one culture to another. Although there has been considerable interest in the cross-cultural study of psychiatric illness and its treatment (see Teicher, 1956; and Benedict and Jacks, 1954), as yet few detailed studies exist either of the course of psychiatric illnesses or of their treatment in various cultures.

The writer believes that in order to make it possible to go beyond the present understanding of the place of cultural influence in psychiatric illness, and in order to gain further perspective on what constitutes a "therapeutic milieu," it is imperative that cross-cultural work be carried out in psychiatric hospitals. Such work should provide a basis for sharper comparisons than heretofore. As indicated in Chapter 13, a number of hospital studies have been carried out in the United States and Europe, but as yet thorough studies of psychiatric hospitals in non-Western cultures have not been done. The writer intends to do his next study in a psychiatric hospital in Japan—hopefully this next study will result in a companion volume to this one.

It is legitimate to raise the question, why should one initiate a study of Japanese psychiatry, or of cross-cultural psychiatry in general? It seems to the writer that three reasons largely motivate anthropologists, and especially those interested in the clinical matters that are the subject of this chapter, to go into the field to make cross-cultural studies—they find it interesting, it gives perspective, and it provides truer cases for comparative purposes. As mentioned earlier in this chapter, a fourth reason should be added in line with the renewed concern in anthropology with what is common to all men—the universals in culture and biology.

The same reasons would apply in particular to the study of Japanese psychiatry. First of all, it is intrinsically interesting in a humanistic sense. Second, it provides a real and meaningful perspective on one's own life and culture. It was for a similar reason that it was suggested in the preceding section that the clinical anthropologist might participate in setting up a training program for psychiatric residents which included, if possible, spending a period of time living and working within another culture. Although much can be obtained from reading, it is no substitute, anthropologically speaking, for actual life in a culture, just as reading about psychiatric case material is no substitute for direct clinical experience. Third, Japanese psychiatry provides a "case," an instance, for cross-cultural comparison in the search to find out more about human similarities and differences. This cannot be done, or can only be done with considerable effort, in a single culture—the variations are not extreme enough, or more cogently, are not set within a sufficiently different matrix of values about what is proper or allowable, good or bad.

Freud (1915, 1930) had a great deal to teach about the vicissitudes of the instincts—about the many and varied ways they can be expressed or reworked—and in clinical cases from any culture it is possible to see a wide variety of defenses and solutions. If these defenses and solutions are talked out or acted out, and if they are not in line with the values of the particular culture in which the doctor and patient are living, then such talking and acting is done in a context which, outside the psychotherapeutic relationship, is disapproving. Without cross-cultural comparison, there is no way of knowing the extent of influence of this context of values—whether approving or disapproving—on the underlying dynamics of the individual's personality. For example, there is much drinking by men in Japan, and a great deal of male dependence and passivity, but still there is little alcoholism as this would be defined in the United States. Some of the aspects of this question may be illustrated by such a simple thing as a whiskey advertisement in *Bungeishunju* (a magazine roughly equivalent to *The Saturday Evening Post*). This ad says a great deal about attitudes in Japanese culture when it shows a pleasant old gentleman smilingly anticipating the pleasure of drinking the six bottles of whiskey he has saved up, while his gray-haired elderly wife kneels on the floor and counts her money—the caption reads: "To each his own happiness." Further understanding is provided by the fact that the wife in the Japanese family manages the money and, circumstances permitting, gives her husband an allowance on which to go out and do his drinking. From this example it would be possible to go on to explore the rhythm and balance in Japanese life between the control necessary to save the whiskey and the release in drinking it; the rhythm and balance between serenity and violence, between *giri* (obligation) and *ninjō* (human feeling). It is not likely that such an ad, or the cultural circumstances represented in it, would occur in the United States, and such an ad draws attention to the question of the influence of the cultural context on the patterning of the dynamics of instinctual gratification.

Not only may the more immediate cultural context exert an influence on the dynamics of the personality, but in a historical or developmental sense, the cultural context may well have influenced how the dynamics were put together. In this regard, the structure and organization of the Japanese family is crucial. In general, for a son, the tie to the mother is not broken as completely as is true in the United States, and the relation between the mother and the eldest son is particularly strong—the more so since the eldest son will bring his bride home to live in the same house as the mother. Younger sons and daughters take their places in descending order in the family, and all have obligations to those above them in a tight hierarchical arrangement.

In Japanese culture there are many types of hierarchy, but the most fundamental are those of age and sex. The authority of the parents continues throughout life, and age carries with it great prestige and power. Women are subordinate to men and traditionally tend to follow the Chinese dictum that a woman obeys her father in her childhood, her husband in middle life, and her son in old age. The discipline of the child is mainly in the mother's hands, the father remaining a somewhat distant figure toward whom the child must show respect. As he grows older a child learns an ever-increasing number of restraints which require subordinating his will to his obligations to family, school, employer, and country. The approval of the outside world becomes exceedingly important, and an individual comes to feel that the eyes of the world are continually upon him (Reischauer, 1957; Babcock and Caudill, 1958).

A description of the social structure of the Japanese family might well begin with the special tie between mother and eldest son. For example, the son's wife is usually chosen for him by his parents (or in any case the marriage is a relationship between two families and never just between two individuals). The wife lives in her husband's family's house, and there is a constant, and usually tense, interplay between the mother, the son-husband, and the wife. In disagreements the son most often sides with his mother against the wife. The wife turns to her first-born son as a source of satisfaction and practical support for her later years, and thus the mother-son relationship moves into another generation.

It would be possible to go on with the analysis of the mother-son relationship much further and to pick up other relationships, such as that between father and daughter, or between father and son's wife, or the roles ascribed to the younger children. Moreover, such a traditional family system is still very tight today, and there are few alternatives to enduring (a term used with much feeling in Japan) and participating in it. Since the end of World War II, however, the still tight family system has shown increasing strain, and today it is both the dynamics of the family in the traditional sense and the strains upon it, which must be considered as factors in the study of psychiatric illness.

With regard to the question of sibling rank, in the small series of male psychiatric cases with which the writer worked in Japan, it seemed that the eldest son was more rigid and constrained, and when he did develop psychiatric difficulties these most often took the form of obsessive-compulsive defenses, depression, and overconformity in general; on the other hand, the younger sons were more outgoing and spontaneous, and when they developed psychiatric difficulties these were more in the nature of impulsive and acting-out disorders. These impressions are in line with the work of others in Japan (Miki and Kimura, 1954) and make sense with reference to the importance attached to the eldest son in the Japanese family and the obligations he is expected to fulfill.

The emphasis placed on close conformity to the rules for behavior in Japanese culture does not mean that the Japanese are an emotionless people. The Japanese are highly emotional, but these feelings are ruthlessly suppressed in important areas of life involving obligations. On the other hand, emotions are freely, even ebulliently, expressed in recreational pursuits, while other ways of release are to turn to nature or to instinctual gratifications available in massage, hot baths, sex, and (mainly for men) alcohol. In Japan, gratification of immediate desire is not a very serious matter, but the fulfillment of obligations is, and in a system that permits little flexibility in this regard, the individual needs a source of support which helps him to find "acceptance" or even "freedom" within his place in the family and in society. Thus, serious use is made by many Japanese of various forms of Buddhism and more recent religious movements (e.g., *Tenrikyō* and *Seichō no Ie*).

A further source of relief from the tensions and obligations of interpersonal relations in Japan is to plead physical weakness or sickness, and a great deal is made of minor ailments and conditions of the body. This is well represented in the use made of the term *senbyōshitsu,* which literally means a tendency of the body to glandular weakness or sickness (more specifically, scrofulosis). This term is often used with pride by parents in referring to their children. For example, something approximately along the lines of, "My child is *senbyōshitsu,* so he cannot go to the school picnic." This statement by one mother to another frequently carries the meaning that my child is more sensitive and talented because he is not "healthy like a pig" as are your children. Possibly owing to the diffusion of ideas, there is a similarity in Japanese and Western thought that the more intelligent and creative a person is, the more likely he is to be physically weak (see Fukuda, 1956; Babcock and Caudill, 1958).

One way of focusing the broad cultural differences which have been alluded to above is to consider briefly some of the differences in the organization of psychiatric hospitals in Japan compared with the United States. For example, the writer's observations in psychiatric hospitals in

Japan indicated that the social structure is tighter and control is more rigidly hierarchical than is generally true for hospitals in the United States. Moreover, the Japanese hospital is organized much more in terms of a "family model," as is also true for many other types of organizations in Japan. This firm control within a family model has many implications for behavior at each level of the hospital. For example, the relations between doctor and patient are clearly, if benevolently, authoritarian. There is no question who is the doctor and who is the patient. Perhaps because of this sharp status difference which provides a sense of security and inevitability, the casual relations between doctor and patient seemed to the writer to be more relaxed and friendly than in American psychiatric hospitals.

In a more dynamic sense, the rhythm of the on-going life in a Japanese hospital seemed different from that of the hospital in the United States. It is not that disturbance did not occur (it certainly did at the time the writer was working in a large hospital: one patient kicked another to death), but rather that violence and emotion tended to erupt quickly and to be dissipated shortly thereafter. Japanese wards do not seem to sustain a level of tension for as long a period as American wards. This is a very interesting area of comparison, which can lead off in many directions. It is useful here to indicate one such direction.

As is well known, and has often been mentioned in this book, Stanton and Schwartz (1954) have reported on the disturbances in three- or four-person systems in the hospital in which the increased agitation of a patient can be linked with an on-going disagreement between members of the staff who exercise authority over the patient. Now it seems quite possible, and this is a hypothesis for further investigation in the study of a Japanese psychiatric hospital, that a certain tacit cultural premise or expectation concerning interpersonal relations underlies the Stanton and Schwartz phenomenon. In terms of American culture, it may be that both staff member and patient are in unspoken agreement that people can be moved quite a distance (consciously and unconsciously influenced in their actions on behalf of another) in human relations. The boundaries of most relationships in American culture are rather fuzzy—to a greater extent than in other cultures it is left up to the individuals concerned how wide a range of action and degree of emotional depth are to be included in a relationship. By contrast, in Japan the boundaries of relationships are very sharp and well known beforehand by participants. Attention was called to this earlier in the relations between doctor and patient, and between *tsukisoi* and patient. To generalize, the potentialities of a relationship in Japan are much more circumscribed, and what one person can do for another is rigidly determined by their relative positions in a tight web of status and obligation. Thus, when a patient and staff member interact in a Japanese hospital they are probably much clearer about the limits surrounding their relationship, and hence feel freer to act spontaneously within these limits, than are a patient and staff member in the United States, but at the same time they are less free to develop the relationship in other directions (Caudill, 1956).

One would not expect then, other things being equal, to find the kind of phenomenon noted by Stanton and Schwartz as evident in Japanese psychiatric hospitals. This is probably one factor, among several, that helps to account for the lesser degree of violence and tension on the wards of hospitals in Japan than in this country, as noted by American psychiatrists (e.g., Cotton and Ebaugh, 1946) visiting in Japan and as experienced by the writer in his own work. The writer's observations, and those of others, were made before the current extensive use of tranquilizing drugs, and this will be an additional factor that must be taken into account in future study.

Work in the psychiatric hospitals of other cultures is often confusing because much of what one sees is overlaid with a Western veneer, since many of the present psychiatrists in non-Western countries have received their training in Europe or the United States. Upon initial impression, much of Japanese psychiatry is similar to that found in Western countries. This similarity is especially true of those aspects of research and treatment based on an organic etiology for psychiatric disorders; in contrast to the United States, however, there is very little emphasis on psychodynamics.

Interwoven with these Western influences on Japanese psychiatry are many aspects of administration and treatment stemming from Japanese culture. One such is the category of nursing personnel, *tsukisoi,* referred to earlier. These women act as personal attendants for patients with all types of illnesses and are employed by general as well as psychiatric hospitals. Differing groups of *tsukisoi* specialize in different categories of illness. When *tsukisoi* are not working on cases in the hospital they live in dormitories scattered throughout the city, which are run somewhat as extended families and are in the charge of an elderly woman who has had much experience in her profession. The writer visited one such dormitory for psychiatric *tsukisoi,* and it is useful to give some of the interview material from this visit, as it serves to emphasize strongly the "family model" that runs throughout the culture of Japan. The head of this dormitory, a woman who previously had spent many years working as a *tsukisoi,* had the following to say about the training necessary for this type of work:

> We had to learn how to get a feeling of mothering others. It is still so at present. These young *tsukisoi* have to learn what is the best way to think of the patient as their own precious and beloved person. We have to keep our eyes on the patient twenty-four hours a day. If we don't, they may start a fire or commit suicide. As you see, these young *tsukisoi* cannot possibly have a feeling of being a mother, so I teach them that they should face their patients with the feeling that they are brothers or sisters. . . . The patients come to depend on the *tsukisoi* if the *tsukisoi* has a strong feeling of serving as to a family member. The patients usually put faith in the *tsukisoi*. . . . For example, the patient often asks the *tsukisoi* about such a small matter as whether it is all right to eat a piece of candy. Also, they cannot stay alone in the room if we have to go out. We build a feeling of love and mercy toward the patient, knowing that they are entirely depending on us. . . . (The writer asked about whether or not the *tsukisoi* took a day off occasionally.) To tell you the truth people in the so-called modern world are quite useless. When I was young I did not lie down for twenty-one days while I was serving one patient. Japanese in the older generation did not consider about themselves and wanted to devote their life to others. In this regard I blame the American Occupation. They taught us only our profession and did not teach us our duty. But it is necessary for *tsukisoi* education to teach the real meaning of sacrificing.

The mention by the head of the dormitory of love, mercy, and sacrifice is interesting, since the name of the dormitory is *Aijinkai,* or "love and mercy organization." One can see here the elements of both helpfulness and tenderness in such an approach, and *also* the real power that is gained thereby over patients, similar to the way in which women in the Japanese family exercise power through sacrifice. Thus, love and sacrifice provide a double-edged sword for *tsukisoi* in a hospital and for members of a family.

The elderly head of the *tsukisoi* dormitory was not merely being old-fashioned when she emphasized the familial role of *tsukisoi.* The writer interviewed a number of *tsukisoi* employed in a small private hospital who were relatively young women. One of these had formed a close relationship with her patient—a very intelligent schizophrenic man, who was in remission and had a strong obsessive-compulsive overlay. This patient had developed a private language with his *tsukisoi* by teaching her his special meaning for words, and over the course of some months, they came to use quite an extensive vocabulary. At one point, the *tsukisoi,* who had come from the country to work in the city, had occasion to visit her family home and was disturbed about doing so because another *tsukisoi* would not be able to care satisfactorily for her patient. Nevertheless, because her family business was pressing, she took the trip. Later, when the writer asked for an example of the patient's private language, she mentioned, among others, what she had said upon returning from her trip:

> After I came back from the country, I described the scenery in the countryside saying, "When the leaves fall down, it is so pretty to see the ripe fruit on the tree."
>
> My patient replied: "It would be so nice if I could eat the ripe persimmon."
>
> (The writer asked what she had replied to this, and she said): "I thought he was pointing to my immatureness."

It is hard to retain the Japanese feeling of the above in translation. It reads much like an exchange of poems between lovers in the *Tales of Genji.* From this, and much additional evidence on this patient's case, the *tsukisoi* would seem to be correct in her feeling that the patient was pointing to her immatureness, and also implying that he would like to eat her up. At the same time, despite this desire, the patient was also referring to the lack of ripeness of the fruit, and hence to the social and psychological distance which separated him from his *tsukisoi.* This matter cannot be analyzed more fully here, but it is hoped that the reader has been able to sense some of the unspoken or only subtly referred to emotional intimacy that existed between these two people without a direct acting out in the sexual sense because of the sharp distinctions between the role of the patient and that of the *tsukisoi,* which are inherent in the tight social structure of the Japanese psychiatric hospital.[3]

One of the most interesting types of treatment that has developed in Japanese culture stems from Dr. Seima Morita's work on a method for the treatment of neuroses. Dr. Morita's influence has been great on Japanese psychiatry, although only a small proportion of psychiatrists use his treatment in unmodified form. During the first week of treatment the patient is isolated in an empty room, and all contact and activity (except eating and eliminating) are prohibited. Following this period, the patient begins to communicate with his doctor through a diary upon which the doctor comments in writing several times a week. Also at this time the patient is set to doing simple manual tasks which will bring him into contact with nature. Emphasis is on the treatment of the patient through

[3] At the time the writer was working in Japan, during 1954–55, there were plans for legislation which would do away with the use of *tsukisoi* in hospitals, and their duties would be divided between graduate nurses and maintenance personnel. This was part of an attempt to raise the professional level of nursing care in the hospital along lines suggested during the Occupation. This is a laudatory aim, but if it were to be carried out in the proposed manner, much of value would be lost, and a type of care that grew out of Japanese culture would be sacrificed to another that was less well suited to the needs of psychiatric patients.

his daily life experiences, and it is felt that a direct approach to the development of the constructive forces within the patient is to be preferred over an analytic approach to the obstructive, pathological aspects of the patient. As Kondo (1953) says: "First is the stress on the curative effects of nature; second is that of manual work; and third is the importance of the attitude called 'acceptance.'" The philosophy behind these procedures has its roots in Zen Buddhism.

Most of the neurotic patients who come for treatment at the various hospitals using Morita's therapy are suffering from obsessive-compulsive symptoms or from hypochondriasis. Beyond this, and in line with the Japanese opinion that their own interpersonal relations are particularly difficult, Japanese psychiatry has created a syndrome which may be translated as anthrophobia (*taijin kyōfushō*). Anthrophobia is manifested by feelings of inadequacy, fear of meeting people, flushing, stuttering, and other signs of anxiety. These symptoms are certainly not unknown in American culture, but we have not, in our psychiatry, focused on them so specifically as to group them in a special disease syndrome.

The writer had the opportunity of working for a few days in one of the psychiatric hospitals specializing in Morita psychotherapy. During this time, a number of "group therapy" sessions were held in which the psychiatrist had in front of him the diaries in which the patients who were attending had been writing. During these sessions, the following sort of exchange was common:

Patient: Doctor, my heart pounds so fast.

Doctor: Anybody has a fast pounding on their heart when they run.

Patient: I feel that I will die because of my fast-pounding heart.

Doctor: How exaggerated, what is the matter with you? You have never died before. You had better not touch a problem you have never experienced. You have already gone to the doctor for an examination for heart trouble. That is it. Do you still want to die?

Patient: I don't have such a feeling any more.

Doctor: That is good. Try to write more on your diary. . . .

Second Patient: I yawned right after I became sick. It was the first yawn I noticed after I became sick, so I wrote about it in my diary. After writing this, I was so depressed by my stuttering. My anthrophobia and stuttering were mixed. I lost all of my memory.

Doctor: You have a great tendency to exaggerate such a small thing.

Patient: I am telling you the truth. I don't remember in what way I came to this hospital.

Doctor: If you don't remember anything, you should not remember your anthrophobia. . . .

Such therapeutic methods may sound authoritarian and repressive to Western ears, yet they have many advantages. Before judging, it would be well for the Western reader to understand something of the philosophical background out of which such therapy has grown (see Watts, 1953). Stunkard (1951) has pointed out the parallel between Western psychotherapy and the interpersonal experiences in the training of a Zen monk. The one indispensable element in this training is the relationship between master and pupil. Beyond this, a number of techniques are also used to advance understanding, such as meditation, the *mondo,* and the *koan.* The *mondo* is a brief dialogue between the master and his disciple, while the *koan* is a problem which is insoluble on an intellectual level and which serves as the subject matter for meditation. For example: "What sound is made by the clapping of one hand?"

The dialogues of which *mondo* are composed sound very similar to the type of exchange which took place in the therapy session cited above. For example, the following is given by Stunkard (1951) as a popular *mondo:*

> Bokuju was once asked: "We have to dress and eat every day, and how can we escape from all that?"
>
> The master replied: "We dress, we eat."
>
> "I do not understand."
>
> "If you do not understand, [put on your] dress and eat your food."

The essential element in the *mondo* is an emphasis on the concrete and continuous confrontation of immediate experience. And for this purpose such techniques as the enigmatic answer in the *mondo* and the slapping, kicking, and ridiculing of the pupil by the master are used. As Stunkard (1951) says: "The slappings and enigmatic answers appear designed to upset the student's expectation or set, and as such must be closely related to psychotherapeutic techniques for dealing with defenses against feeling. This is apparently the sense of the traditional explanation that these replies are attempts to break through intellectual barriers in order to focus upon the concrete immediacy of the occasion." The purpose of all such meditation and the development of a delicate balance between frustration and encouragement in the relation of master and pupil is the sudden flash of enlightenment, or *satori.* This is similar to what is meant by gaining insight in psychotherapy in the West.

Writing in Japanese, Tanaka (1955) has discussed the similarities between Zen and psychoanalysis. His discussion of narcissism and ambivalence is particularly interesting. Tanaka points to the fundamental idea in Buddhism that the universe is a unity and that life is undivided unity. As a result of the state of consciousness in the human individual, life comes to be divided into two parts—that of acting and of observing. In the enlightenment which is reached in the process of Zen these two become blended so that the ego which is observing essentially does not exist. As Tanaka (1955) says: "At this point there is not space even for one hair between will and action." Such a statement of the attempt to do away with the distinction between acting and observing could well be a description of one of the processes in the analysis of defenses in the early stages of psychoanalytic treatment.

The process of Zen is perhaps best presented for the Western reader in the report by a European professor of his experiences with Zen through the art of archery during his six years of work in Tokyo (see Herrigel, 1953). There are also the classic books of Suzuki (e.g., 1938), a good general treatment by Watts (1957), and Benoit (1955) has indicated some of the psychological background in Zen thought. At an earlier date, Alexander (1931) has commented on some of the similarities between certain aspects of Buddhism and psychoanalysis, and Freud (1922) refers to these matters in his discussion of what lies beyond the pleasure principle.

These parallels between an Eastern religion and a Western type of therapy suggest the wider problem of the similarities in the methods that have been developed to help or change people by many cultures. Certainly if the principles which underlie Western psychotherapy are valid, they are so in part because they share in many of the as yet not thoroughly understood processes by which people are affected in their relations with others. The writer has recently had his attention called to two attempts to touch upon this wider problem (Ehrenwald, 1956; Sargant, 1957), but neither approaches the matter from the anthropological and psychodynamic point of view taken in this book. In addition, it is interesting to find many similarities in the processes if not in the ends of psychotherapy and the practice of thought reform in Communist China (Lifton, 1956). And there is much that is thought provoking in the therapeutic use made of dreams among the Negritos in the Philippines (Stewart, 1954).

The time has come to close this book, though such a point is an arbitrary one since the writer has tried to set down here the results of some research which form a part of ideas that are as yet in progress. It is hoped that the reader has received something of value in his journey through one small psychiatric hospital, and that the writer has communicated something of his own excitement about the wider implications of work in such a setting for learning more about the differences and the similarities among human beings in many cultures.

REFERENCES

References

Ackerknecht, Erwin H. (1947). "The Role of Medical History in Medical Education," *Bulletin of the History of Medicine* 21:135–145

Ackerman, Nathan W. (1951). " 'Social Role' and Total Personality," *American Journal of Orthopsychiatry* 21:1–17

Ackerman, Nathan W., and Behrens, M. L. (1956). "A Study of Family Diagnosis," *American Journal of Orthopsychiatry* 26:66–78

Alexander, Franz (1931). "Buddhistic Training as an Artificial Catatonia," *Psychoanalytic Review* 18:129–145

Apple, Dorrian (1956). "The Social Structure of Grandparenthood," *American Anthropologist* 58:656–663

Apple, Dorrian, and Arnason, B. "Some Effects of Status on Patient-Staff Interaction." Unpublished paper

Argyris, Chris (1956). *Diagnosing Human Relations in Organizations: A Case Study of a Hospital.* Studies in Organizational Behavior, No. 2. Labor and Management Center, Yale University, New Haven, Connecticut

Babcock, C. G., and Caudill, William (1958). "Personal and Cultural Factors in the Treatment of a Nisei Man." In Seward, Georgene (editor). *Clinical Studies in Culture Conflict.* New York: Ronald Press (in press)

Bachmeyer, A. C., and Hartman, Gerhard (editors) (1943). *The Hospital in Modern Society.* New York: The Commonwealth Fund

Bales, Robert F. (1950). *Interaction Process Analysis.* Cambridge, Massachusetts: Addison-Wesley Publishing Company

Bales, Robert F. (1956). "Task Status and Likeability as a Function of Talking and Listening in Decision-Making Groups." In White, L. D. (editor). *The State of the Social Sciences.* Chicago: University of Chicago Press

Bales, Robert F., and Slater, P. E. (1955). "Role Differentiation in Small Decision-Making Groups." Chapter Five in Parsons, Talcott, and Bales, Robert F. *Family, Socialization and Interaction Process.* Glencoe, Illinois: The Free Press

Bass, B. M. (1949). "An Analysis of Leaderless Group Discussion," *Journal of Applied Psychology* 33:527–533

Belknap, Ivan (1956). *Human Problems of a State Mental Hospital.* New York: Blakiston Division, McGraw-Hill Book Company

Benedek, Therese (1949). "The Psychosomatic Implications of the Primary Unit: Mother-Child," *American Journal of Orthopsychiatry* 19: 642–654

Benedek, Therese, and Rubenstein, B. B. (1952). *Psychosexual Functions in Women*. New York: Ronald Press

Benedict, Paul K., and Jacks, J. (1954). "Mental Illness in Primitive Societies," *Psychiatry* 17:377–389

Benoit, Hubert (1955). *The Supreme Doctrine*. New York: Pantheon Books

Bettelheim, Bruno (1950). *Love Is Not Enough*. Glencoe, Illinois: The Free Press

Blau, P. M. (1954). "Patterns of Interaction among a Group of Officials in a Government Agency," *Human Relations* 7:337–348

Bowen, E. S. (1954). *Return to Laughter*. New York: Harper and Brothers

Boyd, R. W.; Kageles, S. S.; and Greenblatt, M. (1954). "Outbreak of Gang Destructive Behavior on a Psychiatric Ward," *Journal of Nervous and Mental Diseases* 120:338–342

Brown, Esther L. (1948). *Nursing for the Future*. New York: Russell Sage Foundation

Buell, Bradley, *et al.* (1952). *Community Planning for Human Services*. New York: Columbia University Press

Burling, T.; Lentz, E. M.; and Wilson, R. N. (1956). *The Give and Take in Hospitals*. New York: G. P. Putnam's Sons

Cannon, W. B. (1942). "Voodoo Death," *American Anthropologist* 44: 169–181

Cantril, Hadley (1950). *The "Why" of Man's Experience*. New York: The Macmillan Company

Caudill, William (1949). "Psychological Characteristics of Acculturated Wisconsin Ojibwa Children," *American Anthropologist* 51:409–427

Caudill, William (1952). "Japanese American Personality and Acculturation," *Genetic Psychology Monographs* 45:3–102

Caudill, William (1953a). "Applied Anthropology in Medicine." In Kroeber, A. L. (editor). *Anthropology Today,* pp. 771–806. Chicago: University of Chicago Press

Caudill, William (1953b). "Cultural Perspectives on Stress." In *Symposium on Stress,* March 16–18, 1953, pp. 194–208. Army Medical Service Graduate School, Washington, D.C.

Caudill, William (1955). "Some Effects of Social and Cultural Systems in Reactions to Stress." Paper written as a basis for discussion at a meeting of the Social Science Research Council's Committee on Preventive Medicine and Social Science held in New York in November 1955

Caudill, William (1956). "Perspectives on Administration in Psychiatric Hospitals," *Administrative Science Quarterly* 1:155–170

Caudill, William (1957). "Social Process in a Collective Disturbance on a Psychiatric Ward." In Greenblatt, M.; Levinson, D. S.; and Williams,

R. H. (editors). *The Patient and the Mental Hospital.* Glencoe, Illinois: The Free Press

Caudill, William, and DeVos, G. (1956). "Achievement, Culture and Personality: The Case of the Japanese Americans," *American Anthropologist* 58:1102–1126

Caudill, William; Redlich, F. C.; Gilmore, H. R.; and Brody, E. B. (1952). "Social Structure and Interaction Processes on a Psychiatric Ward," *American Journal of Orthopsychiatry* 22:314–334

Caudill, William, and Stainbrook, Edward (1954). "Some Covert Effects of Communication Difficulties in a Psychiatric Hospital," *Psychiatry* 17:27–40

Clausen, J. A., and Yarrow, M. R. (editors) (1955). "The Impact of Mental Illness on the Family," *Journal of Social Issues,* vol. 11, no. 4 (entire issue)

Coleman, R.; Greenblatt, M.; and Solomon, H. C. (1956). "Physiological Evidence of Rapport during Psychotherapeutic Interviews," *Diseases of the Nervous System* 17:2–8

Cote, F.; Dancey, T. E.; and Saucier, J. (1954). "Participation in Institutional Treatment by Selected Relatives," *American Journal of Psychiatry* 110:831–833

Cotton, H. A., and Ebaugh, F. G. (1946). "Japanese Neuropsychiatry," *American Journal of Psychiatry* 103:342–348

Cumming, Elaine, and Cumming, John (1956). "The Locus of Power in a Large Mental Hospital," *Psychiatry* 19:361–369

Cumming, Elaine, and Cumming, John (1957). *Closed Ranks: An Experiment in Mental Health Education.* Cambridge, Massachusetts: Published for The Commonwealth Fund by Harvard University Press

Dembo, T., and Hanfmann, E. (1935). "The Patient's Psychological Situation upon Admission to a Mental Hospital," *American Journal of Psychology* 47:381–408

Deutsch, K. W. (1952). "Communication Theory and Social Science," *American Journal of Orthopsychiatry* 22:469–483

Devereux, George (1944). "The Social Structure of a Schizophrenic Ward and Its Therapeutic Fitness," *Journal of Clinical Psychopathology* 6:231–265

Devereux, George (1951). *Reality and Dream: Psychotherapy of a Plains Indian.* New York: International Universities Press

Devereux, George (1952). "Psychiatry and Anthropology: Some Research Objectives," *Bulletin of the Menninger Clinic* 16:167–177

Devereux, George (1956). "Normal and Abnormal: The Key Problem of Psychiatric Anthropology." In *Some Uses of Anthropology: Theoretical and Applied,* pp. 23–48. Washington, D.C.: The Anthropological Society of Washington

Devereux, George, and Weiner, F. R. (1950). "The Occupational Status of Nurses," *American Sociological Review* 15:628–634

Dewey, John, and Bentley, A. F. (1949). *Knowing and the Known.* Boston: The Beacon Press

Eaton, J. W. (1956). "The Social Science Content of a Medical Curriculum," *American Sociological Review* 21:614–617
Ehrenwald, Jan (1956). *From Medicine Man to Freud.* New York: Dell Publishing Company
Eliot, T. S. (1943). *Four Quartets.* New York: Harcourt, Brace and Company
Erikson, Erik H. (1950). *Childhood and Society.* New York: W. W. Norton and Company
Fiedler, F. E. (1957). "Non-Fraternization between Leaders and Followers and Its Effects on Group Productivity and Psychological Adjustment," *Proceedings of the Symposium on Preventive and Social Psychiatry* April 15–17, 1957, Walter Reed Army Institute of Research, Washington, D.C. (in press)
Firth, Raymond (1951). *Elements of Social Organization.* New York: Philosophical Library
Fonseca, O. W. (1956). "Emergent Social Structure among Short-Term Psychiatric Patients," *International Journal of Social Psychiatry* 2: 132–140
Frank, L. K. (1951). "Genetic Psychology and Its Prospects," *American Journal of Orthopsychiatry* 21:506–522
Freeman, H. E., and Reeder, L. G. (1957). "Medical Sociology: A Review of the Literature," *American Sociological Review* 22:73–81
French, R. L. (1950). "Verbal Output and Leadership Status in Initially Leaderless Discussion Groups," *American Psychologist* 5:310–311
Freud, Anna, and Burlingham, Dorothy (1944). *Infants without Families: The Case for and against Residential Nurseries.* New York: International Universities Press
Freud, Sigmund (1915). "Instincts and Their Vicissitudes." In *Collected Papers,* vol. IV, pp. 60–83. London: Hogarth Press, 1948
Freud, Sigmund (1922). *Beyond the Pleasure Principle.* London: Hogarth Press
Freud, Sigmund (1930). *Civilization and Its Discontents.* London: Hogarth Press
Fromm-Reichmann, Frieda (1950). *Principles of Intensive Psychotherapy.* Chicago: University of Chicago Press
Fukuda, S. (1956). "Byōjaku Shumi (Hobby of Having a Sickly Body)," *Bungeishunju* October
Gilbert, D. C., and Levinson, D. J. (1956). "Ideology, Personality, and Institutional Policy in the Mental Hospital," *Journal of Abnormal and Social Psychology* 53:263–271
Goffman, E. (1957). "On the Characteristics of Total Institutions," *Proceedings of the Symposium on Preventive and Social Psychiatry,* April 15–17, 1957, Walter Reed Army Institute of Research, Washington, D.C. (in press)
Greenblatt, M.; Levinson, D. J.; and Williams, R. H. (editors) (1957). *The Patient and the Mental Hospital.* Glencoe, Illinois: The Free Press
Greenblatt, M.; York, R. H.; and Brown, E. L. (1955). *From Custodial*

to Therapeutic Patient Care in Mental Hospitals. New York: Russell Sage Foundation

Grinker, Roy R. (1953). *Psychosomatic Research.* New York: W. W. Norton and Company

Hamilton, J. A., *et al.* (1955). "A Study of Turnover and Its Costs," *Hospitals,* vol. 29, May

Hare, A. P.; Borgatta, E. F.; and Bales, Robert F. (1955). *Small Groups: Studies in Social Interaction.* New York: Alfred A. Knopf

Henderson, L. J. (1935). "The Patient and Physician as a Social System," *New England Journal of Medicine* 212:819–823

Henry, Jules (1948a). "Common Problems of Research in Anthropology and Psychiatry," *American Journal of Orthopsychiatry* 18:698–703

Henry, Jules (1948b). "Anthropology and Orthopsychiatry." In *Orthopsychiatry 1923–1948: Retrospect and Prospect,* pp. 263–286. Published by the American Orthopsychiatric Association

Henry, Jules (1954). "The Formal Structure of a Psychiatric Hospital," *Psychiatry* 17:139–151

Henry, Jules (1957). "Types of Institutional Structure," *Psychiatry* 20: 47–60

Henry, Jules, *et al.* (1955). "Projective Testing in Ethnography," *American Anthropologist* 57:245–270

Henry, Jules, and Warson, S. (1951). "Family Structure and Psychic Development," *American Journal of Orthopsychiatry* 21:59–73

Herrigel, Eugen (1953). *Zen in the Art of Archery.* New York: Pantheon Books

Hill, S. R., Jr., *et al.* (1956). "Studies on Adrenocortical and Psychological Response to Stress in Man," *A. M. A. Archives of Internal Medicine* 97:269–298

Hollingshead, A. B., and Redlich, F. C. (1953). "Social Stratification and Psychiatric Disorders," *American Sociological Review* 18:163–169

Honigmann, J. J. (1954). *Culture and Personality.* New York: Harper and Brothers

Howells, W. W. (1955). "Universality and Variation in Human Nature." In Thomas, W. L., Jr. (editor). *Yearbook of Anthropology,* pp. 227–236. New York: Wenner-Gren Foundation

Huxley, Julian S. (1955). "Evolution, Cultural and Biological." In Thomas, W. L., Jr. (editor). *Yearbook of Anthropology,* pp. 3–25. New York: Wenner-Gren Foundation

Hyde, R. W., and Solomon, H. C. (1950). "Patient Government: A New Form of Group Therapy," *Digest of Neurology and Psychiatry* 18:207–218

Johnson, A. M., and Szurek, S. A. (1952). "The Genesis of Antisocial Acting Out in Children and Adults," *Psychoanalytic Quarterly* 21: 323–343

Jones, Maxwell (1953). *The Therapeutic Community.* New York: Basic Books

Kilpatrick, F. P. (editor) (1952). *Human Behavior from the Transac-*

tional Point of View. Hanover, New Hampshire: Institute for Associated Research

Kluckhohn, Clyde (1944). "The Influence of Psychiatry on Anthropology in America during the Past One Hundred Years." In Hall, J. K.; Zilboorg, Gregory; and Bunker, H. A. (editors). *One Hundred Years of American Psychiatry,* pp. 489–518. New York: Columbia University Press

Kluckhohn, Clyde (1951). "The Study of Culture." In Lerner, Daniel, and Lasswell, H. D. (editors). *The Policy Sciences,* pp. 86–101. Stanford: Stanford University Press

Kluckhohn, Clyde (1953). "Universal Categories of Culture." In Kroeber, A. L. (editor). *Anthropology Today,* pp. 507–523. Chicago: University of Chicago Press

Kluckhohn, Clyde; Murray, H. A.; and Schneider, D. M. (editors) (1953). *Personality in Nature, Society, and Culture,* 2nd edition. New York: Alfred A. Knopf

Kluckhohn, Florence Rockwood (1953). "Dominant and Variant Value Orientations." In Kluckhohn, Clyde; Murray, H. A.; and Schneider, D. M. (editors). *Personality in Nature, Society, and Culture,* 2nd edition, pp. 342–357. New York: Alfred A. Knopf

Kondo, Akihisa (1953). "Morita Therapy: A Japanese Therapy for Neurosis," *American Journal of Psychoanalysis* 13:31–37

Kramer, M. (1956). *Facts Needed to Assess Public Health and Social Problems in the Widespread Use of the Tranquilizing Drugs*. Public Health Monograph No. 41. Washington, D.C.: U.S. Government Printing Office

Kroeber, A. L. (1948). *Anthropology*. New York: Harcourt, Brace and Company

Kroeber, A. L. (1952). *The Nature of Culture*. Chicago: University of Chicago Press

Kroeber, A. L. (1955). "History of Anthropological Thought." In Thomas, W. L., Jr. (editor). *Yearbook of Anthropology,* pp. 293–311. New York: Wenner-Gren Foundation

Kroeber, A. L., and Kluckhohn, Clyde (1952). *Culture: A Critical Review of Concepts and Definitions*. Papers of the Peabody Museum, Harvard University, vol. 47, no. 1

Lee, A. M. (1955). "The Clinical Study of Society," *American Sociological Review* 20:648–653

Lifton, Robert J. (1956). " 'Thought Reform' of Western Civilians in Chinese Communist Prisons," *Psychiatry* 19:173–195

Lindemann, E. (1950). "Modifications in the Course of Ulcerative Colitis in Relationship to Changes in Life Situations and Reaction Patterns." In Wolff, H. F.; Wolf, S. G.; and Hare, C. C. (editors). *Life Stress and Bodily Disease,* pp. 706–723. Baltimore: The Williams and Wilkins Company

Mead, Margaret (1949). *The Mountain Arapesh. V. The Record of Unabelin with Rorschach Analysis*. Anthropological Papers of the American Museum of Natural History, vol. 41, part 3

Mead, Margaret (1952). "Some Relations between Social Anthropology and Psychiatry." In Alexander, Franz, and Ross, Helen (editors). *Dynamic Psychiatry,* pp. 401–448. Chicago: University of Chicago Press

Mead, Margaret, and Macgregor, Frances C. (1951). *Growth and Culture.* New York: G. P. Putnam's Sons

Menninger, W. C. (1937). "Psychoanalytic Principles Applied to the Treatment of Hospitalized Patients," *Bulletin of the Menninger Clinic* 1:35–43

Merton, R. K.; Fiske, M.; and Kendall, P. L. (1956). *The Focussed Interview.* Glencoe, Illinois: The Free Press

Miki, Y., and Kimura, Y. (1954). "Elder Brother-Life and Younger Brother-Life," *Japanese Journal of Educational Psychology* 2:69–78

Miller, D. H. (1957). "The Etiology of an Outbreak of Delinquency in a Group of Hospitalized Adolescents." In Greenblatt, M.; Levinson, D. J.; and Williams, R. H. (editors). *The Patient and the Mental Hospital.* Glencoe, Illinois: The Free Press

Mills, T. M. (1953). "Power Relations in Three-Person Groups," *American Sociological Review* 18:351–357

Mills, T. M. (1954). "The Coalition Pattern in Three-Person Groups," *American Sociological Review* 19:657–667

Mills, T. M. (1956). "Developmental Processes in Three-Person Groups," *Human Relations* 9:343–355

Mishler, E. G. (1955). "The Nursing Service and the Aims of a Psychiatric Hospital: Orientations of Ward Personnel to the Care and Rehabilitation of Psychiatric Patients," *American Journal of Psychiatry* 111:664–672

Mishler, E. G., and Tropp, A. (1956). "Status and Interaction in a Psychiatric Hospital," *Human Relations* 9:187–205

Moroney, M. J. (1953). *Facts From Figures,* revised edition. London: Penguin Books

Morse, R. T., and Noble, D. (1942). "Joint Endeavors of the Administrative Physician and Psychotherapist," *Psychiatric Quarterly* 16:578–585

Mosteller, F., and Tukey, J. W. (1949). "The Uses and Usefulness of Binomial Probability Paper," *Journal of the American Statistical Association* 44:174–212

Murdock, George Peter (1949). *Social Structure.* New York: The Macmillan Company

Murray, H. A. (1943). *Thematic Apperception Test (and Manual)*, 3rd revision. Cambridge, Massachusetts: Harvard University Press

Opler, Marvin K. (1956). *Culture, Psychiatry and Human Values.* Springfield, Illinois: Charles C. Thomas

Opler, M. K., and Singer, J. L. (1956). "Ethnic Differences in Behavior and Psychopathology: Italian and Irish," *International Journal of Social Psychiatry* 2:11–22

Papanek, M. L. (1957). "Authority and Interpersonal Relations in the

Family." Unpublished doctoral dissertation, Department of Social Relations, Harvard University

Parsons, Talcott (1951). "Illness and the Role of the Physician: A Sociological Perspective," *American Journal of Orthopsychiatry* 21: 452–460

Parsons, Talcott (1957). "The Mental Hospital as a Type of Organization." In Greenblatt, M.; Levinson, D. J.; and Williams, R. H. (editors). *The Patient and the Mental Hospital.* Glencoe, Illinois: The Free Press

Parsons, Talcott, and Bales, Robert F. (1955). *Family, Socialization and Interaction Process.* Glencoe, Illinois: The Free Press

Parsons, Talcott; Bales, Robert F.; and Shils, Edward A. (1953). *Working Papers in the Theory of Action.* Glencoe, Illinois: The Free Press

Paul, Benjamin D. (editor) (1955). *Health, Culture and Community.* New York: Russell Sage Foundation

Peplau, H. E. (1952). *Interpersonal Relations in Nursing.* New York: G. P. Putnam's Sons

President's Commission on the Health Needs of the Nation (1953). *Building America's Health: America's Health Status, Needs and Resources,* vol. 2. Washington, D.C.: U.S. Government Printing Office

Radcliffe-Brown, A. R. (1952). *Structure and Function in Primitive Society.* London: Cohen and West

Rapoport, R. N. (1956). "Oscillations and Sociotherapy," *Human Relations* 9:357–374

Rapoport, R. N., and Rapoport, R. S. (1957). " 'Democratization' and Authority in a Therapeutic Community," *Behavioral Science* 2:128–133

Redfield, Robert (1953a). *The Primitive World and Its Transformations.* Ithaca: Cornell University Press

Redfield, Robert (1953b). "Relations of Anthropology to the Social Sciences and to the Humanities." In Kroeber, A. L. (editor). *Anthropology Today,* pp. 728–738. Chicago: University of Chicago Press

Redl, Fritz, and Wineman, David (1951). *Children Who Hate.* Glencoe, Illinois: The Free Press

Reischauer, Edwin O. (1957). *Japan and the United States,* 2nd edition. Cambridge, Massachusetts: Harvard University Press

Rice, A. K. (1951). "The Use of Unrecognized Cultural Mechanisms in an Expanding Machine-Shop," *Human Relations* 4:143–160

Riesman, David (1950). *The Lonely Crowd.* New Haven: Yale University Press

Rioch, D. McK., and Stanton, Alfred H. (1953). "Milieu Therapy," *Psychiatry* 16:65–72

Robinson, A. M.; Mellow, J.; Hurteau, P.; and Fried, M. A. (1955). "Research in Psychiatric Nursing," *American Journal of Nursing,* vol. 55, April, May, June

Roethlisberger, F. J., and Dickson, W. J. (1939). *Management and the Worker.* Cambridge, Massachusetts: Harvard University Press

Roseborough, M. E. (1953). "Experimental Studies of Small Groups," *Psychological Bulletin* 50:275–303

Rowland, H. (1938). "Interaction Processes in a State Mental Hospital," *Psychiatry* 1:323–337

Rowland, H. (1939). "Friendship Patterns in a State Mental Hospital," *Psychiatry* 2:363–373

Ruesch, Jurgen (1953). "Synopsis of the Theory of Human Communication," *Psychiatry* 16:215–243

Ruesch, Jurgen, and Bateson, Gregory (1951). *Communication: The Social Matrix of Psychiatry*. New York: W. W. Norton and Company

Sapir, Edward (1949). *Selected Writings of Edward Sapir*. Edited by Mandelbaum, D. G. Berkeley: University of California Press. The article referred to in Chapter 14 was originally published as "Psychiatric and Cultural Pitfalls in the Business of Getting a Living," *Mental Health,* Publication No. 9 of the American Association for the Advancement of Science, 1939 (out of print)

Sargant, William (1957). *Battle For the Mind*. New York: Doubleday and Company

Saunders, Lyle (1954). *Culture Difference and Medical Care*. New York: Russell Sage Foundation

Schaffer, L., and Myers, J. K. (1954). "Psychotherapy and Social Stratification," *Psychiatry* 17:83–93

Schoenfeld, H. (1952). "Why People Work in Hospitals," *Hospitals,* vol. 26, December

Schwartz, Charlotte G. (1953). *Rehabilitation of Mental Hospital Patients*. Public Health Monograph, No. 17. Washington, D.C.: U.S. Government Printing Office

Schwartz, Morris S., and Shockley, Emmy L. (1956). *The Nurse and the Mental Patient*. New York: Russell Sage Foundation

Sheimo, S. L.; Paynter, J.; and Szurek, S. A. (1949). "Problems of Staff Interaction with Spontaneous Group Formations on a Children's Psychiatric Ward," *American Journal of Orthopsychiatry* 19:599–611

Simmel, E. (1929). "Psychoanalytic Treatment in a Sanatorium," *International Journal of Psychoanalysis* 10:70–89

Simmons, L. W., and Wolff, H. G. (1954). *Social Science in Medicine*. New York: Russell Sage Foundation

Simmons, O. G.; Davis, J. A.; and Spencer, K. (1956). "Interpersonal Strains in Release from a Mental Hospital," *Social Problems* 4:21–28

Sivadon, Paul D. (1957). "Techniques of Sociotherapy," *Proceedings of the Symposium on Preventive and Social Psychiatry,* April 15–17, 1957, Walter Reed Army Institute of Research, Washington, D.C. (in press)

Smith, Harvey (1949). "Sociological Study of Hospitals." Unpublished doctoral dissertation, Department of Sociology, University of Chicago

Smith, Harvey (1955). "Two Lines of Authority Are One Too Many," *The Modern Hospital* March

Spiegel, John P. (1954). "New Perspectives in the Study of the Family," *Marriage and Family Living* 16:4–12

Spiegel, John P. (1956). "A Model for Relationships among Systems." In Grinker, Roy R. (editor). *Toward a Unified Theory of Human Behavior,* pp. 16–26. New York: Basic Books

Spiegel, John P. (1957). "The Resolution of Role Conflict within the Family," *Psychiatry* 20:1–16

Spiro, M. E. (1951). "Culture and Personality: The Natural History of a False Dichotomy," *Psychiatry* 14:19–46

Stainbrook, Edward, and Wexler, M. (1956). "The Place of the Behavioral Sciences in the Medical School," *Psychiatry* 19:263–269

Stanton, Alfred H. (1956). "The Study of the Psychiatric Hospital as a Therapeutic Society," *Centennial Papers, Saint Elizabeths Hospital,* Washington, D.C., pp. 143–152

Stanton, Alfred H., and Schwartz, Morris S. (1954). *The Mental Hospital.* New York: Basic Books

Stewart, Kilton (1954). *Pygmies and Dream Giants.* New York: W. W. Norton and Company

Straus, R. (1957). "The Nature and Status of Medical Sociology," *American Sociological Review* 22:200–204

Strodtbeck, F. L., and Mann, R. D. (1956). "Sex Role Differentiation in Jury Deliberations," *Sociometry* 19:3–11

Stunkard, Albert (1951). "Some Interpersonal Aspects of an Oriental Religion," *Psychiatry* 14:419–431

Sullivan, H. S. (1931). "Socio-Psychiatric Research: Its Implications for the Schizophrenia Problem and for Mental Hygiene," *American Journal of Psychiatry* 10:977–991

Suzuki, D. T. (1938). *Zen Buddhism and Its Influence on Japanese Culture.* Kyoto: Eastern Buddhist Society

Szurek, S. A. (1947). "Dynamics of Staff Interaction in Hospital Psychiatric Treatment of Children," *American Journal of Orthopsychiatry* 17:652–664

Tanaka, Tadao (1955). *Zen to Gendaijin* (Zen and People in the Modern World), 2nd edition. Tokyo: Gengensha

Teicher, M. I. (1956). "Comparative Psychiatry: Some References in Ethnopsychiatry," *Revue Internationale d'Ethnopsychologie Normale et Pathologique,* vol. I, nos. 1 and 2

von Bertalanffy, L. (1950). "The Theory of Open Systems in Physics and Biology," *Science* 111:23–29

von Foerster, Heinz (editor) (1953). *Cybernetics: Circular Causal and Feedback Mechanisms in Biological and Social Systems.* Transactions of the Ninth Conference, March 20–21, 1952. New York: Josiah Macy, Jr. Foundation

Watts, Alan W. (1953). "Asian Psychology and Modern Psychiatry," *American Journal of Psychoanalysis* 13:25–30

Watts, Alan W. (1957). *The Way of Zen.* New York: Pantheon Books

Wessen, A. F. (1951). "The Social Structure of a Modern Hospital." Unpublished doctoral dissertation, Department of Sociology, Yale University

Williams, R. H. (1953). "Psychiatric Rehabilitation in the Community," *Public Health Reports* 68:1231–1236

Wilson, A. T. M. (1950). *Hospital Nursing Auxiliaries: Notes on a Background Survey and Job Analysis*. London: Tavistock Publications

Wolfenstein, Martha (1957). *Disaster: A Psychological Essay*. Glencoe, Illinois: The Free Press

Woodward, J. (1950). *Employment Relations in a Group of Hospitals*. London: The Institute of Hospital Administrators

World Health Organization (1953). *Expert Committee on Mental Health, Third Report*. Technical Report Series, No. 73. Geneva, Switzerland

INDEX

Index